Gay, Straight, and the Reason Why

Gay, Straight, and the Reason Why

The Science of Sexual Orientation

SECOND EDITION

SIMON LeVAY

OXFORD
UNIVERSITY PRESS

OXFORD
UNIVERSITY PRESS

Oxford University Press is a department of the University of Oxford. It furthers
the University's objective of excellence in research, scholarship, and education
by publishing worldwide. Oxford is a registered trade mark of Oxford University
Press in the UK and certain other countries.

Published in the United States of America by Oxford University Press
198 Madison Avenue, New York, NY 10016, United States of America.

Library of Congress Cataloging-in-Publication Data
Names: LeVay, Simon, author.
Title: Gay, straight, and the reason why : the science of sexual orientation / Simon LeVay.
Description: Second edition. | Oxford ; New York : Oxford University Press, [2017] |
Includes bibliographical references and index.
Identifiers: LCCN 2016006377 (print) | LCCN 2016014053 (ebook) |
ISBN 9780190297374 (pbk. : alk. paper) | ISBN 9780190297381 (UPDF) |
ISBN 9780190297398 (EPUB)
Subjects: LCSH: Sexual orientation. | Sex (Psychology) | Sex (Biology)
Classification: LCC BF692 .L476 2017 (print) | LCC BF692 (ebook) | DDC 155.3/4—dc23
LC record available at http://lccn.loc.gov/2016006377

This material is not intended to be, and should not be considered, a substitute for medical or other
professional advice. Treatment for the conditions described in this material is highly dependent on
the individual circumstances. And, while this material is designed to offer accurate information
with respect to the subject matter covered and to be current as of the time it was written, research
and knowledge about medical and health issues is constantly evolving and dose schedules for
medications are being revised continually, with new side effects recognized and accounted for
regularly. Readers must therefore always check the product information and clinical procedures
with the most up-to-date published product information and data sheets provided by the
manufacturers and the most recent codes of conduct and safety regulation. The publisher and the
authors make no representations or warranties to readers, express or implied, as to the accuracy or
completeness of this material. Without limiting the foregoing, the publisher and the authors make
no representations or warranties as to the accuracy or efficacy of the drug dosages mentioned in the
material. The authors and the publisher do not accept, and expressly disclaim, any responsibility
for any liability, loss, or risk that may be claimed or incurred as a consequence of the use and/or
application of any of the contents of this material.

3 5 7 9 8 6 4
Printed by Sheridan Books, Inc., United States of America

CONTENTS

PREFACE TO THE SECOND EDITION

The five years that have passed since the publication of the first edition of this book have seen considerable progress in our understanding of how sexual orientation develops. Molecular geneticists have come closer to identifying "gay genes." Brain scientists have probed deeper into the neural wiring that underlies sexual attraction. Psychologists have given us a clearer view of the cognitive and personality traits that distinguish gay people from straight people. They have also helped us better understand how a trait as counterintuitive as homosexuality can persist over the generations and why it exists in most human cultures. To cover these advances I have added mention of over 170 research papers that have appeared since I wrote the first edition.

In general, the recent studies strengthen the idea that gay people differ from straight people in more than the direction of their sexual feelings. There is great diversity among lesbians and gay men, to be sure, but in general homosexuality is part of a collection of gender-atypical traits, just as heterosexuality is part of a collection of gender-typical traits. These different "packages" arise because the sexual differentiation of the brain goes forward differently in individuals destined to become gay adults as compared with their same-sex heterosexual peers. Differences in genes, sex hormones, and their interactions with the developing brain are what cause this divergence.

Some of the recent findings are pointing in interesting new directions, however. There is increasing evidence, for example, that sexual orientation is affected by epigenetic processes. These are processes that involve chemical alterations to the genome but not to the DNA base sequence itself—the "letters" of the genetic code. Another area of active inquiry is the "older-brother effect"—the observation that boys with older brothers have an increased likelihood of becoming gay men. Canadian researchers believe that they are homing in on the biological basis for this effect.

Perhaps most significantly, it's becoming obvious that there is much more to sexual attraction than "gay" and "straight." Bisexuality, asexuality, attraction to different age groups,and the various kinds of gay sexuality indicated by the colloquial terms "butch," "femme," "top," and "bottom"—all these have begun to attract the attention of biologically oriented researchers. So has transexuality, which has some features in common with homosexuality. I have added a new chapter, titled "Beyond Gay and Straight" (Chapter 11), that is devoted to these other important aspects of sexuality and gender.

The University of Lethbridge, Alberta, hosts a conference every few years under the title "The Puzzle of Sexual Orientation." The 2015 conference, organized by Paul Vasey, Kelly Suschinksy, and Jean-Baptiste Leca, attracted many of the leading researchers in the field. In this book I mention some of the research findings presented at the conference. It is expected that most of these presentations will be published in a special edition of *Archives of Sexual Behavior* sometime in 2016.

INTRODUCTION

In August of 1991, when I was a neuroscientist working at the Salk Institute for Biological Studies in San Diego, I published a short research paper in the journal *Science*. The article was titled "A Difference in Hypothalamic Structure Between Heterosexual and Homosexual Men." It attracted a great deal of interest from the media, the general public, and the scientific community, and it helped trigger a wave of new research into an age-old question: What makes people straight or gay?

The *hypothalamus** is a small region at the base of the brain that helps regulate several of our instinctual drives, including our sex drive. In my study, I took specimens of the hypothalamus from men and women who had died and were undergoing autopsy. About half of the men were gay. I focused on a region at the front of the hypothalamus that is known to be involved in regulating the sexual behaviors typically shown by males. Within this region lies a rice-grain-sized collection of nerve cells named *INAH3*, which is usually larger in men than in women. I confirmed this basic sex difference. In addition, however, I found that INAH3 was significantly smaller, on average, in the gay men than in the straight men. In fact, there was no difference in size between INAH3 in the gay men and the women in my sample. I interpreted this finding as a clue that biological processes of brain development may influence a man's sexual orientation.

I was certainly not the first person to have thought about sexual orientation from a biological perspective. A hundred years ago a German physician and sex researcher, Magnus Hirschfeld, proposed that brain development followed different paths in fetuses destined to become gay adults and those destined to become straight. Just a year before I published my study, a Dutch group reported that another cluster of cells in the hypothalamus, the *suprachiasmatic*

---

* Most technical terms are italicized at first mention and are defined in the Glossary.

nucleus, differed in size between gay and straight men. And during the mid-1980s psychiatrist Richard Pillard of Boston University had reported evidence that homosexuality clustered in certain families, raising the possibility that genes running in those families might be influencing the sexual orientations of family members.

But my report differed in significant respects from most earlier ones. For one thing, by studying a brain region that is known to help regulate our sexuality I was, perhaps, cutting closer to the heart of the matter than earlier studies had done. Also, many of the earlier studies had talked about homosexuality as if it was an abnormality or problem, while heterosexuality was something so normal that it barely needed to be mentioned. Many were framed around the spoken or unspoken question, what's wrong with gay people?

There's nothing wrong with gay people. I'm gay myself, and happy to be so. There are some differences between us and the rest of humanity, certainly, as I'll discuss in this book. Some of those differences are trivial, and some may influence people's lives in interesting ways, making being gay or straight more than just a matter of "who we love." But pathology doesn't come into it.

Whatever the exact reason, my 1991 study received a lot more attention from the media and from the public at large than had earlier studies. On the day of publication most of the leading US newspapers carried front-page stories about it. Because I was hometown talent, the *San Diego Union-Tribune* actually gave my report top billing, relegating what was probably a more significant news item on that day—the collapse of the Soviet Union—to a humbler position on the page.

Gay people reacted more favorably to my report than they had done to earlier studies. Some gay academics did exhibit a certain hostility—I recall psychologist John De Cecco of San Francisco State University denouncing my paper as "another example of medical homophobia" in a television interview. More commonly, though, gay people told me that my finding validated their own sense of being "born gay" or being intrinsically different from straight people. This they perceived as a good thing, because people with anti-gay attitudes often portray homosexuality as a lifestyle or a choice that people make—and by implication a bad choice.

My own position is this: The scientific knowledge currently available does bolster the idea that gays and lesbians are distinct "kinds" of people who are entitled to protection from discrimination, especially by governments, rather in the same way that racial minorities are. But I also believe that there would be plenty of reasons why gay people should be accepted and valued by society even if being gay were proven to be an outright choice.

I wrote extensively about the social implications of this kind of research in my earlier book *Queer Science* (LeVay, 1996), so I will not revisit that theme in the present book, except for a few closing remarks. Rather, my intent here is simply to give some idea of where the science stands today, a quarter-century after my *Science* paper appeared.

That paper was followed by a welter of new research. Not by myself, because I left my position at the Salk Institute in 1992. Since then I have occupied myself as a writer and teacher, but I have maintained a close interest in the field that I had worked in. Much of the new research has been done by a younger generation of scientists—neuroscientists, endocrinologists, geneticists, and cognitive psychologists—in laboratories across the United States, in Canada, and overseas.

My study and the publicity it generated helped trigger much of this new work, but it certainly wasn't the whole inspiration. Pillard, for example, along with psychologist Michael Bailey of Northwestern University, published an important genetic study on sexual orientation in late 1991, just a few months after my *Science* paper appeared. Their study had been completed before my paper came out and was in no way influenced by it. Pillard and Bailey's work led to further studies by their own research groups, and it helped draw molecular geneticists and other specialists into the field.

Taken together, the multitude of research studies published since 1991 have greatly strengthened the idea that biological factors play a significant role in the development of sexual orientation, in both men and in women. More than that, they tend to bolster a particular kind of biological theory. This is the idea that the origins of sexual orientation are to be sought in the interactions between sex hormones and the developing brain. These interactions are what predispose our developing minds toward some degree of "masculinity" or "femininity." In other words, this theory places sexual orientation within the larger framework of gender, but gender as seen from a very biological perspective.

The idea that the interaction between sex hormones and the fetal brain might be an important factor in the development of sexual orientation is not new. In fact, Hirschfeld suggested as much in the early 20th century. But now there is evidence, and that evidence is what much of this book is about.

The first chapter of the book discusses the meaning of terms like *sexual orientation, homosexual, bisexual, heterosexual, gay,* and *straight,* and it reviews what we know about the prevalence of different sexual orientations, both in contemporary Western society and across cultures and historical periods. It also examines how stable a person's sexual orientation is over her or his lifetime. My conclusion from this review is that sexual orientation is indeed a fairly stable aspect of human nature, and that straight, gay, and bisexual people have existed across most, though perhaps not all, cultures. I also conclude that we need to think somewhat differently about sexual orientation in men and in women, and that cultural forces greatly influence how homosexuality is expressed in different societies and across the span of history. There are limits, in other words, to what we may hope to explain with biological ideas.

The second chapter is a brief review of *non-biological* theories of sexual orientation. These include traditional Freudian theories that focus on parent–child relationships, as well as behaviorist ideas that see a person's sexual orientation as the end product of a learning process. The chapter will also consider the idea, espoused by some Christian conservatives as well as by a few gay activists, that a person's sexual orientation is the result of a conscious and voluntary choice. I'll conclude that all such theories fail to adequately explain the diversity in people's sexual orientations. This failure makes the search for biological factors all the more compelling.

Chapter 3 outlines a biological theory of sexual orientation. It describes what we know about other aspects of sexual development and how they are regulated: by a cascade-like sequence of interactions among genes, sex hormones, and the cells of the developing body and brain. These processes don't go forward in complete isolation from the outside world—there is the potential for interactions between internal biological programs and environmental factors, and such interactions likely increase as development goes on. As a result of genetic differences between individuals, as well as the random variability of biological processes and perhaps feedback effects from the environment, these biological processes go forward differently in different individuals, leading to diversity in sexual orientation. I lay out how these ideas will be tested in the remaining chapters of the book.

Chapter 4 asks, Are there differences between gay and straight people when they are still children—that is, before their sexual orientations become apparent to themselves or others? The answer is, yes, there are. Retrospective studies, as well as prospective studies that follow children through to adulthood, are in agreement: Children who eventually become gay adults—I'll call them *pre-gay children*—are different, at least on average, from those who become straight. Pre-gay children are, to a variable extent, atypical or nonconformist in a number of gender-related traits, meaning that these traits are shifted toward the norms for the other sex as compared with children of the same sex who grow up to become straight. The differences are not necessarily as marked as some popular stereotypes would suggest. Still, they do indicate that sexual orientation is influenced by factors operating early in life. And because there is evidence that biological factors influence these gendered childhood traits, the finding that pre-gay children are gender-nonconformist in these traits is consistent with a biological model of sexual orientation.

What about adulthood? Even though many gender-nonconformist children grow up into gay adults, they often become more gender-conformist in the process. Nevertheless, as is discussed in Chapter 5, psychologists have amassed a great deal of evidence about psychological differences between gay and straight adults. Most, though not all, of these differences concern traits that typically differ between men and women, and the differences are usually such that gay people are shifted toward the other sex compared with heterosexual individuals of their own sex. It is difficult to explain these shifts in gay people as the *result* of being gay. Rather, it seems likely that they reflect differences in the early sexual development of the brain, differences that affect a "package" of gendered psychological traits including sexual orientation.

Chapter 6 investigates the role of sex hormones in the development of sexual orientation. I review experiments in which researchers have artificially manipulated the sex hormone levels of animals during development. These manipulations can cause animals that would otherwise have become heterosexual to mate preferentially with animals of their own sex. Though such experiments cannot be undertaken in humans, there are "experiments of nature" that accomplish something similar. There are also observations on certain anatomical markers, such as finger lengths, that say something about the hormonal environments to which gay and straight people were exposed before birth. From these studies we can conclude that in humans as in animals, sex hormone levels during development influence a whole variety of gendered traits, including sexual orientation.

In Chapter 7 I discuss the evidence that a person's genetic endowment influences her or his ultimate sexual orientation. Much of this evidence comes from family and twin studies. These studies indicate that *genes* exert a significant, though not all-dominating, influence on sexual orientation. There is now evidence as to where in the genome some of these "gay genes" are located. Alterations to genes that don't affect the DNA sequence may also play a role. (These are known as *epigenetic effects*.) Molecular-genetic studies in animals, especially in the fruit fly *Drosophila*, also give clues about how sexual orientation is regulated. Lastly, I consider how genes predisposing to homosexuality might persist in the population even though gay people have relatively few children. It turns out that there are robust mechanisms capable of keeping such genes in circulation.

In Chapter 8 I turn to my own area of expertise, the brain. Several studies, including my study on INAH3, point to structural differences between the brains of gay and straight men. Similar differences have been described in one animal species—the domestic sheep, in which a minority of males (rams) are sexually oriented toward other males. Differences between the brains of lesbian and straight women have also been reported. The brains of gay people don't just look different from those of straight people; they function differently, too. The chapter reviews a range of functional studies, including one that reports on different activity patterns in the hypothalami of gay and straight people when these people are exposed to odors that are thought to act as human pheromones or chemosignals.

The bodies of gay and straight people are not obviously different—if they were, telling them apart would be much easier than it is. Still, as Chapter 9 describes, there have been reports of subtle anatomical differences. These include differences in the relative proportions of the limbs and trunk and differences in facial structure. There also are differences in the lateralization (or sidedness) of brain structure and function. There are subtle but objectively detectable differences in unconscious behaviors such as walking style and voice quality as well. Recognizing these subtleties is the basis of *gaydar*—the sometimes fallible sense of whether a person one meets is gay or straight.

Chapter 10 discusses an intriguing finding by a Canadian research group: A boy's birth order in his family affects his likelihood of becoming a gay man. Specifically, a boy who has older brothers is more likely to grow up gay than a boy who does not. The Canadian researchers have produced evidence that this effect of older brothers is a result of biological interactions between pregnant women and their fetuses.

Chapter 11 goes beyond the gay–straight dichotomy that is suggested by the book's title. It reviews the controversial topic of bisexuality in men and in women, as well as other aspects of sexual and gender expression such as asexuality, pedophilia, and transexuality.

The final chapter represents my attempt to draw the various lines of evidence together into a coherent theory of sexual orientation. I argue that the same processes that are involved in the biological development of our bodies and brains as male or female are also involved in the development of sexual orientation. Nevertheless, I also emphasize our inability to explain in a precise way why any particular individual becomes gay or straight, let alone bisexual. Much remains to be discovered, and I point to various promising directions for future research.

Gay, Straight, and the Reason Why

1

What Is Sexual Orientation?

Sexual orientation has to do with the sex of our preferred sex partners. More specifically, it is the trait that predisposes us to experience sexual attraction to people of the same sex as ourselves (*homosexual, gay,* or *lesbian**), to people of the other sex (*heterosexual* or *straight*), or in some varying degree to both sexes (*bisexual*). In this chapter I explore the implications of this definition.

Sexual orientation, as just defined, is just one aspect of a person's sexuality; there are plenty of others.[1] In popular (sometimes derogatory) discourse it is common to hear terms like *asexual, poly, pansexual, swinger, monogamous, tranny, tranny chaser, fag hag, chubby chaser, sadist, masochist, sex maniac, nymphomaniac, frigid, butch, femme, bear, twink, rice queen, top, bottom, hooker, john, cougar, cougar bait, child molester,* and *rapist.* The familiarity of these terms speaks to a widespread concern with aspects of sexuality other than sexual orientation. I will delve briefly into one or two of these other aspects in Chapter 11, but for the most part this book is concerned with sexual attraction to males and females and how these attractions come to be.

Criteria for Sexual Orientation

We usually judge sexual orientation based on a person's sexual *attraction* to men and to women—that is, on her or his *feelings*—as expressed in answers to direct questions such as "Are you sexually attracted to men, to women, or to both men and women?" The question doesn't refer to interviewees' feelings of sexual attraction at the very instant of being asked, of course, but to the trait that predisposes them to experience such feelings over some extended period, perhaps their entire adult life.

---

* I use *homosexual* and *gay* interchangeably, but the two terms have different connotations. *Homosexual* has the flavor of a label applied to a set of people; *gay* is the self-chosen identifier that has largely replaced it. I also use *gay woman* and *lesbian* interchangeably; some other writers have drawn distinctions between the two terms.

Some studies, such as the pioneering work of Alfred Kinsey in the 1940s and 1950s, have taken into account sexual *behavior*—that is, the extent to which a person actually has sexual contacts with men or women—in defining sexual orientation. The problem with that approach is that sexual behavior is influenced by many factors that have nothing to do with a person's basic sexual feelings and that are changeable over time. Is a woman in prison a lesbian simply because she has sex with the women she is locked up with? Probably not. Is a man straight simply because he follows his church's teaching to "be fruitful and multiply"? Probably not.

The factors that influence the choice of actual sex partners include the availability of partners, the person's moral sense, the desire to conform or to have children, curiosity, financial incentives, and so on. It's true that, on occasion, actions may speak louder than words—as, for example, when a self-declared heterosexual man is observed seeking sexual contacts in men's toilets. People don't always tell the truth about themselves; they may not even know what the truth is. Still, in describing people's sexual orientation, we generally do best to listen to what they tell us about their sexual feelings.

Attraction may not be a single, unitary phenomenon. There is *physical attraction*, meaning the desire to engage in actual sexual contact, and *romantic* or *emotional attraction*, which is a desire for intimacy that is not necessarily expressed in sexual contact. Romantic attraction shades off into forms of close friendship that have nothing to do with sex. For this reason many researchers consider physical attraction to be the more reliable criterion for sexual orientation. In this book, in fact, I use "sexual attraction" to mean physical attraction.

Although sexual attraction is usually assessed simply by asking people who they are attracted to, there are also methods that sidestep verbal communication. For example, people tend to look longer at photographs of people they find sexually attractive. Thus the measurement of viewing time while a subject peruses photographs of semi-nude men and women can give a good indication of sexual orientation.[2]

Sexual orientation may work in part by unconscious mechanisms that can be accessed in the laboratory. Two groups of researchers showed their subjects photographs of naked men and women on a computer monitor, but prevented these images from reaching the subjects' consciousness.[3] (They did this by presenting the images very briefly to one eye while masking the images with high-contrast visual noise presented to the other eye.) Immediately thereafter, the subjects had to perform a visual discrimination task, which involved judging the orientation of a line. Although the subjects denied having seen any human figures, they performed the discrimination task better when the line was at the location previously occupied by their preferred target (e.g., a naked woman if the subject was a heterosexual man) and worse when the line was at the location of their non-preferred target (a naked man in the same example). This result shows that the subjects unconsciously attended to the targets they found more attractive, and the visual discrimination task revealed which sex those targets were.

As another alternative to feelings or behavior, researchers sometimes use *arousal* as a criterion for sexual orientation. Sexual arousal means being "turned on" sexually: It is the temporary state of excitement that a person may experience in the presence of an attractive partner, while viewing erotic images, or while imagining or engaging in actual sexual contacts. One way to measure arousal is to monitor physiological responses to erotic stimuli in the laboratory. For men, this method can make use of a transducer placed around the penis that measures the degree and rate of penile erection while the subject, say, views erotic images. For women, an analogous device can measure color changes in the walls of the vagina as they become engorged with blood during sexual excitement. Vaginal lubrication also can be used as an indicator of arousal.

Genital phenomena of this kind are probably closely related to physical attraction, in men at least, and measuring them may circumvent any reluctance a subject may have to speak frankly about his or her feelings. For that reason, genital measures are sometimes used to assay the sexual feelings of persons accused or convicted of child molestation. Monitoring genital arousal is too time-consuming and invasive of privacy to be of widespread use in sex research, but I will mention some studies that use this technique.

Another aspect of physiological arousal involves changes in the size of the pupils of the eyes. Pupils dilate for many reasons, but one of these is sexual arousal. Pupils dilate more when people view images of persons of their preferred sex than when viewing images of the other sex,[4] and these differences can be measured in a laboratory setting. I will mention the use of this technique, as well as yet other physiological measures of sexual arousal, in several chapters of this book.

There is an inner, subjective state of sexual arousal that precedes and accompanies genital arousal or that may occur without any genital arousal. Some researchers ask people to indicate their degree of sexual arousal— by pushing or pulling a lever, for example—while viewing various kinds of potentially arousing images or videos. Others have attempted to access subjective arousal by the use of functional brain imaging techniques. I am not convinced, however, that there is much difference between subjective arousal and the state of experiencing sexual attraction (as opposed to the trait of sexual orientation).

Sexual Orientation in Men and Women

As sketched in Figure 1.1, we can think about sexual orientation in men and women in two alternative ways. The usual terminology of sexual

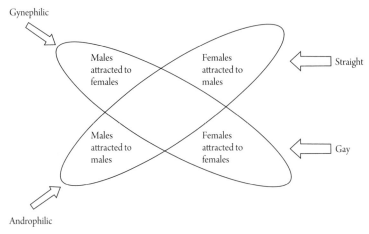

Figure 1.1 Alternative conceptions of sexual orientation: either in terms of the specific sex of the persons to whom an individual is attracted (as seen by reading within each diagonally oriented oval) or in terms of whether the individual is attracted to persons of the same or the opposite sex (as seen by reading horizontally across the figure).

orientation—heterosexual, bisexual, and homosexual—emphasizes the equivalence of sexual orientation in the two sexes. In both men and women, heterosexuality means attraction to the other sex, homosexuality means attraction to the same sex, and bisexuality means attraction to both sexes. This usage makes sense culturally, because in both sexes heterosexual people are the majority, who are commonly perceived as normal, and in both sexes homosexual (and perhaps bisexual) people form a small and sometimes stigmatized minority.

But does this usage make sense when we are trying to understand causation? In other words, when considering what makes people heterosexual or homosexual, should we be looking for similar causes in men and women?

One can certainly construct developmental models that work the same way in both sexes. Let's consider a couple of hypothetical examples. In one model, we could imagine that the development of heterosexuality involves a psychological process in early life in which we first establish a sense of our own sex as male or female and then exclude people of this sex from the realm of attractive sex partners. Thus we are left with people of the other sex as potential objects of attraction. Both male and female homosexuality, in this model, could result when children identify themselves as belonging to the other sex than the one to which they belong anatomically. In a second, equally hypothetical model, heterosexuality results from a "conformist" trait that causes both men and women to accept the cultural norms for their sex, while homosexuality results from a "rebellious" trait that causes both males and females to reject those norms. In either model, a single process or trait would explain the development of homosexuality in both sexes.

In contrast with such ideas, one can emphasize the equivalence of heterosexuality in men and homosexuality in women—because, after all, both are defined by sexual attraction to *women*. Similarly, heterosexuality in women is in a sense equivalent to homosexuality in men—both are defined by sexual attraction to *men*. Sex researchers sometimes use special terms when they want to emphasize this way of looking at things: *gynephilic* (woman–loving) when referring to straight men and gay women, and *androphilic* (man–loving) when referring to straight women and gay men.[†]

It's just as easy to construct developmental models that fit this point of view. For example, one could speculate that a certain gene mediates sexual attraction to the look, voice, smell, or behavior of women, and that this gene is switched on in straight men and gay women but switched off (or absent) in straight women and gay men—and vice versa for a gene mediating attraction to the look, voice, smell, or behavior of men. Another hypothetical model of this kind might invoke the rewarding effect of sexual pleasure as a causal agent, such that regardless of one's own sex, one becomes permanently oriented toward the sex of the partner with whom one first has sex. Thus people who initially happen to have sex with females become gynephilic (straight men and gay women), and those who initially have sex with males become androphilic (straight women and gay men). I hasten to add that I don't actually believe this model, but it is one that has been put forward in the past to explain the development of sexual orientation, particularly homosexuality, as we'll see in Chapter 2.

It's also possible to construct hybrid models that incorporate elements of both kinds of models just described. But the general point is this: We need to be careful not to assume that the same processes necessarily cause homosexuality (or heterosexuality) in both sexes. It is quite possible that a single factor might promote homosexuality in one sex and heterosexuality in the other—or indeed that the factors influencing sexual orientation are completely unrelated in the two sexes.

Stability of Sexual Orientation

Calling sexual orientation a trait implies that it is stable over time. Obviously, most of us believe that sexual orientation is stable, because we use terms like "a lesbian" or "a straight man" to describe individuals. This usage wouldn't make much sense unless sexual orientation was a reasonably durable attribute of a person.

[†] *Androphilic* and *gynephilic* are usually understood to mean attraction specifically to adult males or females, whereas *homosexual* and *heterosexual* define attraction to same- or opposite-sex persons without regard to their age. This distinction is not particularly relevant to the theme of this book.

Surprisingly few studies have actually followed people over time to see whether their sexual orientations remain the same or change. In one study, published in 2012, Steven Mock and Richard Eibach (of the University of Waterloo, Canada) analyzed data from the National Survey of Midlife Development in the United States.[5] In this survey about 2500 women and men, mostly in their late 30s, were asked questions about their sexual orientation, and they were asked the same questions 10 years later. Of those people who identified as heterosexual at the initial interview, very few (1.4% of the women and 0.8% of the men) reported a different sexual orientation at the 10-year follow-up. The men who identified as homosexual were somewhat more likely to change: 2 out of 21 individuals (9.5%) did so, one to bisexual and the other to heterosexual. The identities of individuals in the other three groups—bisexual men, bisexual women, and homosexual women—were much less stable: 47%, 65%, and 64%, respectively, reported a different sexual orientation at the second interview. Similar findings were reported in an earlier, smaller study conducted in New Zealand, in which men and women were interviewed at 21 years of age and again five years later.[6]

Another study, by psychologist Lisa Diamond of the University of Utah, focused on 89 young women whose sexual attractions were non-heterosexual at the start of the study.[7] When reinterviewed 10 years later, all but 8 of these women were still non-heterosexual. There were often more-subtle shifts within the broad category of "non-heterosexual," however, and there were more changes in the *labels* that the women applied to themselves than in the actual direction of their attractions.

Diamond believes that women in general—and perhaps men too—are much more fluid (capable of change) in their sexual orientations than is usually believed.[8] Still, she did not include heterosexual women in her study, and as mentioned above such women are very unlikely to become bisexual or lesbian, at least over a 10-year time span.

It seems fair to conclude from these and other studies that people's basic sexual orientation doesn't commonly undergo major shifts. This is in line with the common belief that it's appropriate to label people (including oneself) as straight, bisexual, or gay/lesbian.

It does sometimes happen that men and women "come out" as gay or lesbian later in life—in their 40s, 50s, or even later, often after many years of heterosexual marriage. I have met quite a number of such people, and in discussing their life histories with them I have been struck by a major difference between the sexes. The men regularly say that that they were aware of having a same-sex attraction throughout their adult lives. They did not act on it (or did act, but were not open about doing so) and may not even have considered themselves gay, for reasons such as shame, religious teaching, or the desire to have a conventional family. US Congressman Robert Bauman, who was married to a woman for two decades before coming out as gay, gave this account to historian Eric Marcus:

> It was nearly twenty years later that my wife and priest confronted me. I was already a congressman by this time, drinking heavily, involved with hustlers, and in and out of gay bars. . . . All through this period I was thoroughly convinced that I wasn't gay. I wasn't a homosexual. I couldn't be a person like that. People wonder how I could have convinced myself of that, but from an early age it was a matter of building certain walls within my mind. . . . [I]t took almost three years of religious and psychiatric counseling for me to acknowledge that I was gay.[9]

The women I've spoken with give much more diverse accounts, but quite commonly they will say that they were completely unaware of having a sexual attraction to women until they met a specific woman or went through a significant life event, such as divorce, later in life. Here's how comedian Carol Leifer put it in an online interview:

> [I]t was like my life threw me a surprise party. I really didn't have any clue, and in fact, had very good physical relationships with men. It was around when I turned 40 that I had this really intense desire to have an affair with a woman. It just kind of overtook me, kind of like when you feel like you're on a mission.[10]

Thus my informal impression is that at the level of conscious awareness of sexual attraction, some women but few men gravitate toward an authentically new homosexual orientation later in life.

There has been a long-running debate about whether gay people who want to become heterosexual can do so through some kind of intervention. Methods that have been promoted as helping people achieve this goal include psychoanalysis, other forms of psychotherapy, conditioning, and religion-based group programs.[11] The majority viewpoint among mental-health professionals is that these so-called *conversion therapies* or *reparative therapies* have little if any chance of success and can cause significant harm by reinforcing the gay person's negative self-image.[12]

Prevalence of Different Orientations

Kinsey devised a seven-category scale of sexual orientation running from 0 (exclusive heterosexuality) to 6 (exclusive homosexuality), with the intervening numbers representing various degrees of bisexuality. This is the famous *Kinsey scale*.[13] Contemporary researchers often use fewer categories—five or even three. In the case of three categories, orientations are often defined as "heterosexual," meaning exclusive or near-exclusive attraction to the other sex; "bisexual," meaning significant attraction to both sexes; and "homosexual," meaning exclusive or near-exclusive attraction to one's own sex.

The distribution of sexual orientations in the population has been studied by means of large-scale random-sample surveys conducted in the United States and elsewhere.[14] Fairly typical are the findings of the National Survey of Family Growth (NSFG) conducted in the United States between 2006 and 2008.[15] In this study, 97.2% of men and 95.2% of women reported heterosexual attraction (attraction only or mostly to the opposite sex); 0.5% of men and 2.8% of women reported bisexual attraction (equal attraction to both sexes), and 1.9% of men and 1.4% of women reported homosexual attraction (attraction only or mostly to the same sex). The NSFG data are plotted in Figure 1.2, which uses a five-point scale of sexual orientation.

Although the numbers vary somewhat, most studies agree on several points. First, heterosexuality is far and away the most common orientation among both men and women. Second, with regard to non-heterosexual people, there is a difference between the sexes. Very few men say that they are equally attracted to both sexes; most place themselves at or near one or the other end of the scale. Women don't fall so clearly into two groups, because there are more women who say that they are equally attracted to both sexes than who place themselves at or near the homosexual end of the scale. This sex difference appears in survey after survey, often more markedly than in the NSFG.

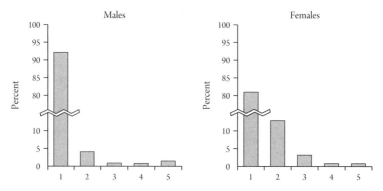

Figure 1.2 Distributions of sexual orientations for US males and females ages 18–44 years, based on data from the 2006–2008 National Survey of Family Growth. Group 1: attracted to opposite sex only; group 2: attracted mostly to opposite sex; group 3: attracted to both sexes; group 4: attracted mostly to same sex; group 5: attracted to same sex only.

It may be that these national surveys underreport the prevalences of gay people and perhaps bisexual people. Such underestimates could happen if some respondents are reluctant to acknowledge same-sex attraction—a trait that is still stigmatized in some quarters. To investigate this issue a group of economists at Ohio State University[16] used a survey method that made it unnecessary for respondents to disclose their sexual orientation at all.[‡] With this approach the prevalence of same-sex attraction was found to be significantly greater than that derived from direct questioning.

Christian Rudder, cofounder of the OkCupid dating site, performed a demographic analysis to estimate the true prevalence of homosexuality in the United States.[17] He showed that the prevalences of self-declared gay people in US states are strongly correlated with the levels of gay tolerance in each state—both are low in Mississippi and both are high in Hawaii, for example. But the actual prevalence of gay people (or gay men at least) doesn't appear to vary between states, because the percentages of Internet porn searches that are for gay male porn are nearly the same in all states—about 5%.[18] What's more, an analysis of birthplace and current residence shows that gay people are no more likely than straight people to move from, say, Mississippi to Hawaii, so differential migration doesn't explain the state-to-state differences. Therefore, Rudder argues, the low prevalence of self-declared gay people in conservative states is simply the result of their reluctance to admit to same-sex attraction. If so, the true prevalence of homosexuality in the United States would be somewhere near its reported prevalence in the gay-friendliest states, namely, in the 4–5% range.

Many gay and bisexual people are convinced that that the true prevalence of same-sex attraction is greater than surveys suggest. They can cite some recent surveys, such as two surveys conducted by the Internet-based market research company YouGov in the United States and Britain, which found same-sex attraction to be much commoner than previously thought—22% and 23% of respondents in those surveys said that they were not completely heterosexual.[19] Those numbers are probably unreliable, however, because the respondents were not randomly chosen from the entire population. In addition, the numbers may be distorted by cultural trends that have elevated the "coolness value" of a bisexual identity, especially among young people. All the same, the weight of the evidence points to a true prevalence of non-heterosexual orientations that is somewhat higher than estimates derived from the earlier national surveys.

[‡] In this "veiled elicitation method" respondents had to state how many items in a set of statements were true, only one of which asked about sexual attraction. The researchers could not determine the sexual orientation of any single individual from the data obtained this way, but they could apply statistical procedures to determine the distribution of sexual orientations within the entire sample.

Bisexuality is a complex and controversial topic, and researchers don't agree on how to define or measure it. Very often, scientific studies of sexual orientation exclude bisexual people altogether or lump them with gay people as "non-heterosexual." For that reason I am postponing a detailed discussion of bisexuality until Chapter 11.

Are There Categories?

On the face of it, the findings described so far suggest that sexual orientation in men can be described to a first approximation in terms of two categories—straight and gay—whereas sexual orientation in women has more of a *dimensional* quality, being distributed in a continuum across the spectrum of orientation, so that dividing women into two (or even three) categories might be more of a semantic convenience than an objective reality.

A set of objective statistical procedures called *taxometric analysis* can be used to assess whether a psychological trait, however dimensional it may appear in raw data, actually has an underlying categorical structure. A category identified by such a procedure is called a *taxon*. Several research groups have applied this methodology to the analysis of sexual orientation.[20] The most recent and largest of these studies was based on a survey of over 33,000 subjects; it was conducted by Alyssa Norris of Washington State University and her colleagues. They found that both male and female homosexuality constituted taxons. The male taxon comprised 3% of the male subjects and included not just the gay-identified men but also nearly all men who declared any degree of bisexual attraction. The female taxon comprised 2.7% of the female population. However, this taxon included less than half of all the women who declared some degree of same-sex attraction; the remainder fell outside the taxon. This result suggests that women as a group show some sexual fluidity, but not enough to blur out the categorical nature of female sexual orientation.

If this analysis is correct, it might be appropriate to ask what causes homosexuality in both men and women, but the answer to this question would provide a less complete understanding of sexual orientation in women than in men.

Sexual Orientation Across Cultures

Has homosexuality existed across different cultures and historical periods? And if so, have the relative numbers of gay people been the same as what we see in contemporary Western society?

The answer to the first question is, possibly not. According to a survey of the anthropological literature by Julien Barthes and colleagues at the University of Montpellier, France, male homosexuality is absent from the majority of non-stratified human cultures—meaning cultures, often made up of hunter-gatherers or pastoralists, that lack social classes.[21] By male homosexuality here is meant not simply homosexual behavior but the existence of adult men who have a lasting preference for male sex partners, even when female partners are available. Such men might of course escape notice, especially when they are "the only gay in the village" (the proud boast of Daffyd, hero of the BBC comedy series *Little Britain*) and never visit other villages except on raiding expeditions. Still, based on current knowledge, there is little justification for claiming that male homosexuality is a human universal or that it was a feature of ancestral human populations. This issue is discussed further in Chapter 7. The existence of female homosexuality in non-stratified cultures is not well documented either.

In stratified or westernized cultures, on the other hand, there seems to have always been a minority of homosexual individuals, and their proportions may not vary much around the globe. Sociologist Fred Whitam conducted informal surveys of male sexual orientation in several less-westernized countries such as Guatemala and the Philippines.[22] He concluded that in such cultures, about 5% of the male residents of large cities are gay, which roughly matches the estimated prevalence of male homosexuality in large Western cities such as London.

With regard to the question of homosexuality's presence in past historical periods, the problem is that sexual orientation was rarely conceptualized or described in the same way as it is today. The term *homosexual*, for example, was introduced in the 1860s. In earlier Western culture, most people thought of homosexuality not as an attribute of a distinct group of people but as a sinful or criminal behavior ("sodomy") that anyone might be tempted to engage in. To the extent that there was any recognition of a distinct group of people characterized by same-sex desire, it focused on a subset of what we would now call gay men and women—namely, gay men who were extremely feminine in manner and social role, and gay women who were extremely masculine.

The term *molly*, for example, was used in 18th-century London to refer to homosexual men who socialized in "molly-houses," where they affected women's dress and manners and entered into same-sex liaisons that they termed "marriages."[23] It seems likely that homosexual men who played more-conventional gender roles existed at that time but chose to maintain their anonymity. After all, voluntarily outing oneself as a homosexual man would hardly have been an attractive option in 18th-century England, where sodomy was still a capital offense.

In some cultures, unmarried women were sequestered and thus were invisible to men and unobtainable to them as sex partners. In such environments, adult men, especially young unmarried men, often sought male adolescents as sex partners. Ancient Greece is a particularly well-known example—so much so that "Greek love" has long been used as a colloquial term for homosexuality.[24] A more recent example was the same-sex culture that existed in Afghanistan under the Taliban, when all women were hidden behind their burkas. "I like boys, but I like girls better," one Kandahar resident was quoted as saying in a *Los Angeles Times* article. "It's just that we can't see the women to see if they are beautiful. But we can see the boys, and so we can tell which of them is beautiful."[25] About half of all men in Kandahar engaged in sex with boys at one time or another, according to one local medical professor interviewed for that article.

In such cultures, the choice of adolescent boys as partners probably reflects the fact that these youths, lacking beards and adult musculature, are closer to women in appearance than are adult men. Thus it would be quite wrong to assert that many or most men in ancient Greece or in Afghanistan were homosexual in the sense of having a strong preference for males when given the choice of sex partners. What these cultures do demonstrate is the degree to which sexual desire and sexual behavior accommodate themselves to a restricted range of options, just they may do in prisons and other single-sex environments today.

Yet even in ancient Greece there was awareness that some men and women did have an authentic preference for same-sex partners. This comes across most clearly in Plato's *Symposium,* in which one of the participants at a drinking party extemporizes a creation myth to explain the existence of homosexual and heterosexual men and women. Plato's account could be interpreted as the first genetic theory of sexual orientation.[§] In fact, two of the participants at that party, Pausanias and Agathon, were a male couple who are known to have stayed together well into their adult lives—an arrangement suggesting that these men were homosexual in the modern sense. But their long-lasting partnership seems to have been unusual. We have no way of knowing what the actual prevalence of homosexuality in the modern sense was in ancient Greece, other than that it existed.

---

§ Plato put the account into the mouth of the comic playwright Aristophanes, who described how humanity originally existed as double creatures, like pairs of present-day humans stuck together. Some of these pairs consisted of two males, some of two females, and some were male–female hybrids. In punishment for their transgressions an angry god cut them all into halves. Sexual attraction, Aristophanes said, is the desire to be reunited with one's ancestral other half. Thus the three kinds of original creatures gave rise to gay men, lesbians, and heterosexual men and women, respectively. Plato may have created the story by expanding on a preexisting myth of the creation of men and women by division of a single ancestral creature; such stories existed in Egyptian mythology (with the god Geb and the goddess Nut), Judaic mythology (where Eve was formed from Adam's rib), and possibly Babylonian mythology.

Anthropologists have established that sexual relationships between males and between females have occurred widely in non-Western cultures. In one particularly common arrangement, boys who have been feminine since childhood may choose as adults to adopt the gender role of a female or of some combination of female and male, and they may enter into sexual relationships or marriages with conventionally masculine men.[26] In many Native American cultures these individuals were given specific names, such as *winkte* in the Lakota language, and they were considered to be *two-spirit people* who took on special roles in society. One Lakota man offered a "biological" explanation for the origin of *winktes*. "We think that if a woman has two little ones growing inside her, if she is going to have twins, sometimes instead of giving birth to two babies they have formed up in her womb into just one, into a half-man/half-woman kind of being."[27]

Similarly, there are accounts in various non-Western cultures of women taking on male or male/female roles and partnering with conventionally feminine women. Walter Williams cites a 16th-century account of such women living in northeastern Brazil: "They wear their hair cut in the same way as the men, and go to war with bows and arrows and pursue game, always in company with men; each has a woman to serve her, to whom she says she is married, and they treat each other and speak with each other as man and wife."[28] Explorers named Brazil's great waterway the "river of the Amazons" because of the similarity of these local women to the warrior women of Greek mythology.

Two-spirit people and Amazons were clearly homosexual in the sense that they were consistently attracted to persons of the same anatomical sex as themselves. They were also, however, what we would call *transgender*, which is not the case for most contemporary gay men and women. There are some people in our society—very feminine gay men and very masculine gay women—who occupy a zone of overlap between a homosexual and transgender identity. A possible US example is that of LGBT activist Chaz Bono, who was born female and who identified as a lesbian for many years. In 2009 Bono announced that she was changing her sex to male. The two-spirit people and Amazons may be thought of as occupying that same territory.

What about the conventionally gendered individuals who partnered with two-spirit people or with Amazons? Were they the counterparts of today's conventional gay men and women? Very possibly some of them were, but they were not usually recognized as anything different from regular men or women. Lakota men who entered a relationship with a *winkte*, for example, quite commonly took up with anatomical women before or after that relationship. In the distant past, when the Lakota people practiced polygamy, these men often had a *winkte* and a female wife at the same time. Although men who partnered with *winktes* were commonly subject to some ridicule for doing so, they were not thought of as a different *kind* of person in the same way that *winktes* were.

To assert that they were in fact homosexual would be to claim far more under-standing of their mental lives than we possess.

Thus what we learn from different times and cultures is somewhat paradox-ical. On the one hand there is widespread evidence of homosexual relationships, as well of homosexual individuals who could be thought of as transgender. But the majority of gay men and women in our own culture—those who iden-tify with their anatomical sex and have an enduring preference for same-sex partners—don't seem to have numerous and obvious counterparts in non-Western cultures. And the homosexual relationships that we think of as typical today—relationships between pairs of fairly similar, conventionally gendered men or women of like age—seem in other cultures to have been much less com-mon or less visible than relationships characterized by differences in age or in gender. To use the terminology applied by sociologist Stephen Murray, *age-stratified* and *gender-stratified* relationships have been the dominant forms of homosexual bonding in other cultures, while *egalitarian* relationships are the most visible form in our own.[29]

Do these differences between cultures undermine the effort to understand sexual orientation in biological terms? Probably not, for several reasons. For one thing, the differences may not be as great as they seem. Both gender-conformist and gender-nonconformist gay people may well have existed in all cultures, but with differing visibility. Just among American lesbians of the last hundred years or so, there have been marked swings between a cultural em-phasis on gender nonconformity (e.g., as represented by "diesel dykes") and on gender conformity and between an emphasis on egalitarian relationships and on those that are gender stratified (so-called butch–femme relationships—see Chapter 11).[30] Yet these swings, driven by social forces such as the women's liberation movement of the 1960s and 1970s, probably mask a more or less con-stant underlying reality, which is that there is a spectrum of gender diversity within the category of gay women; the same reality holds for gay men.

A biological theory of sexual orientation needs to explain not only why there is a link between homosexuality and a broader gender nonconformity but also why there is such diversity in gender-related traits among gay people. Biologists also have to acknowledge that much that is important about sexual orientation—especially the diverse ways that homosexuality and heterosexu-ality are conceived of and acted out in different societies—lies outside of the arena of biological investigation.

2

Why We Need Biology

Almost everyone has some opinion about what determines sexual orientation. Often they frame their ideas in terms of what went wrong in the lives of gay people. Some hypotheses are little more than old wives' tales.* Others offer at least the semblance of scientific credibility. In this chapter I review the principal *non-biological* theories that have been presented over the years. Each of these theories has significant shortcomings. Collectively, their weakness spurs the search for other, *biological* explanations.

Psychoanalytic Theories

Most of us think of the sex drive as something that makes its first appearance at or after puberty, when raging sex hormones transform the body and mind of a meek-mannered child into those of a horny adolescent. The founder of psychoanalysis, Sigmund Freud (1856–1939), took a very different view. He proposed that the erotic instinct, or *libido* as he called it, is already fully active at birth and undergoes several radical transformations during childhood.[1] A newborn infant's libido, Freud claimed, is focused on the mouth and is satisfied by suckling at the mother's breast. The libido then moves to the child's anus, where it is satisfied by defecation. At about two years of age the libido becomes focused on the *phallus* (penis or clitoris), where it can be satisfied by masturbation.

Freud spelled out what happens next more explicitly for males than females, perhaps because the majority of his patients were men. At around the same time as the libido becomes focused on the phallus, it also begins to be directed externally, toward other people. In boys the libido is directed toward other males, because they also possess a penis. This is therefore a homosexual phase, but one of which adult men (whether straight or gay) have repressed all memory.

---

* I've been told at various times that homosexuality is caused by the consumption of spoiled food, by the exposure of pregnant women to fluorescent light, or by the failure to chant "HU" for 20 minutes per day.

15

At about three years of age a boy's libido transfers to his mother. This is the famous *Oedipal phase*, named for Oedipus, the character in Greek mythology who unwittingly married his own mother. The boy remains sexually fixated on his mother for two or three years. Then his libido enters a period of latency in which it is largely inactive, to be awoken again after puberty in the form of adult heterosexuality. This sequence is the developmental process that Freud considered normal.

Homosexuality in adult men resulted, according to Freud, from a disruption of this process. In *pre-Oedipal homosexuality*, the libido failed to enter the Oedipal phase and simply remained stuck for a lifetime in the early homosexual phase. In *Oedipal homosexuality*, the libido did enter the Oedipal phase but failed to leave it, so the boy remained erotically fixated on his mother.

Freud placed much more emphasis on Oedipal than on pre-Oedipal homosexuality. This raised a problem: Why would remaining erotically fixated on one's mother make a boy grow up to be sexually attracted to men? Wouldn't it be more likely to make him heterosexual, given that his mother was a woman?

To get around this problem, Freud proposed that the growing boy, unable to shake off his attraction to his mother but equally unable to satisfy that desire, resolves the dilemma by identifying with his mother and seeking sex partners who represent himself. In other words, when he enters sexual relationships with other men he is psychologically re-establishing the Oedipal bond, but with roles reversed.[†]

That left the question, what caused a boy to remain erotically focused on his mother and thus to become homosexual? The reason, Freud said, was that his mother was too closely attached to and involved with him, or even seductive, and thus prevented him from breaking away. Alternatively (or additionally), the father might be distant or hostile, generating in his son an irrational fear of castration and thus forcing him into an excessively close relationship with his mother.

In constructing this theory, Freud was probably influenced by what gay men told him about their childhood relationships with their parents. As has been documented more recently in statistical studies of large numbers of subjects, gay men do indeed describe their relationships with their mothers as closer, and their relationships with their fathers as more distant or hostile, than straight men do.[2] As with most other such claims in this book, this is a statement about averages, and it's not true for everyone: There are plenty of gay men who got on famously with their fathers, and plenty of straight men who didn't. Still,

---

[†] In a later formulation, Freud proposed that homosexuality results when the boy is so identified with his mother that he seeks to take her place in her sexual relationship with his father (the "negative Oedipal complex"). In that model, adult homosexuality is the re-enactment of the desired relationship with the father.

this significant difference, on average, between gay and straight men demands some explanation, and Freud provided one.

The problem is that there are other possible explanations, some of which are more plausible or straightforward than Freud's. The simplest one is that boys who become gay (pre-gay or pre-homosexual boys) and those who become straight (pre-straight or pre-heterosexual boys) differ from each other in ways that parents pick up on. As pointed out by the late Richard Isay, a gay-affirmative psychoanalyst, if pre-gay boys have traits that fathers dislike and mothers like, then this would set up the same relationships that Freud described, but with the direction of causation reversed.[3] Rather than a mother's closeness or a father's hostility making their son gay, it would be the son's "gayness" making his mother close and his father hostile.

In Chapter 4 I'll present evidence that pre-homosexual boys do indeed differ from pre-heterosexual boys in a number of traits—traits that can be summarized with the term *gender nonconformity*. Thus it's very plausible that some fathers might reject their pre-homosexual sons on account of what they perceive as "sissiness" or a lack of interest in the typically masculine activities that fathers often like to engage their sons in. Conversely, some mothers might actually like such traits in their sons. Even if they don't, they might become unusually protective of a son who they see being exposed to teasing or hostility from the father or from other children.

Over the course of the 20th century Freudian theory had a lot of its raw sexual content watered down or excised. Some later analysts, such as Carl Jung, thought of the libido as a more general motivating force within the psyche rather than an explicitly sexual urge. And the Oedipal complex became a simple desire for emotional closeness with the mother rather than a lust for sexual intercourse with her. But that change didn't undermine the role in many psychiatrists' minds of the mother–son bond in the development of homosexuality. "You've got to get these mothers out of the way," said UCLA psychiatrist Richard Green to a couple who feared that their gender-nonconformist son would become homosexual. He recommended that the father spend more one-on-one time with the boy.[4]

Green himself has since changed his views about the development of sexual orientation, but other therapists—especially those purporting to offer advice on preventing or "curing" homosexuality—continued to emphasize the crucial role of the Oedipal complex. The late Charles Socarides, a psychoanalyst who claimed to have helped many men get the "monkey of homosexuality off their backs,"[5] attributed male homosexuality to "a lifelong persistence of the original primary feminine identification with the mother, and a consequent sense of deficiency in one's masculine identity."[6] Joseph Nicolosi, who is one of the best-known "reparative therapists" currently active, writes that "if [a father] wants his son to grow up straight, he has to break the mother–son connection that is proper to infancy but not in the boy's interest after the age of three."[7]

What about sexual orientation in women? Freud believed that a young girl, like a boy, goes through an early Oedipal fixation on her mother, but when she finds out that her mother lacks a penis she redirects her sexual desire toward her father. Thus the girl begins to compete with her mother for her father's love. In the one case of female homosexuality that Freud described in detail, this relationship was damaged by the birth of a younger brother when the girl was 16. "It was not *she* who bore the child, but her unconsciously hated rival, her mother," wrote Freud. "Furiously resentful and embittered, she turned away from her father and from men altogether."[8] Instead, she fell in love with a woman, who (in Freud's view) represented both her (hated) mother and another brother, older than herself, whose penis had made a "strong impression" on her when she was 5 years old. Thus psychologically it was really a bisexual relationship rather than a strictly homosexual one.

Byzantine accounts like this one—and I've omitted most of the details—were Freud's stock in trade. They raise the question, How did Freud figure all this out, and what evidence did he present to persuade us that he was right? For the most part, there *was* no evidence: We just have to trust that Freud's insights were correct. And that's the general problem with psychoanalytical theories.[9] It's not that they've been proven wrong; it's just that there's no good reason to think they're right. In that situation, their implausibility and complexity counts against them. They're like the theory that unidentified flying objects are alien spacecraft: They could be—but why believe that when there's no evidence to support it, and more-mundane explanations exist?

Learning Theories

Influence of Early Sexual Experiences

In stark contrast to this psychoanalytic perspective, learning theorists (especially those who fall under the heading of *behaviorists*) have taken a much simpler view of the mind. In behaviorist thought, the minds of babies are pretty much blank slates, though they come supplied with the ability to form mental associations, to seek pleasurable experiences, and to avoid unpleasant ones. A person's tendency to seek male or female sex partners, from this perspective, is simply the consequence of innumerable "carrots" and "sticks" that have shaped his or her sexual feelings during childhood and adolescence.

According to a simple behaviorist theory, popular in the 1960s and 1970s, the major "carrot" influencing sexual orientation is the pleasure of sex itself, especially orgasm. If a person's first sexual contact is with a woman, he or she will desire further contacts with women; if it is with a man, he or she will desire further contacts with men. Thus a person who starts off with no particular preference in sex partners gradually develops an ingrained attraction to one sex or the other.[10] This theory led to the idea that male homosexuality results from sexual contact with an older male—a stranger or an older brother—during childhood or adolescence.[11] Although the contact might be a one-time experience, the boy may evoke memories of it during solitary masturbation, thus strengthening its influence.[12]

According to one study, both gay men and lesbians are indeed far more likely than heterosexuals to have had sexual contact with an older person of their own sex during childhood or adolescence.[13] On the face of it, this finding could be taken to support the idea that the sex of one's first sex partner influences a person's ultimate sexual orientation. For this to be true, however, we would have to assume that the children or adolescents were sexually passive targets for molestation by their elders. In reality, it is likely that many of them, especially the adolescents, already felt sexually attracted to same-sex partners. If so, they might have initiated the contacts or responded willingly to the older persons' advances. Even if they did not, the older persons might have picked up on cues that were indicative of the children's future sexual orientation and selected them on that basis.

Cross-cultural evidence also speaks against the notion that the sex of the first sex partner influences a person's ultimate sexual orientation. In some non-Western cultures, such as that of the Sambia of New Guinea, all boys are required to engage in sexual contacts with older male youths for several years before they have any access to females, yet most if not all of these boys become heterosexual men.[14] Similarly, homosexual behavior is common among British children and adolescents who attend single-sex boarding schools, yet adult Britons who attended such schools are no more likely to engage in homosexual behavior than those who did not.[15]

Finally, many (probably most) young people in our own culture develop an awareness of their sexual orientation while they are still virgins or before they have had any sexual experiences with partners of their preferred sex. These people's sexual orientation could not have been determined by the sex of their first partners.

Childhood Abuse

Gay men and lesbians are more likely than straight people to report having experienced physical or sexual abuse during their childhood.[16] While this heightened risk of abuse results at least in part from the reaction of parents and others to the children's gender nonconformity, this factor accounts for only about one-third of the increased risk, according to a study led by Andrea Roberts of Harvard University's School of Public Health.[17]

Roberts's group concluded that some of the additional risk comes about because childhood abuse itself makes children more likely to become gay adults.[18] This conclusion depended on the use of an unusual statistical technique, and a controversy arose about whether the Roberts study had used the technique correctly.[19] In addition, as pointed out by Judith Andersen (of the University of Toronto) and John Blosnich, the great majority of abused children do not become gay or bisexual adults, and many gay and bisexual adults have no childhood history of abuse.[20]

A recent study conducted by a Chinese group found evidence supporting the original idea—that the increased rate of childhood abuse among pre-gay boys is entirely a response to their gender-nonconformist behavior.[21] In fact, the gender-nonconformist boys in the Chinese study who became straight men were just as likely to report childhood abuse as those who became gay. Thus the weight of the evidence does not support the notion that childhood abuse is a causal factor in the development of homosexuality.

Gender Learning

Because so many people become aware of their sexual orientation before they have had sexual contact with their preferred partners or before they have had any experience of partnered sex, theorists have looked for other ways in which people might "learn" their sexual orientations. The most commonly expressed idea is that sexual orientation develops out of a broader process of gender learning.

Gender is the set of mental and behavioral traits that differ, to a greater or lesser degree, between males and females. An example of a gendered trait shown by children is engagement in rough-and-tumble play: In most or all human cultures boys engage in more such play than girls. (I will have more to say about childhood gender characteristics in Chapter 4 and about adult gender characteristics in Chapter 5.)

According to the *standard social science model*,[22] gender differences are learned. The learning might take place directly, for example by parents' rewarding sons who engage in rough-and-tumble play and punishing daughters who do so. Alternatively, the child might take a more active role—first establishing a sense of his or her own sex and then acquiring other gender characteristics through imitation of same-sex role models and other forms of social interaction.[23]

John Money, a well-known sex researcher at the Johns Hopkins School of Medicine who died in 2006, was the leading proponent of the idea that a person's sexual orientation develops as part of this process of gender learning.[24] As evidence in favor of his theory, Money cited a remarkable and ultimately tragic case history. This concerned a child named Bruce Reimer. Bruce was born a normal boy, but he suffered the destruction of his penis during a botched circumcision procedure when he was seven months old. Money told the parents that such a young boy would not yet have acquired a definitive gender or sexual orientation, and he therefore advised them have the boy's testicles removed also and to raise him as a girl. This they did. Over the ensuing years, Money reported, the change of gender was a great success, with the child—whose name was changed to Brenda—developing a suite of girlish characteristics and looking forward to marrying a man.

In reality, Brenda never accepted a female gender identity, hated her developing breasts, and ultimately demanded and received medical treatment to turn her back into a male. He then adopted a new name, David. As an adult man David was sexually attracted to women, contrary to Money's prediction. Money never divulged the true story; the facts were revealed after some detective work by sexologist Milton Diamond of the University of Hawaii[25] and by journalist John Colapinto, who wrote a book about the case.[26]

One case history by itself should not make or break a theory. Still, other cases also had outcomes that refute the notion that sexual orientation develops as a part of the process of gender learning. Another boy who, like Bruce Reimer, lost his penis in infancy (at two months of age) and was reassigned as a girl did successfully adopt a female gender identity that lasted into adulthood. However, she was predominantly attracted to women and was partnered with one at the most recent follow-up.[27] According to Money's learning theory of sexual orientation, having learned a female gender identity, she should also have learned to be sexually attracted to men.

In a similar vein, medical scientists at the Johns Hopkins Medical Institutions studied 14 genetic males who were reassigned as female when they were babies because severe congenital malformations of the pelvic area had left them without functional penises.[28] As they grew up, most of these individuals chose to revert to the male sex, but regardless of whether they did or not, those who were old enough to report a sexual orientation said that they were sexually attracted to females. These results again suggest that sexual orientation is not learned but inborn.

Looking at all these cases together, it seems that gender identity may be somewhat more susceptible to social influence than is sexual orientation. Here too, however, nature usually trumps nurture.

If role modeling played an important part in the development of sexual orientation, we'd expect that the sexual orientation of a child's parents would be a strong influence on that child's ultimate sexual orientation. In fact, however, the vast majority of gay people have straight parents. This may be an unfortunate fact, in that it means that gay children are generally deprived of the support that gay parents would be most able to give them. Nevertheless, it argues against an important influence of role modeling or parental teaching in the development of sexual orientation.

Of course, some gay people are parents themselves, so what about *their* children? Do they grow up gay under the influence of parental role modeling? The answer is no, not usually. Children raised by gay parents don't differ in sexual orientation (or in any other significant characteristics) from those raised by straight parents, according to a review[29] of numerous studies.[†]

Role modeling might also operate during the teen years to influence adolescents' sexual orientation. In this case peer networks would likely be an important conduit for such modeling. A group at Rosalind Franklin University, led by psychologist Tiffany Brakefield, conducted a study that addressed this issue.[30] They used data from the National Longitudinal Study of Adolescent Health, which not only asked teens about their sexual feelings and behaviors but also had them list the names of their friends in order of closeness. The researchers used statistical methods to determine whether close friends shared a variety of traits and behaviors. They found that an adolescent and his or her friends (and friends of friends) did indeed show a significant tendency to share sexual activity levels and the degree to which they desired a romantic relationship. No such tendency was found, on the other hand, for sexual orientation, making peer role modeling an unlikely influence on this trait.

Is Sexual Orientation a Choice?

As recently as 2004, one-third of Americans believed that being homosexual was a "lifestyle preference," according to a *Los Angeles Times* poll.[31] Beliefs may have changed somewhat since then (see Chapter 12), but the concept of homosexuality as a choice is still widespread, especially among political conservatives.[32]

If sexual orientation is a choice, gay people should remember having made it. But by and large, they don't. In the mid-1990s Janet Lever (then at the RAND Corporation) analyzed the responses of gay men and lesbians to a questionnaire in *The Advocate*, a leading gay magazine. Only 4% of gay men and 15% of lesbians said that choice had anything to do with why they were gay.[33] In contrast, 90% of the gay men and 50% of the lesbians said that they felt they were "born gay." (The remainder of the women mentioned factors such as childhood experiences.)

If people choose to be gay, they presumably could also choose *not* to be gay. Yet very few if any gay people who have attempted to become straight—often at enormous financial and psychological cost—have succeeded in doing so.[34]

[†] Girls who are the biological children of lesbians may have an increased likelihood of becoming bisexual or lesbian, perhaps on account of genes running in those families (see Chapter 7).

Why is there such a striking difference of opinion between the general population and gay people on whether being gay is a choice? The explanation may have to do with the *level* at which people conceptualize sexual orientation. Among the general population, especially those people who do not have gay friends or relatives, it seems natural to view sexual orientation in terms of people's actual sexual behavior, the communities they join, and the identities they claim for themselves. At these levels, choice certainly does play an important role.

Among gay people themselves it seems more natural to conceptualize sexual orientation in terms of sexual attraction, because sexual attraction is the wellspring of motivation that guides (but doesn't dictate) all their behavioral choices. To a large extent, then, people who argue about whether being gay is a choice or not are talking past each other. As discussed in the previous chapter, I agree with most sex researchers in taking the direction of sexual attraction as the key criterion for sexual orientation, and like most sex researchers I doubt that people choose to experience sexual attraction to one sex or the other.

The Biological Alternative

Researchers have turned to biological ideas about the origins of sexual orientation in part because other theories have failed to provide persuasive explanations. In addition, however, biological research has advanced to the point that it can offer ideas about the development of traits that used to fall squarely within the province of psychology. *Biological psychology* (or *psychobiology*) is the name of the hybrid discipline that has grown up around these ideas.

With regard to sexual orientation, biological psychologists have made a variety of important observations:

- Homosexual behavior is common among *nonhuman animals*. In at least one species—domestic sheep—individual animals have a durable preference for same-sex partners.
- Both in childhood and during adult life, gay people differ from straight people of the same sex in a variety of mental traits that fall under the general label of *gender*.
- There is evidence that the levels of *sex hormones* circulating during fetal life influence these gendered traits.
- There is evidence that *genes* influence sexual orientation and other aspects of gender.
- There are structural and functional differences between the *brains* of gay and straight people. To judge from animal experiments, these are caused by differences in prenatal levels of sex hormones or in the way that the brain responds to those hormones.

- There are differences in the structure and function of the *bodies* of gay and straight people.
- *Birth order* influences sexual orientation in men, and this influence appears to operate through biological mechanisms rather than social ones.

The following chapters lay out the evidence for these statements and attempt to tie them together to form a coherent biological theory of sexual orientation.

3

The Outline of a Theory

Humans are animals. We cannot fully understand ourselves without acknowledging our kinship with other species and learning from what they have to teach us. Observations on nonhuman animals, and experiments that make use of them, are fundamental to human biology, and they should be fundamental to psychology and sociology too.

That's not to say that humans are the *same* as other animals. Every species is the product of its own evolutionary history and is therefore unique—otherwise it would not be a species. Humans differ markedly in bodily appearance from our closest nonhuman relatives. A chimpanzee—even wearing a tuxedo—doesn't risk being mistaken for a person. Our human minds mark us off even more clearly from chimpanzees and other primates. We are unique in our highly developed capacities for toolmaking, language, empathy, foresight, art, science, and spirituality.[1] Some aspects of our minds and behaviors have close parallels among nonhuman animals; others do not.

Male and Female Brains

Where does our sexuality stand in this respect? Let's start with some anatomy. Across all mammalian species, including ourselves, there are consistent differences between male and female bodies. These differences are most obvious in the genitals and in secondary sexual characteristics such as mammary glands (breasts), but equally important and consistent are differences in the internal reproductive organs: Males have testes, a prostate gland, and some other sexual glands, along with the tubing to connect them, while females have a vagina, a uterus, oviducts (fallopian tubes), and ovaries.

Although less obvious at a casual glance, there are also anatomical differences between male and female brains. Neuroanatomist Roger Gorski and his colleagues at UCLA made a key discovery in the late 1970s.[2] They were studying the hypothalamus, an ancient region at the base of the brain that plays an important role in the regulation of many basic behaviors such as feeding and drinking as well as reproductive behaviors. Using rats as their animal model, Gorski's group focused on a region at the front of the hypothalamus called the medial preoptic area, which was known to be involved in the generation of sexual behavior typically shown by male animals, such as mounting of females. Within the medial preoptic area they noticed a cluster of cells that was much larger in male than in female rats. They named this cluster the *sexually dimorphic nucleus of the preoptic area*, or SDN-POA. (*Sexually dimorphic* means differing in structure between males and females. A *nucleus*, in neuroanatomical parlance, is a consistently recognizable aggregate of *neurons* at a certain location within the brain.)

Since the time of Gorski's discovery, comparable cell groups have been described in the hypothalami of other mammals, including primates.[3] The comparable cell group in the human hypothalamus is the third interstitial nucleus of the anterior hypothalamus, or INAH3. INAH3 is typically about two to three times larger in men than in women.[4]

We now know that INAH3 is just one out of numerous sexually dimorphic structures in the human brain.[5] Considered individually, most of these structures show considerable overlap in size between men and women.[6] But when the sizes of several of these structures are considered collectively, using what is called *multivariate analysis*, it is possible to tell the sex of a brain with a high degree of confidence.[7]

Sex differences exist not only in the relative sizes of brain regions[8] but also in brain connections,[9] synaptic architecture, and the distribution and amounts of neurotransmitters (signaling molecules used in neuron-to-neuron communication) and receptors (molecules that detect and respond to neurotransmitters and hormones).[10] Not surprisingly, then, brain activity patterns also differ between males and females, even when they are engaged in similar mental tasks. These differences can, for example, involve the lateralization of cerebral functions—that is, the extent to which a mental task engages one side of the brain more than the other.[11]

Sex differences are most marked for brain circuits that are involved in sexual functions, such as the hypothalamus and some other structures that are connected with it; these include structures named the amygdala and the bed nucleus of the stria terminalis.[12] Comparing these regions in a male and female brain, an expert would have a good chance of telling which sex was which. In other regions of the brain, whose functions may not be directly concerned with sexual behavior, the differences are more subtle. Nevertheless, most of the brain is "gendered" in one way or another.

Male and Female Behaviors

Given these biological differences between male and female brains, it's not surprising that there are mental and behavioral differences between the sexes.

Male and female animals usually show fairly robust differences in sexual behavior: Most commonly, males seek female sex partners, whereas females seek males, and the actual behaviors that male and female animals display during courtship and mating differ in stereotypical ways. A female rat, for example, will solicit sex from a male by repeatedly approaching and retreating from him while wiggling her ears in a provocative fashion. The male follows the female and attempts to mount her from the rear. The female raises her rump and moves her tail to the side, thus exposing her genital area (the *lordosis reflex*). The male briefly penetrates the female, the pair separate, and the mating is repeated several times until the male ejaculates. Guiding these behaviors are sensory cues such as the distinct odors, vocalizations, visible movements, and tactile stimuli generated by male and female rats. Males and females respond to these cues in distinct ways.

Besides these sex differences in partner choice and the behavioral patterns associated with courtship and mating, male and female rats differ in a range of other behaviors, such as aggressiveness, exploratory behavior, navigation, and behavior toward pups. In other words, there is a constellation of *gendered* or *sex-biased* traits in rats and other animals, some closely connected with reproduction and some less so.[13]

Development of Sex Differences in Animals

How do these behavioral differences come about? Starting with the pioneering studies of the French endocrinologist Alfred Jost in the mid-20th century, biologists have discovered a chain of causal events that lead from genes to sexually differentiated mental or behavioral traits.[14]

The chain begins with sex chromosomes. Male mammals, including human males, possess an *X chromosome* and a *Y chromosome*, whereas females possess two X chromosomes. The Y chromosome carries only a very small number of genes, but one of them, called *SRY* (gene names are italicized by convention), is a master gene that initiates male development and inhibits female development.[15] It does so by instructing two small patches of embryonic tissue to develop into testes—the male reproductive glands that produce sperm and that also secrete testosterone, the principal sex hormone in males, as well as a variety of testosterone-like hormones. (These hormones, along with testosterone, are collectively called *androgens*, from Greek roots meaning "male-makers.") Testosterone in turn drives the development of the rest of the body and the brain in a male-typical direction.

In females, which are free of the inhibitory influence of *SRY*, other genes instruct those same patches of embryonic tissue to develop into ovaries—the female reproductive glands. The ovaries produce ova and also secrete two hormones that are important in female development and physiology, estrogen and progesterone. But these hormones are not secreted in significant amounts during prenatal or early postnatal development: They only come into their own at puberty. Thus during fetal life, the key distinction between males and females is that males have high levels of circulating testosterone and other androgens, secreted by the testes, whereas female have low levels of these hormones. (The androgens that are found in female fetuses are secreted by the adrenal glands.[16])

This sex difference is not absolute, however. When researchers took blood samples from a large number of male and female human fetuses at mid-pregnancy, they found a slight overlap in the testosterone levels of males and females.[17] In other words, it is not possible to identify a fetus's sex with complete certainty on the basis of a one-time testosterone measurement.

Testosterone plays the leading role in the sexual differentiation of the brain. The evidence for this statement comes from experiments in which the levels of testosterone have been artificially manipulated.[18] For example, lowering the levels of testosterone (by castration) or blocking testosterone's effects (with chemical antagonists of testosterone) in developing rats leads to the development of an SDN-POA that is smaller and contains fewer nerve cells than in untreated males. Conversely, *adding* testosterone to developing female rats (by injection) leads to the development of an SDN-POA that is larger and contains more nerve cells than in untreated females and is about the same size as in untreated males.

Although SDN-POA is the "model system" that has been studied most extensively, these hormonal manipulations actually affect the development of many sexually differentiated systems in the brains of rats and other animals. And it is not always the case that high testosterone levels lead to *larger* structures. Another cell group in the rat hypothalamus, called *AVPv*, is involved in the regulation of the female reproductive cycle and maternal behavior.[19] AVPv is sexually dimorphic in the reverse direction from SDN-POA: It is larger in females than males. In this case, high testosterone levels during development cause AVPv to end up *smaller* and to contain *fewer* cells than it otherwise would.[20]

Although hormonal manipulations can greatly alter the sexual development of the brain, the *timing* of these manipulations is very important. In the case of the rat's SDN-POA, the most-dramatic effects are seen if testosterone is added or removed during a *critical period* of development. The critical period begins abruptly on the 18th day of fetal life (which is about four days before birth) and tapers off gradually a few days or weeks after birth.[21] Castration of adult male rats has no effect on the size of SDN-POA, although it does cause some shrinkage of individual neurons within this structure.[22]

What is happening during the critical period? In male rat fetuses, the testes secrete a surge of testosterone, beginning about the 15th day of fetal life. The surge reaches a peak on the 18th day and gradually declines thereafter, with a secondary peak immediately after birth.[23] This surge does not normally occur in females. Thus castration of males (or the use of testosterone blockers) prevents the surge (or blocks its effects), whereas adding testosterone to females mimics the normal male surge.

The normal testosterone surge in males affects the ultimate size of sexually dimorphic cell groups such as SDN-POA and AVPv. It does so not by influencing how many nerve cells are created but by influencing how many die.[24] In the normal course of development, immense numbers of young neurons die without ever becoming functionally integrated into brain circuits. This *programmed cell death*, though seemingly wasteful, actually helps to sculpt the complex cellular architecture and connections of the mature brain.[25] In the case of SDN-POA and AVPv, about the same number of nerve cells are created in males and females, but in the first few days after birth testosterone reduces the rate of cell death in SDN-POA but accelerates the rate of cell death in AVPv.[26] Thus SDN-POA ends up larger in males, whereas AVPv ends up larger in females. If this cell death is prevented (by eliminating one of the genes responsible for it), then males and females end up with similar numbers of cells in these sexually dimorphic cell groups, in spite of differences in testosterone levels.[27]

Testosterone doesn't just influence neuronal survival, however. At later stages of development it also influences the growth of neurons, their synaptic connections with other neurons, their sensitivity to hormones, and their activity patterns. In other words, testosterone has a pervasive influence on brain structure and function.

The early effects of testosterone on the rat's developing nervous system are referred to as *organizational effects*, because they influence the basic layout of neuronal systems in a more or less permanent way. Organizational effects by themselves are not sufficient for adult sexual function. Hormones are also necessary in adulthood to facilitate and sustain sexual behavior. These are called *activational effects*, because they "turn on" functional systems whose basic structure developed much earlier in life. Activational effects are generally not permanent: The continued presence of hormones is required, or the behavior will cease. In male rats, for example, removal of testosterone by castration quickly extinguishes male-typical sexual behavior. In female rats, estrogen and progesterone have important activational effects, controlling the periodic onset and cessation of the rat's sexual receptivity around the estrous cycle. They do this by modifying the excitability of neurons in certain parts of the hypothalamus[28] and by causing synaptic connections to form and dissolve in a cyclical fashion.[29]

Although the concepts of organizational and activational effects of sex hormones have proven useful, the distinction between the two may not always be as clear-cut as was once thought.[30] For example, organizational effects may occur not merely during early development but also at puberty, when the sexual differentiation of the brain continues beyond what was accomplished during the early developmental period. Both testosterone (mainly in males) and estrogen (mainly in females) drive this second wave of brain differentiation.[31]

At least one sexually dimorphic brain structure has been shown to change size in rodents in response to hormonal manipulations even after puberty has been completed.[32] This adult plasticity apparently reflects changes in the size of neurons, however, and not their number.[33] Why some brain systems seem to be "set in concrete" after the completion of early development, whereas others remain somewhat malleable, is not yet understood.

Given that testosterone levels early in development have long-lasting effects on the organization of sexually dimorphic brain regions such as SDN-POA, it's hardly surprising that they also affect sexual functioning in adulthood. A great deal of research has been done, for example, on the two key behaviors involved in mating by rodents: mounting (shown most commonly by males) and the lordosis reflex (shown most commonly by females).

William C. Young and his colleagues at the University of Kansas performed the key studies in this area in the 1950s.[34] They found that female guinea pigs that were exposed to testosterone prenatally were much more likely to mount other animals in adulthood and less likely to display lordosis when mounted than untreated females. Conversely, adult males deprived of testosterone during the critical period were less likely to mount other animals and more likely to display lordosis than untreated males. In other words, the disposition to perform mounting or lordosis in adulthood is a consequence of the organizing effect of high or low testosterone levels, respectively, during early brain development.

These early findings have since been extended to other behaviors and other species. For example, Young's graduate student Robert Goy went on to direct a many-year study of rhesus monkeys at the University of Wisconsin, starting in 1971. In rhesus monkeys, pregnancy lasts 166 days, compared with only 22 days in rats. Goy's group found that during a rhesus monkey's fetal life there are several distinct critical periods, during which different aspects of sex-differentiated behavior are organized.[35]

Sexual Partner Preference in Animals

The aspect of behavior that is most relevant to the topic of this book is the preference most animals show for sexual contact with opposite-sex partners. Is this preference "organized" by sex hormones during development? The answer is yes—to a degree. If newborn female rats are briefly exposed to testosterone, for example, they will prefer female sex partners in adulthood—the opposite of the usual preference for males.[36] Conversely, male rats that are deprived of testosterone by castration around the time of birth and then treated with female hormones in adulthood will prefer males as sex partners.[37] Simply treating an adult male rat with female hormones has no such effect.

Similar findings have been made in a variety of other species. Female zebra finches that are treated with masculinizing hormones while still in the egg or while they are nestlings prefer to form lifelong pair bonds with other females in adulthood, rather than with males.[38] Male pigs that are castrated soon after birth and given estrogen injections in adulthood prefer to approach other males and perform sexual solicitations to them, even in the presence of potential female partners. Male pigs that were hormonally intact in early life do not show such behavior, even if in adulthood they are castrated and given estrogens.[39]

Still, there are some caveats that need to be expressed. For one thing, these organizing effects of hormones may interact with social factors. In zebra finches, for example, the full masculinizing effect of early hormone treatment on the partner preference of female birds occurs only if those birds are also deprived of social contact with males while they are juveniles.[40]

A second important point is that the actual hormones involved differ between species.[41] In birds, such as zebra finches, estrogen rather than testosterone is the circulating hormone that masculinizes the brain during development. In rodents and carnivores, testosterone plays a significant role in brain masculinization,[42] but some of its actions require its conversion to estrogen by an enzyme named *aromatase* once it enters the brain.[43] In fact, male rats that are treated with an aromatase-blocking drug during prenatal life commonly exhibit a same-sex partner preference when they are adult and may show female-typical sex behavior when paired with an untreated male.[44]

In primates, on the other hand, testosterone by itself seems to be the principal hormone needed for masculinization. Aromatase can also convert testosterone to estrogen in the primate brain, but blocking aromatase has much less dramatic effects in primates than it does in other mammals. In humans, in fact, genetic mutations that render aromatase completely nonfunctional seem to leave male psychosexual development unaffected.[45] In other words, applying the lessons of one species to another can be tricky.

Testosterone-Independent Effects

Testosterone and estrogen may not be the only hormonal players influencing the sexual differentiation of the brain. A male-specific hormone called *anti-müllerian hormone* (AMH) is secreted by the testes during both pre- and postnatal life; its best-known function is to suppress the development of the female reproductive tract. In rodents, AMH also plays a role in the sexual differentiation of SDN-POA, and its presence is necessary for the development of some behavioral sex differences.[46] What role AMH may play in human sexual development is not yet known.

It is also possible that some aspects of the sexual differentiation of the brain do not depend on hormones at all. Every cell in an animal's body contains a copy of that animal's entire *genome* (its complete genetic endowment) in its nucleus, including its sex chromosomes. Thus all brain cells "know" the sex of the animal that they are part of. Do they make any use of that intrinsic information? Apparently so, because many genes are expressed more strongly (i.e., are more active) in the developing neurons of one sex or the other, even before these neurons are exposed to any sex hormones. When developing neurons in females are exposed to testosterone, their pattern of gene expression is shifted partially in a male-typical direction; some aspects of gene expression, however, remain female-typical even in the presence of testosterone, suggesting that this hormone is not the sole driver of male-typical brain development.[47]

Molecular geneticists have produced mice in which the "intrinsic sex" of brain cells differs from the anatomical and hormonal sex of the entire animal. Study of these animals has shown that the intrinsic sex of brain cells does indeed influence the sexual differentiation of the brain and sexually differentiated behaviors such as aggression.[48] These effects are less dramatic than the well-established effects of sex hormones, but that they can be demonstrated at all should make us cautious about attributing each and every sex difference in brain and behavior to differences in hormone levels, whether during development or in adult life.

Origins of Variation Within Each Sex

I've outlined above what we know about the chain of events that leads, in non-human animals, from sex chromosomes to early hormone exposure to brain differentiation and finally to differences in behavior between male and female adults. What factors might modify this chain of events so as to produce a diversity of outcomes among adults of the *same* sex?

One such factor is *genetic variation* among individuals of the same sex. For example, male animals are typically more aggressive than females, but individual males differ in aggressiveness. To study the biological basis for this variability, Dutch researchers bred two strains of mice, one of which was reliably more aggressive than the other. They found that there were consistent biological differences between males of the two strains, including higher circulating testosterone levels during early development in the more aggressive mice.[49]

In another study, a research group at Brigham Young University found that male rats from two different strains had different-sized SDN-POAs. The rats from the strain with the larger SDN-POAs engaged in more-aggressive sexual behavior than those from the other strain.[50] The difference between the strains seems to have been caused by genetic differences in the sensitivity of the rats' brains to sex hormones.

Another approach to studying the influence of genes on sex-differentiated behavior is to remove a particular gene of interest using the techniques of molecular genetics. University of Virginia researchers, for example, produced female mice lacking one of the genes responsible for the animals' sensitivity to estrogen. These females did not perform lordosis under any circumstances.[51] Such artificial experiments do not necessarily explain the variability in sexual behavior within a natural population, but they do offer avenues for exploring the roots of such variability.

Another factor that probably plays a greater role than is commonly realized is sheer *random variability*—variability that is not controlled by genes but rather is the product of some kind of biological "dice-throwing" during development. When we consider that mammals, including humans, possess only 20,000 genes or so, and that these genes have to regulate the development of billions of brain cells and all their synaptic connections, along with the entire remainder of the body, it's obvious that brain organization cannot be genetically specified in precise detail. Rather, genetic instructions produce trends and tendencies that allow for some diversity in outcome.

Here's one example illustrating the significance of such random variability. In species where pregnant females carry multiple fetuses at the same time—which is to say, in most mammals—both male and female fetuses are likely to be present in the same uterus, but chance dictates how many there are of each sex and how they are positioned relative to one another. In rats and mice, the uterus consists of two tube-like "horns," and the fetuses are strung out along each horn like peas in a pod. Fetuses (of either sex) that happen to be located between two males develop higher levels of testosterone in their blood than fetuses of the same sex that lack any male neighbors.[52] That's because they pick up some testosterone that has crossed the short space between adjacent fetuses, either by simple diffusion or by transport in blood vessels. The extra dose of testosterone has a long-lasting effect on the size of the animals' SDN-POAs and on their sexual behavior.[53] This particular effect is irrelevant to the majority of humans who are singletons, and even women who have male twins show little evidence of having been influenced by their brothers' hormones.[54] Still, there are likely to be numerous other ways in which nature throws dice to produce diversity in gendered traits.

Finally, *environmental factors* can influence the chain of developmental processes so as to produce variability in brain organization and gender-related behavior among animals of the same sex. One environmental factor that operates prenatally is stress. When pregnant rats or mice are severely stressed during the critical period mentioned earlier, the stress is communicated via hormonal channels to their fetuses. As a consequence, testosterone levels in male fetuses are much lower than usual from the 18th day of pregnancy onward (i.e., during the critical period).[55] These prenatally stressed males have smaller SDN-POAs than unstressed males do, and their sexual behavior in adulthood is demasculinized (they are less likely to show mounting behavior) and feminized (they are more likely to show the lordosis reflex). When given a choice of sex partners, they prefer males.[56]

Postnatal environmental factors that can influence sexual behavior include social conditions during rearing. I mentioned one example earlier: Depriving young female zebra finches of contact with males intensifies the effects of early hormone treatment on their partner preference in adulthood. Goy's group studied the effect of being reared in single-sex groups on the play-sex behavior of juvenile rhesus monkeys.[57] Generally speaking, juvenile males and females display both mounting behavior (the typical sexual behavior of adult males) and presenting behavior (the posture adopted by an adult female who is soliciting a mount), but juvenile males show more mounting and juvenile females show more presenting. Depriving young monkeys of the company of opposite-sex peers, however, increased the likelihood that they would show play-sex behaviors typical of the other sex.

Yet another example of the effect of social conditions comes from the work of Bradley Cooke (now at Georgia State University) and colleagues. They reported that rearing male rats in isolation after weaning reduces the adult size of some sexually dimorphic structures in their brains (the SDN-POA and a region within the amygdala) and leaves them deficient in some male-typical sexual behaviors.[58] Cooke and colleagues suggested that these effects occur because early social isolation reduces testosterone levels in males.

In Figure 3.1 I've sketched the bare bones of the pathway that appears to control the development of sexual partner preference and other gendered

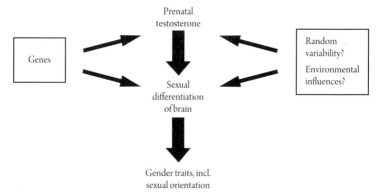

Figure 3.1 Basic elements of a prenatal hormonal theory of the development of sexual orientation.

traits in a variety of nonhuman animals that have been studied in the laboratory. Differences in levels of circulating sex hormones—usually testosterone—
during one or more critical periods of development cause the brain to develop
in a more male-like or more female-like direction, and these differences influence a spectrum of gendered traits in juvenile life and adulthood, including the
preference for male or female sex partners. Genetic differences, random variability, and environmental factors influence this pathway by changing early sex
hormone levels or by modifying the strength or nature of the brain's responses
to sex hormones.

Relevance to Human Sexual Orientation

The remainder of this book is an exploration of the idea that this same causal
pathway is the principal route by which humans acquire their sexual orientations. This is not a new idea. In fact, its roots can be traced back to biologically focused sex researchers of the early 20th century, such as the German
gay-rights pioneer Magnus Hirschfeld and the Austrian endocrinologist Eugen
Steinach.[59] In the latter part of the 20th century, the German neuroendocrinologist Günter Dörner promoted a prenatal hormonal theory of human sexual
orientation based in part on experiments in rats.[60] Other researchers have put
forward similar ideas.[61]

   Two things have changed in recent years. First, a great deal of new and detailed research has been done, both on humans and on experimental animals,
that has helped strengthen, modify, and flesh out the theory. This new research
will be presented in the following chapters.

   In addition, attitudes have changed over time. Dörner, for example, began
his research with the point of view that homosexuality was a mental disorder
that had a biological cause. He suggested a method to prevent homosexuality
in men, which would be to administer extra testosterone to male fetuses that
were at risk of becoming gay adults.[62] Later in his career, Dörner presented
his research in a very different way: He said that it demonstrated the natural,
non-pathological nature of homosexuality and that homosexuality should
therefore be deleted from the World Health Organization's list of mental
disorders.[63]

   Dörner's change of heart paralleled a broader change in views about homosexuality in academe and among the general public over the last several
decades. Although the issue of "what makes people gay" still has some social,
political, and legal resonance, most researchers now view sexual orientation
as worth studying simply because it is a significant aspect of the diversity that
makes us human. That is how I aspire to cover the topic in the remaining chapters of this book.

Sexual Orientation in Nature

Before I abandon my focus on nonhuman animals, however, it's worth taking a brief look at the question of sexual orientation in nature. What I've discussed up to this point has been, for the most part, how hormonal, genetic, or other methods can influence sexual behavior, including sexual partner preference, in laboratory animals. This research could be read as bolstering a pathological view of homosexuality, because it seems to show that it takes a syringeful of drugs to produce homosexual behavior. That's not how I view the matter: I see these interventions simply as probes into the workings of a natural process. But to get away from the laboratory and all it implies, let's take a brief look at the wider world of animal sexuality.

Sexual contacts and partnerships between animals of the same sex have been described in hundreds of species, according to an encyclopedic survey by Bruce Bagemihl.[64] Many of these descriptions are casual or anecdotal; nevertheless, such behaviors have been closely studied by *ethologists* (scientists who study animal behavior in nature) in quite a few species, ranging from birds to primates.[65]

For the most part, what has been described is not homosexuality in the sense of a durable preference for sexual contacts or relationships with same-sex partners. Rather, it is same-sex contacts by animals that also engage in heterosexual contacts or would do so if given the chance. Thus it could be read as illustrating a broad bisexual potential in the animal kingdom.

Sometimes, homosexual partnerships have the quality of "second best" choices that are forced on individuals by circumstances. That seems to be true for two species of birds that have been closely studied, graylag geese (*Anser anser*) and western gulls (*Larus occidentalis*). A research group at the Konrad Lorenz Research Station in Austria has observed a flock of free-ranging (but non-migratory) graylag geese over many years.[66] These geese form sexual pair bonds that typically last two or three years. At any time, some fraction of the pairs in the flock consists of male–male pairs. This phenomenon is related to the fact that there is usually an excess of males in the flock, because females are more frequently killed by predators. In years when the excess of males is high, the number of male–male pairs can rise to more than 20% of all pairs; in years when males and females are present in approximately equal numbers, it falls to 10% or so. The males who form these partnerships tend to be older birds, who may be forced into same-sex partnerships because they are rejected by females. Male–male partnerships often break up if females become available. Although the males in a pair bond engage in sexual contact, they don't do so very amicably. Usually, both birds struggle to take the "top" position—the one adopted by the male in heterosexual matings.

According to the Austrian researchers, males who lack partners have low rank in the flock and may therefore be disadvantaged in a variety of ways, such as being pushed to the outside of the flock, where they are exposed to predation. Thus the adaptive value of these same-sex relationships may be that they help males retain some social status. It is possible that some of the males have a lifelong preference to bond with other males, but this has not been clearly established so far.

Somewhat similar observations were made on western gulls by ecologist George Hunt and his colleagues at the University of California, Irvine.[67] During the 1970s, gull colonies on the Channel Islands off the coast of Southern California had a marked excess of females, because males had been weakened by exposure to pesticides. Up to 14% of all nesting pairs during that period consisted of female–female pairs. These birds behaved very like male–female pairs, sexually and otherwise. Later, when the source of pollution was controlled and the sex ratio returned to equality, the number of female–female pairs fell dramatically.[68] In the mid-1990s I was part of a group of observers who scoured one island in search of female–female pairs, but we found none.

Female–female pairs in gulls are not necessarily non-reproductive, because individuals in these relationships frequently have sexual contacts with male partners outside the pair bond. Thanks to such behavior, many of the female–female gull pairs successfully hatch their eggs and cooperate in raising their chicks. Thus homosexual relationships may not be as maladaptive in evolutionary terms as they seem at first glance. It's not known whether male graylag geese who engage in male–male relationships father offspring by sex with females outside their pair bonds.

Turning to primates, one species well known for homosexual behavior is our oversexed relative the bonobo, or pygmy chimpanzee (*Pan paniscus*). Male and female bonobos engage in frequent sexual contacts with both same-sex and opposite partners; no individuals exhibit exclusively homosexual or exclusively heterosexual behavior. Homosexual contacts (as well as many heterosexual contacts) appear to serve the purposes of conflict resolution and alliance formation, according to primatologists who have made careful observations of bonobos.[69] Female alliances in particular, which are cemented by frequent sexual contacts, have allowed females to assert greater dominance in bonobo society than is seen among other great apes.

Paul Vasey, who is an ethologist and anthropologist based at the University of Lethbridge in Canada, has focused on same-sex behavior among female Japanese macaques (*Macaca fuscata*).[70] Nearly all the females observed by Vasey mounted other females on frequent occasions, in addition to engaging in sexual contacts with males. According to Vasey, the female–female mounting serves no evolutionarily adaptive function such as conflict resolution or alliance formation. Rather, he suggests that females simply "discovered" the pleasurable nature of mounting in the course of mounting males—a behavior they some-times engage in to stimulate reluctant males into sexual activity. Because males don't always tolerate being mounted by females, the females switched to more-cooperative, female partners. Vasey's hypothesis is not proven, but it does illustrate a point worth emphasizing: Not every behavior has to have an explicit value in terms of survival or reproductive success. Some behaviors are accidental byproducts of evolutionary adaptations and are not adaptive in themselves.

Homosexuality in the sense of a durable preference for same-sex partners has not been widely described among nonhuman animals. In fact, there is only one species in which it has been shown to occur with any regularity, and that is the domestic sheep (*Ovis aries*).[71] About 8% of rams, when given the choice of rams or ewes as sex partners, mate preferentially with rams. Aside from their atypical partner choice, the sexual behavior of these homosexual rams is typ-ical: They go through the same series of behaviors that heterosexual rams per-form when approaching and mounting females—including the characteristic head-raised, lip-curling behavior known as the *flehmen response*, which helps with the detection of sex chemosignals—but they penetrate their partners anally rather than vaginally. Whether homosexual rams also occur among wild sheep is not known. A great deal of male-on-male mounting does occur in wild sheep species, however.[72]

Because rams, like men, can be rather cleanly divided into homosexual and heterosexual groups on the basis of their preference for male or female sex partners, sheep have become the focus of a research effort to explain what determines an individual's sexual orientation. The findings of this research will be presented in later chapters. For now, it's simply worth mentioning that the sexually dimorphic cell group in the sheep's hypothalamus that is equiva-lent to the rat's SDN-POA is larger in heterosexual rams than in homosexual rams.[73] This finding suggests that some aspect of the developmental pathway involving sex hormones and the brain differs between rams of different sexual orientation, in line with the ideas developed earlier in this chapter on the basis of experiments on laboratory animals.

The observation of homosexual behavior among nonhuman animals sug-gests that the capacity for such behavior could have evolved for a variety of different reasons, some of which have been mentioned above. Of course, these reasons could be relevant to humans too. I will revisit this issue in Chapter 7, in connection with a discussion of genetic influences on human sexual orientation.

4

Childhood

This chapter and the next one lay out evidence for the idea that gay and straight people differ from each other in more aspects of their psychology than just their sexual orientation. To some extent, homosexuality is part of a "package" of mental traits, many of which can be considered gender-variant or gender-nonconformist, whereas heterosexuality is part of a package of gender-typical or gender-conformist traits. The present chapter discusses this idea with regard to children, and the following chapter discusses it with regard to adults.

On the face of it, this excursion into psychology is quite a departure from the biological issues discussed in the previous chapter, and it may not be immediately obvious what the topic has to do with the central theme of this book, which is how sexual orientation develops. In reality, however, there is a close connection. The idea will be put forward, partly in these two chapters and partly later in the book, that the association between sexual orientation and other gendered traits arises because all these traits differentiate under the influence of a common biological process—the sexual differentiation of the brain under the influence of sex hormones.

Obviously, this point of view carries a risk of stereotyping. As has been confirmed by many surveys over past half-century, the general population views gay men as relatively feminine and lesbians as relatively masculine.[1] These beliefs—especially when reduced to stereotypical descriptors such as "queeny" or "mannish"—have not exactly been helpful in promoting respect for gays and lesbians. They can also make it hard for men and women who don't seem to match those stereotypes to accept that they are gay, even if they are conscious of same-sex attraction or engage in homosexual behavior.

There is a great deal of diversity in the gender-related traits of gay men and of lesbians, as there is among heterosexual people. This diversity may turn out to be quite important in understanding the mechanisms by which sexual orientation develops, and I will revisit this issue in Chapter 11. Most research studies have not taken this diversity into account, however, and have simply compared samples of gay and straight people as defined by their self-declared attraction to women or men. Thus for the greater part of this book I will be treating gay women and men as homogeneous groups.

Development of Gendered Childhood Traits

With regard to the topic of this chapter, it's important first of all to point out that children, like adults, have a gender. In other words, there are fairly consistent differences in mental and behavioral characteristics between boys and girls.[2] Here are some examples of traits that are gendered in childhood. Boys are more active than girls, and they engage in more rough-and-tumble play.[3] Boys and girls have different toy preferences: Boys prefer toy vehicles, toy weapons, balls, and construction toys; girls have broader preferences, but tend to prefer dolls and household items such as toy kitchen implements.[4] Girls are more interested in infants than are boys.[5] Boys have better throwing accuracy, but girls have better control of fine hand movements.[6] Boys do better than girls at a range of visuospatial tasks, such as targeting (as with throwing accuracy) and *mental rotation* (deciding whether two objects seen from different viewpoints are identical or not).[7] Girls have better verbal fluency (ability to quickly come up with words that match a certain category) than boys.[8] Girls are more people oriented; boys are more thing oriented.[9] Boys prefer the company of boys; girls prefer that of girls.[10] Girls' and boys' voices are recognizably different, even though there is no difference in the pitch of their voices before puberty.[11] All these statements are statements about averages, of course, and don't necessarily apply to individual children.

Although there is considerable agreement that childhood gender differences exist, there are diverse opinions as to how they arise. The traditional feminist perspective attributes them principally to parental encouragement, role modeling, peer pressure, and other forms of socialization. There is little doubt that those forces do indeed have an effect. In one study, infants whose parents reinforced traditional gender-typed behavior came to exhibit more such behavior.[12] And in a very large study of three-year-old British children, the average gender characteristics of boys and girls who had an older sibling were found to be shifted in the direction of the sex of that sibling, presumably as a result of role modeling.[13] Even so, these socialization effects are quite small; in the latter study, for example, boys with older sisters were far more masculine than any girls, even those girls who had older brothers.

There is a great deal of evidence that biological factors play an important role in children's gender development. For one thing, some of these gendered characteristics exist in nonhuman animals, where socialization effects are likely to be less strong, if they exist at all. The greater participation in rough-and-tumble play by males, for example, has been observed in the young of apes, monkeys, rodents, and other mammalian species.[14] Newborn female monkeys are more likely than males to look at the faces of conspecifics and to show other signs of social interest.[15] The toy preferences of male and female monkeys are uncannily similar to those of boys and girls, even when the monkeys are tested with human children's toys that they have never seen before.[16] And juvenile female rhesus monkeys spend more time with infants than do juvenile males.[17]

Another reason for suspecting that biological factors are at work is that some of these gendered traits arise very early in life. The people/thing difference, for example, appears to be present on the day of birth: Newborn girls prefer to look at faces, whereas newborn boys prefer to look at mechanical mobiles, according to a study by Simon Baron-Cohen's group at Cambridge University.[18] (This study has been criticized on technical grounds.[19]) The male superiority in mental rotation is evident by three to five months of age, before socialization factors could plausibly have influenced this trait.[20] Differences in toy preference are evident at three to eight months of age.[21]

Finally, there is evidence that prenatal hormones influence at least some of these gendered traits. With experimental animals, it's a fairly straightforward matter to demonstrate this. For example, the administration of testosterone to female rhesus monkeys during fetal life increases their participation in rough-and-tumble play when they are juveniles.[22] In sheep, the same treatment causes juvenile ewes to behave more aggressively toward other juveniles. This permits them to rise higher in the female dominance hierarchy than ewes who were not exposed to testosterone prenatally.[23]

In humans, this kind of intentional experiment would be unethical, but "experiments of nature" provide something similar in the form of genetic conditions that affect the hormonal environment during fetal life. One such condition is *congenital adrenal hyperplasia*, or CAH (earlier called adrenogenital syndrome). In CAH, a genetic mutation knocks out one of the enzymes involved in the manufacture of corticosteroid hormones (hormones produced in the adrenal gland). As a byproduct of this condition, the adrenal glands secrete higher-than-normal levels of androgens (testosterone-like hormones). The condition is generally recognized at birth and corrected; thus the period of abnormal androgen exposure is mainly before birth, although the exact period and degree of exposure are not usually known. (In recent years it has proven possible to treat fetuses at risk for CAH well before birth, but doing so raises some ethical concerns.[24])

In boys, these extra androgens do not have obvious effects, because all male fetuses are awash in testosterone secreted by their own testes. In girls, however, the effects can be quite marked. In severe cases, the girls' genitals are partially masculinized. In milder cases there may be few or no genital abnormalities.

Several groups have investigated whether CAH girls' exposure to unusually high levels of androgens has any effect on their gendered traits during childhood.[25] It does. CAH girls are, on average, more active and aggressive than unaffected girls, engage in more rough-and-tumble play, and choose playmates (of either sex) who engage in such play. They have toy preferences similar to those of boys, are better than other girls at some visuospatial tasks (such as targeting), are less interested in infant care or doll play, are less certain that they want to be mothers when they grow up, and are more likely to have a masculine gender identity. These effects tend to be greater in girls who have the more severe forms of the condition and who therefore probably had more exposure to androgens.

Biosocial investigator Rebecca Jordan-Young has argued that these differences result from indirect effects of CAH on girls, such as traumatizing medical interventions, and not from the actual androgen exposure.[26] Jordan-Young's arguments are unconvincing, in my opinion. Nevertheless, parental treatment may have some influence on the gendered behavior of CAH girls, just as it does on the gendered behavior of children in general.[27]

The CAH studies strongly suggest that prenatal androgen levels influence a variety of gender traits in childhood. Still, CAH is a special case, and the question remains, do prenatal androgens help generate the diversity in gender characteristics among the general population of healthy girls (or boys)?

Melissa Hines and her colleagues at London's City University approached this question by measuring testosterone levels in the blood of several hundred pregnant women and then studying the children who resulted from those pregnancies.[28] (Sampling the mothers' rather than the fetuses' blood is less than ideal, but obtaining fetal blood samples is too invasive for this kind of study. Maternal testosterone levels do give some idea of the testosterone levels to which the fetus is exposed.) Among the girls born of those pregnancies and studied at three years of age, gender characteristics were strongly related to prenatal testosterone: The higher the prenatal testosterone levels, the more masculine were the girls' gendered traits. In contrast, these traits appeared to be unaffected by a variety of potential socialization forces, such as the presence or absence of a man in the home. More recently, Hines's group, in collaboration with Baron-Cohen and his colleagues, have measured testosterone in amniotic fluid rather than in the mother's blood. With this improved sampling method, the researchers were able to show that higher prenatal testosterone levels were associated with more-masculine play behavior in both girls and boys.[29] Another study, by Baron-Cohen's group, found that *lower* prenatal testosterone levels were associated with greater empathy at six to eight years of age.[30]

I don't want to leave readers with the impression that everything is cut and dried and that all findings support the simplest model, which is that high prenatal testosterone leads to masculine traits and low levels lead to feminine traits. It's not that simple. For example, although girls with CAH are better at targeting than other girls, they are not better at mental rotation, according to a study by Hines's group.[31] And CAH *boys* actually performed worse at mental rotation than other boys—the opposite of what one would predict on the basis of the simplest model. This anomalous finding was supported by another study, in which high prenatal testosterone in *normal* boys was related to slightly lower performance on a mental rotation task at age seven.[32]

Such anomalous findings are no reason to abandon the general hypothesis, but they do suggest that there are complexities that need to be explored. For example, a full accounting will probably require more attention to the *timing* of testosterone exposure (mental rotation might be organized postnatally rather than prenatally, for example) and to *nonlinear effects* (meaning that testosterone might have its greatest masculinizing effect on a trait at some intermediate level, with lesser effects at both lower and higher levels). I will return to these issues later in the book.

Childhood Traits Associated with Adult Sexual Orientation

Retrospective Studies

Do children who become gay adults (pre-gay children) differ from children who become straight adults (pre-straight children)? There's one major obstacle to answering this question, which is that neither children themselves nor the people who nurture them or study them can know for sure what the future sexual orientation of any particular child will be. So how can we study the characteristics of pre-gay children and compare them with those of pre-straight children if we don't know which children are which?

The most obvious and widely used method is retrospective. Adults remember their childhoods (though not infallibly), and many have provided descriptions of what they were like as children. Here, for example, are extracts from two men's published autobiographies:

> [My father] loved power tools and guns, old Cadillacs, pickup trucks, and campers. I didn't. He liked to build houses, hunt deer, and tinker with engines, and he would have enjoyed having me working and playing at his side, but while he was out in the shop painting, plumbing, or rewiring, I was lying on the living room floor, listening on the radio to Milton Cross narrate Texaco's "Saturday Morning at the Opera."

> I grew up in the projects with a small group of friends, and we spent all our time thinking, talking, and playing sports. . . . [My father] taught me how to throw a curve, and he often got us bleacher seats for Red Sox games at Fenway Park. These games were the most exciting part of my youth. . . . I felt I belonged in the game. It was as if somebody had injected baseball into my veins, and from then on it was always in my blood.

Which of these two narratives was written by a gay man and which by a straight man? The answer, actually, is that *both* were written by gay men. The first was written by Mel White, the well-known gay clergyman and activist.[33] The second was written by Dave Pallone, the National League baseball umpire who came out as gay after he left the sport.[34] Individual recollections by gay men, then, are quite diverse, as are those of lesbians, straight women, and straight men. Some accounts match stereotypes; some don't.

Psychiatrists who have seen many gay men in their practices do report that such men consistently speak of having been gender-nonconformist during their childhoods. Thus Richard Isay wrote as follows:[35]

> Each of the several hundred gay men I have seen in consultation or treatment over the past 30 years has described having had one or more gender-discordant traits during childhood. Most frequently, they report a lack of interest in "rough-and-tumble" or aggressive sports; many speak of having preferred to play with girls rather than other boys.... Almost all recall that as children they felt a close bond with their mothers, with whom they shared many interests.

Reports such as this suggest that the stereotypes are correct, but still, there is reason for caution in interpreting them. Typically, these reports deal with gay men, not lesbians. And they may not be representative of all gay men: Boys who are strongly gender-nonconformist are more likely than other boys to experience anxiety and depression in adulthood,[36] and for this reason may be more likely to come to the attention of psychiatrists. Finally, such studies are not quantitative and they lack control groups of non-gay subjects.

To get beyond these potential problems, researchers have interviewed large numbers of gay and straight adults about their childhoods and applied statistical tests to the results. In a 1983 study using this method, for example, Ray Blanchard and his colleagues concluded that pre-gay boys are less physically aggressive than pre-straight boys.[37] In another study from the same period, UCLA psychologists gave questionnaires to 792 subjects—198 gay men, 198 lesbians, 198 straight men, and 198 straight women—who were recruited from the general population.[38] The questionnaires asked about 58 play and sports activities in earlier and later childhood. The responses for one activity—participation in baseball at ages five to eight—are shown in Figure 4.1. Overall, the study documented very sizable and statistically significant shifts in the gender-typed behaviors of pre-gay children, both boys and girls, compared with pre-straight children of the same sex. Pre-gay children participated less in gender-typical activities and more in gender-atypical activities. Still, not all children—whether they ended up gay or straight—conformed to these patterns.

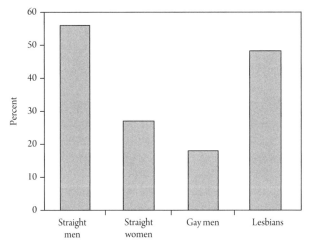

Figure 4.1 Sports participation and sexual orientation. Bars show the percentages of straight and gay men and women, interviewed around 1980, who said they played baseball between ages five and eight. If the study were repeated today it might well show smaller differences between straight men, straight women, and lesbians, given the increased participation in sports by girls. Data from Grellert et al. (1982).

In the mid-1990s Michael Bailey and Kenneth Zucker reanalyzed the data from 41 retrospective studies of this kind.[39] They confirmed that differences exist between the gender characteristics of pre-gay and pre-straight children, always in the direction of gender nonconformity among the pre-gay children. These differences were very sizable and statistically significant for both pre-gay boys and pre-gay girls, but were larger for boys than for girls. In other words, based on these retrospective data, gender nonconformity in childhood is more predictive of adult homosexuality for boys than for girls.

Several further studies of this kind have been carried out since the time of Bailey and Zucker's meta-analysis, with similar results.[40] One study, for example, focused on the question of how consistently pre-gay boys differ from pre-straight boys across different cultures.[41] Several hundred gay and straight men in Turkey, Brazil, and Thailand were questioned about their childhood characteristics. The findings were very consistent: In all three cultures, pre-gay boys were less aggressive and less interested in sports than pre-straight boys. They were more likely to have associated with girls and to have participated in typical girls' activities. The study also included samples of self-identified bisexual men. These men reported childhood characteristics that were intermediate between those reported by gay and straight men, but they were generally closer to those of the straight men.

Another recent study, carried out by a Finnish group led by Katarina Alanko, focused on twins.[42] This study confirmed the association between childhood gender nonconformity and adult homosexuality and again found that this association, though present in both sexes, was stronger for males than for females. The study also used the twin paradigm to investigate genetic effects underlying the association. I'll discuss that aspect of the study in Chapter 7.

Further bolstering the findings of these studies are reports by anthropologists who have studied a variety of non-Western cultures. In most cases, these studies have focused on men who, in adulthood, take on feminine or mixed-gender roles and who partner sexually with conventionally gendered men. As already mentioned in Chapter 1, such individuals usually have a history of marked femininity during childhood.[43] The anthropological literature on women is much more limited, but to the extent that it exists it supports the relationship between cross-gendered behavior in childhood and adult homosexuality. The Mohaves of the American West, for example, recognized a group of girls called *hwame*, who "threw away their dolls" and, in adulthood, married women.[44] Because the anthropological literature focuses for the most past on homosexual adults who are gender-nonconformist or even transgender, it leaves unclear whether there have been more-conventionally gendered homosexual adults in non-Western cultures, and if so what their childhood characteristics may have been.

With all retrospective studies there is the potential problem that recollections may be inaccurate or biased. To get around this problem, researchers from Bailey's group at Northwestern University, led by Gerulf Rieger, recruited gay and straight men and women who possessed videos of themselves as children.[45] The researchers prepared short clips from these videos and showed them to judges, who were also gay and straight men and women. Although the judges were not told the subjects' sexual orientations, they nevertheless rated the pre-gay children as far more gender-nonconformist than the pre-straight children, consistent with the findings of the retrospective studies just discussed. What's more, the observers' judgments of the videos correlated quite well with the subjects' own descriptions of their childhood characteristics, suggesting that such self-recall is fairly accurate. The differences between the pre-gay and pre-straight children began to emerge at about three years of age and increased over the following few years. I will return to this study in Chapter 9 when I discuss the topic of "gaydar."

Prospective Studies

The ideal method to pin down the relationship between childhood traits and adult sexual orientation would be to recruit a large group of children, study them in as much detail as possible, and then follow them over a decade or more to determine their sexual orientations. Several such prospective studies have been done. The best known was conducted between the late 1960s and early

1980s by psychiatrist Richard Green while he was at UCLA.[46] Green later became research director of the Gender Identity Clinic at London's Charing Cross Hospital; he is the life partner of Melissa Hines, whose research on gender development was discussed earlier in this chapter.

Green recruited 66 feminine boys as well as 56 boys who were matched to this first group on a number of demographic variables but were unselected for gender traits. (They were not specifically chosen to be masculine.) The feminine boys were not just slightly unmasculine: Most said that they would have preferred to be girls, and some came across almost like miniature transexuals. They often expressed *gender dysphoria* (severe dissatisfaction with their biological sex). Here is part of an interview with a five-year-old boy, "Richard," whose parents brought him to Green on account of his persistent cross-dressing and avoidance of male playmates:

Green: Have you ever wished you'd been a girl?
Richard: Yes.
Green: Why did you wish that?
Richard: Girls, they don't have to have a penis.
Green: They don't have to have a penis?
Richard: They can have babies. And—because they—it doesn't tickle when you tickle them here.
Green: It doesn't tickle when you tickle them here? Where your penis is?
Richard: Yeah. 'Cause they don't have a penis. I wish I was a girl.
Green : You wish you were a girl?
Richard: You know what? I might be a girl.

Green interviewed the boys, and their parents, repeatedly during the boys' childhood and adolescence. The results were striking: Of the 35 boys in the control group whom Green was able to follow through to adolescence or young adulthood, all were heterosexual; of the 44 feminine boys whom Green was able to follow, only 11 were heterosexual, while 33 were homosexual or bisexual. In other words, the markedly feminine boys were likely to become gay or bisexual adults. Still, there were exceptions. "Richard" was one of them: Interviewed at age 18, he gave every indication of being heterosexual both in feelings and actual sexual behavior.

Several other prospective studies, most less ambitious that Green's, have reached similar conclusions: Extremely feminine boys often become gay men.[47] Similarly, extremely masculine girls often become lesbian women.[48] A minority of extremely gender-conformist boys and girls become transgender or transsexual adults.[49]

Because these studies started off with clinical samples of very unusual children, they don't allow us to assess the overall strength of the connection between childhood gender nonconformity and adult homosexuality. In 2013, however, a Dutch group led by Thomas Steensma published the results of a study of 897 girls and boys, aged 4 to 11, who had been recruited from the general population of Holland.[50] The children were not studied directly; rather, their parents were asked whether their children behaved like the other sex or expressed a wish to be the other sex. Any child who was reported to exhibit either of these behaviors at least some of the time was designated as gender-variant.

Twenty-four years later the same subjects, now mostly in their early 30s, were asked about their sexual orientations. Of the subjects who had been described as gender-variant, 10–12% reported a homosexual orientation, as compared with less than 2% of the other subjects. This was a very significant difference, bolstering the statistical association between childhood gender nonconformity and adult homosexuality. The association, however, was not nearly as strong as one might have concluded from the studies by Green and others—probably because most of the children designated gender-variant in the Dutch study were only moderately so, as compared with the extremely gender-nonconformist children who were the subjects of the earlier research.

Looking at all the studies, it seems that the "average" gay adult has a history of moderate rather than extreme gender nonconformity, yet many children who are moderately gender-nonconformist become straight adults. Thus the value of these studies is not to demonstrate that children's gendered behavior is predictive of their future sexual orientations—it may be for a few children, but for most it is not. Rather, the point is that there is a statistically very significant association between childhood gender traits and adult sexual orientation. That association requires some explanation.

Contrasting Models

Two general kinds of explanation have been put forward. In one, childhood gender characteristics, whatever their origin, are a causal link in the development of adult sexual orientation—a link that involves social interactions of some kind. To give a concrete example, psychologist Daryl Bem of Cornell University proposed what he called the "exotic becomes erotic" theory of sexual orientation.[51] This theory proposes a five-step causal sequence leading to an adult's sexual orientation:

1. Biological factors such as prenatal hormones influence a child's personality, especially gendered traits such as aggressiveness.
2. These personality traits induce the child to prefer certain gender-conforming or gender-nonconforming activities and therefore to socialize with same-sex or opposite-sex peers.

3. Children come to feel similar to the children with whom they usually associate and different from the children with whom they do not usually associate.
4. The sense of difference causes children to experience psychological arousal (antipathy or apprehension) in the presence of children with whom they do not usually associate.
5. This psychological arousal later becomes transformed into sexual attraction. Thus gender-conforming girls develop sexual attraction to males, and gender-nonconforming girls develop sexual attraction to females, and vice versa for boys.

Because theories such as Bem's propose that biological factors such as genes and sex hormones have direct effects only on nonsexual childhood gender traits and not on sexual orientation, they imply that a child's psychosexual outcome as gay or straight will depend not only on these biological factors but also on the proposed intervening social factors.

Before Bem proposed his theory, another model of the same general kind was put forward by Green.[52] He suggested that femininity in boys triggers rejection from fathers and male peers, leading to a yearning for close contact with males ("male-affect starvation," in Green's phrase). This yearning might cause the adolescent to seek sexual relationships with males and to derive satisfaction from such relationships. As with Bem's model, Green's model implied that interventions to reduce a boy's femininity or to improve his relationships with his father and male peers would decrease the likelihood of his becoming a gay adult. (These ideas don't correspond to Green's thinking today.)

In a second kind of explanation, childhood gendered traits are linked to adult sexual orientation not through a "socialization loop" of the kind proposed by Bem and Green, but because they are both components of a package of gendered traits that tend to develop in a more sex-typical or sex-atypical direction under the influence of common biological drivers such as genes and hormones. This explanation appeals to the concept, outlined earlier on the basis of animal experiments, that levels of androgens during early development organize the brain circuits that mediate a wide variety of gendered traits, including sexual orientation, even though these traits may emerge at quite different times in postnatal life. Under this kind of model there is no particular reason to think that early interventions of the kind just described would change a child's ultimate sexual orientation.

Choosing between these two kinds of explanations requires more information than I've presented so far, and I'll postpone discussion of which kind has greater merit until Chapter 12. As a general comment, though, it's worth pointing out a widespread misperception. This is the idea that biological factors such as genes and hormones exert their effects only at the beginning of life—giving the individual a hefty kick in a certain direction, as it were—and that socialization and the general vicissitudes of life take over thereafter. In reality, genes and hormones exert a sustained or even growing influence over the life span. For example, the *heritability* of many psychological traits—the fraction of the variability in these traits that can be attributed to genetic differences between individuals—actually *increases* from childhood into adulthood.[53] Thus there is no reason to conclude that social processes help decide whether a person becomes gay or straight simply by virtue of the many-year gap between birth and the awakening of same-sex or opposite-sex desire.

Characteristics of Gay and Straight Adults

For the most part, adults are aware of the direction of their sexual feelings and therefore know what their sexual orientations are. Thus the central problem of the previous chapter—identifying the pre-gay and pre-straight children—doesn't arise when studying the characteristics of gay and straight adults. It's usually sufficient to recruit samples of adults who are willing to give information about themselves in the confidential setting of an interview, written questionnaire, or Internet-based survey. Thus a large number of studies have focused on what differences or similarities may exist between people of different sexual orientation. More such studies are added every year.

Gendered Traits in Adulthood

I'll start with a brief summary of traits that differ, *on average*, between men and women, without regard to sexual orientation.[1] Some of these are simply the continuations of the gendered traits of childhood or could be thought of as adult versions of those traits (for example, actual aggression versus play-fighting). Others, especially in the area of sexuality, seem to arise for the first time at puberty.

In the area of cognition, women perform better than men at some memory tasks, including episodic memory (memory of events), verbal memory, and memory of the locations of objects. They are also better at tests of verbal fluency and some other verbal skills, at face recognition, and at behavioral tasks requiring fine hand movements. They perform better than men in most tests of the sense of smell.[2] Men perform better than women at a variety of visuo-spatial tasks, such as mental rotation, targeting accuracy, and navigation (especially when navigating by distant landmarks or compass directions rather than by local cues). Men are slightly more likely than women to be left-handed or mixed-handed.[3]

Sex differences in personality and social behavior are the subject of a recent review by Marco Del Giudice.[4] Women score higher than men on measures of expressiveness, sociability, empathy, openness to feelings, altruism, and neuroticism. (This last item includes the tendency to depression, anxiety, self-consciousness, and low self-esteem.) Men score higher than women on measures of assertiveness, competitiveness, aggressiveness, and independence. (These "getting things done" traits are sometimes referred to collectively as *instrumentality*.) Men prefer thing-oriented activities and occupations (e.g., carpenter), whereas women prefer people-oriented activities and occupations (e.g. social worker). Women have better-developed aesthetic interests and less-developed technological interests than men.[5] And as one might expect, when asked to place themselves on a scale of masculinity–femininity, men rate themselves more masculine and women rate themselves more feminine.[6] Simon Baron-Cohen and colleagues have argued that *systemizing*—interest in rule-governed systems outside the social domain, such as computers—is a basic quality of the male mind.[7]

None of these differences are absolute, of course—women and men overlap to a greater or lesser degree in all of them. Still, when these personality features are measured collectively by multivariate analysis, there is only about 10% overlap between women and men, which is similar to the overlap in multivariate measures of facial structure. In other words, people's personalities can tell you which sex they are about as reliably (though not as fast) as looking at their faces.

Marked sex differences exist in the area of sexuality.[8] Men are more interested than women in casual or uncommitted sex, have more-accepting attitudes toward such behavior, and make more attempts to engage in it. Men have a greater desire for variety in their sex lives, including a greater interest in having multiple partners. There are sex differences in jealousy: Men are more likely than women to experience *sexual jealousy* (fear that their partner is having sex with another person), whereas women are more likely than men to experience *emotional jealousy* (fear that their partner is becoming emotionally involved with another person).[9] Men are far more likely to have unusual sexual interests (such as fetishisms) and to suffer from *paraphilic disorders* (sexual interests or practices that are sufficiently distressing or harmful to be deemed pathological).[10] They are also more likely to engage in sexual aggression.[11]

Men and women differ to some extent in the criteria they use to judge sexual attractiveness. Men focus more than women on the youthfulness and physical attractiveness of their potential long-term partners, whereas women focus more than men on nonphysical attributes such as personality, wealth, and power.[12]* Men are more interested in visual sexual stimuli, including pornography.[13] Men masturbate more than women.[14]

---

* When seeking short-term or casual relationships, both women and men focus primarily on physical attractiveness (Schmitt et al., 2012).

There is of course the basic difference in sexual orientation, with men more likely to experience attraction to women (gynephilia—see Chapter 1), and women more likely to experience attraction to men (androphilia). This difference carries along with it more-specific attractions to physical characteristics of the other sex, such as breasts or a muscular physique. Other differences related to sexual orientation include a greater prevalence of exclusive homosexuality among men and a greater prevalence of bisexuality among women. There is also a clearer association between genital arousal and self-declared sexual orientation in men than in women. These issues were discussed in Chapter 1.

Origin of Gendered Traits

As with childhood traits, the gendered traits of adults appear to be influenced by biological factors such as genes and sex hormones. Among the evidence for this influence is that many of the sex differences exist widely across countries and cultures, in nonliterate populations as well as among the well educated, and in societies that enforce traditional gender roles as well those that are more egalitarian.[15] In fact, contrary to what one might expect on the basis of a simple socialization model, gender differences in personality seem to become *more* marked as societies cast off traditional expectations about the roles of men and women.[16]

Several of the traits that are gendered in humans are also gendered in non-human primates and other mammals. For example, males and females of other mammalian species, such as rats, differ in their navigational skills and in the cues they use while navigating, and these differences mimic quite closely those described in humans.[17] Even male and female cuttlefish, which are invertebrates related to squid, use different strategies to navigate[18]; these differences could hardly result from socialization, because cuttlefish parents pay no attention to their offspring after hatching.[19]

Genes help establish the diversity in gendered traits seen among individuals of the same sex. This conclusion comes mainly from studies of twins—specifically, from the observation that *monozygotic* ("identical") twin pairs, who possess the same genes, are more similar to each other in gendered traits than are same-sex *dizygotic* ("fraternal") twins, who share only about half their genes. Estimates of the heritability of gendered traits range around 40–50%, values that are quite similar to the heritability of a wide range of other psychological traits.[20]

I mentioned in the previous chapter that girls affected by congenital adrenal hyperplasia, who were exposed to unusually high levels of androgens before birth, are shifted in the masculine direction on a variety of gendered traits. This shift remains evident through adolescence into adulthood, affecting self-assessed masculinity–femininity as well as specific *cognitive* skills such as targeting.[21] Still, not all gendered traits are shifted to the same degree: Whereas childhood toy preferences are very strongly affected, pushing CAH girls most of the way toward boys' preferences, the position of adult CAH women on the continuum of self-assessed masculinity–femininity is shifted only a small part of the way toward men's average position. What's more, there can be interactions among the various traits. For example, the increased spatial skills of women with CAH may result in part from their more frequent engagement in male-typical activities.[22]

The findings on CAH women don't necessarily tell us whether differences in prenatal hormone levels contribute to the variability in gendered traits among healthy women or among healthy men. Ideally, this question would be studied by measuring testosterone levels in a sample of healthy fetuses and then examining those individuals' gendered traits when they are adults. This approach is difficult, however, on account of the long waiting time that would be involved.

There are less-direct ways of probing the relationship between prenatal androgen exposure and adult gender, however. These involve finding markers—measurable anatomical or physiological characteristics—that are believed to give some indication of an individual's exposure to androgens before birth. The characteristics that are thought to serve as markers include such things as the relative lengths of different fingers, bodily asymmetries, and certain functional properties of the auditory system. I will discuss these markers in more detail in later chapters. For now, it's just worth pointing out that studies of these markers do offer support for the idea that prenatal androgen levels influence the variability in gendered traits among healthy adults of the same sex, but the findings are sometimes weak or inconsistent between studies.[23]

In line with the idea that sex hormones exert both organizational effects during development and activational effects in adulthood, variations in *adult* sex hormone levels may also contribute to variability in gendered traits. This influence is most obvious with radical changes such as the profound drop in testosterone levels in adult men whose testicles are removed. Such castrated men experience a major reduction in sex drive and aggressiveness over time. More interesting and subtle are the psychological changes that accompany the rise and fall of sex hormone levels around a woman's menstrual cycle. These include changes both in cognitive skills and in sexual feelings and behaviors. For example, heterosexual women experience a shift in partner preference toward more-masculine-looking men near the time of ovulation.[24] Some popular accounts have represented this as a dramatic swing in sexual preferences—from nurturing sweeties to square-jawed hunks and back—but in reality it's only a quite modest shift.

Differences in hormone levels might also help generate the diversity of cognitive abilities among individual adults. For example, according to some studies, women with higher testosterone levels tend to perform better at visuospatial tasks, as if testosterone is important both as an organizer and an activator for visuospatial abilities. Men, on the other hand, may show the opposite relationship: In some studies, *lower* testosterone levels have been associated with better visuospatial performance.[25] This is reminiscent of the paradoxical findings in CAH boys mentioned in the previous chapter: Those boys, who were exposed to unusually high testosterone levels prenatally, performed worse at visuospatial tasks than other boys. Thus it seems that the optimal testosterone levels for visuospatial abilities may lie somewhere in the low masculine range, rather than at the top of the masculine range as one would intuitively guess. In other words, there might be a nonlinear relationship between testosterone levels and visuospatial ability, both during early development and during adult life.

The variations in testosterone levels found among healthy adults of the same sex may in part reflect variations in the same hormone during development. In other words, there could be an organizational effect of prenatal testosterone on adult testosterone levels. However, environmental factors such as stress and nutrition also can affect adult levels of testosterone and other sex hormones in dramatic ways, and sex hormone levels decline with aging in both sexes.

Cognitive Traits

Visuospatial Abilities

I now turn to research on cognitive differences between gay and straight people, starting with visuospatial skills. The visuospatial test that shows the most consistent and large sex difference is the mental-rotation test, in which men outperform women.[†] At least six research groups have conducted sizable studies comparing performance on this task between gay and straight men. Five of these studies—one of them employing an Internet-based test taken by several hundred thousand subjects from around the world (see Figure 5.1)— reported that gay men perform less well than straight men.[26] The sixth study failed to find any difference.[27]

With regard to women, three studies found a shift in the opposite direction— that is, lesbians performed better on the task than straight women.[28] One study found no difference.[29] The mental-rotation skills of both gay men and lesbians are probably shifted toward those of the other sex, but the shift in lesbians is smaller and doesn't show up so reliably.

[†] According to one study, men's superior performance results from their greater confidence rather than from any difference in spatial skills per se (Estes & Felker, 2012).

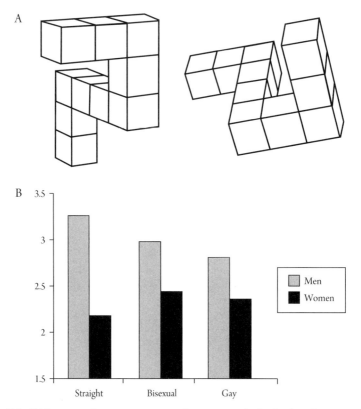

Figure 5.1 (A) In mental-rotation tests, subjects are asked whether figures such as these are the same object viewed from different angles. (B) Mental-rotation scores for straight, bisexual, and gay men and women in an Internet-based study (Peters et al., 2007). Gay men performed worse than straight men, and lesbians performed better than straight women, but gay men still performed better than lesbians. The scores for bisexual men were intermediate between those for straight and gay men; the scores for bisexual women were not significantly different from those for lesbians.

Although mental rotation is the visuospatial task that's been investigated most closely, there are also numerous reports of gay/straight differences in other spatial tasks.[30] All in all, there is considerable evidence that gay people's visuospatial abilities are shifted, on average, in the direction of the other sex.

Verbal Fluency

As mentioned in Chapter 4, verbal fluency refers to the ability to generate responses quickly when asked to name words that fit a given category. Women tend to outperform men in verbal fluency and some related verbal skills, although the sex differences are not generally as large or consistent from study

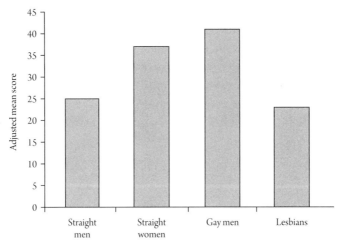

Figure 5.2 Verbal fluency and sexual orientation. Bars show the average scores of straight and gay men and women on test questions such as "In one minute, list as many words as you can that begin with the letter 'd.'" Data from Rahman et al. (2003).

to study as they are for mental rotation. In 2003 Qazi Rahman and colleagues measured verbal fluency in 240 individuals—60 straight men, 60 straight women, 60 gay men, and 60 lesbians.[31] The findings are summarized in Figure 5.2: The gay men performed significantly better than the straight men and about as well as the straight women, while the lesbians scored significantly worse than the straight women and about as poorly as the heterosexual men.

These particular data suggest a complete gender "inversion" in verbal fluency among gay men and women compared with their heterosexual peers. If we look at all the studies on this topic, however, the picture is mixed. Some studies have reported a gay/straight difference similar to that just described.[32] Some have reported a smaller difference in the same direction[33] or a difference between gay and straight men but not between lesbian and straight women.[34] Some have not found differences in verbal fluency but have found differences on another verbal task, verbal association (coming up with as many synonyms for a given word as possible in a given time).[35] Thus the weight of the published research suggests that gay men and women's verbal fluency is indeed shifted in the direction of the other sex, but this shift may not be as complete or consistent as suggested by the particular data set shown in Figure 5.2.

Memory Tasks

Few studies have compared gay and straight people's performance on memory tasks, but Rahman's group has examined object-location memory, a trait that generally favors females. In tests of object-location memory, the subject is shown a display of many different items; the display is then hidden and the subject is asked to recall as many items as possible, as well as their locations. Sometimes the subject is shown two displays, one after the other, and asked which items have changed between the displays. The Rahman group found that gay men outperformed straight men on this kind of task and in fact did as about well as straight women. They did not find a significant difference between lesbians and straight women, however.[36]

Intelligence

One early review of the literature concluded that both lesbians and gay men are more intelligent than their same-sex peers, even when matched for age, educational level, and other factors.[37] Those early studies may have suffered from "volunteer bias," such that only relatively intelligent gay people were available for study. In 2012, however, Satoshi Kanazawa of the London School of Economics reported on an analysis of three large-scale random-sample studies conducted in the United States and Britain. Kanazawa found that in both males and females, high intelligence in childhood was associated with a greatly increased likelihood of being gay in adulthood.[38] While this approach avoided the problem of volunteer bias, it may have been subject to another kind of problem: Smarter gay people might have been more open about their sexuality than those who were less intelligent. Still, Kanazawa's findings are suggestive of a link between homosexuality and intelligence.

Handedness

Findings on the relationship between handedness and sexual orientation differ somewhat from the results discussed above. Comparing men and women in general (without regard to their sexual orientation), men are slightly more likely to be non-right-handed (i.e., left-handed or mixed-handed) than women.[39] I'll describe this difference by saying that men are slightly "left-shifted" with respect to women. If this is a basic sex difference resulting from an early developmental process, and if sexual orientation is influenced by the same process, we would predict that gay men will be *right-shifted* with respect to straight men, whereas lesbians will be *left-shifted* with respect to straight women. In fact, however, a meta-analysis of numerous studies concluded that *both* gay men and lesbians are left-shifted with respect to their same-sex counterparts,[40] although some individual studies have failed to detect this shift[41] or have detected it only in one sex.[42]

Richard Lippa has argued, based on the results of a large-scale study, that there is *no* basic sex difference in handedness between heterosexual men and heterosexual women.[43] The reported greater prevalence of non-right-handedness among men than among women, Lippa says, is simply due to the fact that random samples of men include more gay men than lesbians, because homosexuality is commoner in men than women, and it is these gay men who shift the average male handedness slightly toward the left end of the handedness spectrum.

Another interesting fact about handedness and sexual orientation is that in some studies, handedness predicts whether or not gay people resemble straight people in cognitive performance, as if there are two different kinds of gay people. For example, Cheryl McCormick and Sandra Witelson of McMaster University in Ontario, Canada, reported that right-handed gay men scored much worse than right-handed straight men at a certain visuospatial task, whereas the non-right-handed gay men did about the same as the non-right-handed straight men.[44]

Anthony Bogaert of Brock University in Ontario has also produced data supporting the idea that gay men can be divided into two groups on the basis of handedness.[45] His findings have to do with birth order, and I will discuss this issue further in Chapter 9.

Olfaction

A Czech group tested the sense of smell in straight and gay men and women.[46] They found that while straight women and lesbians performed better than straight men (consistent with a basic sex difference that had been reported previously[47]), olfactory performance was sex-atypical in gay men. I'll return to this study in Chapter 11, because it provides some evidence for there being different kinds of gay men.

Personality Traits

Masculinity–Femininity

When we ask, "What are gay people like?" it is personality traits rather than cognitive skills that first come to mind. This is the area where stereotypes about feminine gay men and masculine lesbians are most prevalent. What's the reality?

One way to investigate this question is simply to ask gay and straight people how masculine or feminine they consider themselves to be. In 2005 the British Broadcasting Corporation ran an Internet-based survey that was taken by

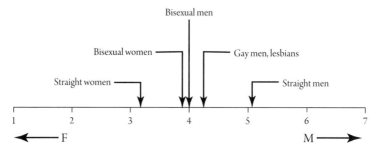

Figure 5.3 Masculinity–femininity and sexual orientation. This plot shows the average self-assessed masculinity–femininity of UK subjects on a seven-point scale. All four non-heterosexual groups cluster near the middle of the scale. The data are from a large Internet-based study (Lippa, 2008b).

nearly half a million individuals worldwide.[48] The survey asked respondents to classify themselves as "heterosexual (straight)," "bisexual," or "homosexual (gay, lesbian)." It also asked them to assess their own masculinity or femininity on a seven-point scale. As shown in Figure 5.3, gay and bisexual men assessed themselves (on average) as far more feminine than did straight men, and gay and bisexual women assessed themselves as far more masculine than did heterosexual women. All four non-heterosexual groups clustered fairly near the middle of the masculine–feminine spectrum, about halfway between the average positions of the straight men and straight women.

The results shown in the figure are for British respondents, but the results from other regions of the world were almost identical. (Of course, given that the respondents had to have access to a computer and had to understand English, they must all have been westernized to some degree.) In other words, homosexuality and bisexuality are associated with a very robust and significant shift in self-perceived masculinity–femininity toward the other sex, but not with a complete gender inversion. These findings confirm a wealth of smaller studies that have yielded similar results.[49]

Occupational Preferences

Another area that reveals a relationship between sexual orientation and gendered personality traits is that of occupational preferences. There has long been a stereotype that people who take up gender-atypical occupations (male nurses, female soldiers, etc.) are likely to be gay. Anecdotal evidence supports the stereotype. Here's one such anecdote, told by World War II veteran and lesbian activist Johnnie Phelps:

> One day I got called in to my commanding general's office—and it happened to be Eisenhower at the time—and he said: "It's come to my

attention that there may be some lesbians in the WAC [Women's Army Corps] battalion. I'm giving you an order to ferret those lesbians out. We're going to get rid of them." And I looked at him and I looked at his secretary standing next to me, and I said, "Well, sir, if the General pleases, sir, I'll be happy to do this investigation for you, but you have to know that the first name on the list will be mine." And he was kind of taken aback, and then this woman standing next to me said, "Sir, if the General pleases, you must be aware that Sergeant Phelps's name may be second, but mine will be first." And then I looked at him and I said: "Sir, you're right, there are lesbians in the WAC battalion. And if the General is prepared to replace all the file clerks, all the section commanders, all the drivers, every woman in the WAC detachment"— there were about nine hundred and eighty–something of us—"then I'll be happy to make that list." And he said, "Forget the order!"[50]

Phelps's anecdote is just a personal recollection and, even if true of its time, it doesn't necessarily mean that women in today's military are unusually likely to be lesbian, because military service has become a much more "ordinary" occupation for women than it was in the 1940s. But according to an analysis by researchers at the RAND Corporation,[51] lesbian or bisexual women are indeed much more prevalent in the military (10.7%) than in civilian occupations (4.2%), whereas gay or bisexual men are slightly *under*represented (2.2% versus 3.2%).†

In 1997, Michael Bailey and Michael Oberschneider published a study that focused on one occupation in which gay men are usually assumed to be overrepresented—professional dance.[52] They asked a large number of dancers about the prevalence of gay people among their colleagues. The results suggested that nearly 60% of male dancers are gay—an extraordinary degree of enrichment, considering that gay men make up no more than about 3–4% of the overall male population (see Chapter 1). The same study concluded that only about 3% of female dancers are lesbian, which is at most a small increase over the percentage in the general female population. Whether so many male dancers are gay because dance is a feminine activity, because it is a form of aesthetic expression (see below), or for some other reason is not completely clear.

Military service and professional dance are two extremes in terms of stereotypes about "gay" occupations for women and men. Whatever the proportion of people in these occupations who are gay, it's obvious that the vast majority of lesbians are not in the military and the vast majority of gay men are not

† The study used data from the National Longitudinal Study of Adolescent Health, which followed over 20,000 adolescents into their adult careers.

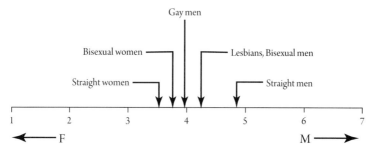

Figure 5.4 Occupational preferences and sexual orientation. This plot shows the average preferences for "gendered" occupations of UK subjects on a seven-point scale. Positions of groups of differing sexual orientation correspond well with those shown in Figure 5.3 for self-assessed masculinity–femininity. Data from Lippa (2008b).

professional dancers. What's more, people's actual occupations are not as informative about personality as are their occupational *preferences*. That's because people don't necessarily work in the field they would most prefer or that would best suit their talents.

To address occupational preferences in the general population, the BBC Internet study asked about respondents' interest in eight occupations that—as shown by preliminary testing—were much more attractive to one sex than to the other.[53] The occupations preferred by men were car mechanic, builder, electrical engineer, and inventor; those preferred by women were costume designer, dance teacher, florist, and social worker. (Note that all the "masculine" occupations were thing oriented, whereas at least three of the "feminine" occupations were people oriented.) Figure 5.4 shows that as with masculinity–femininity, all the gay and bisexual groups had gender-shifted preferences, and again these shifts were similar no matter where in the world the respondents lived. With minor exceptions, the occupational preferences of the various groups corresponded quite well to their self-assessed masculinity–femininity.

Sexuality

Given that sexual orientation is an aspect of sexuality, one might expect that gay people would differ from their same-sex peers most strongly in the facets of personality that are also sexual in nature. Yet that turns out not to be the case, at least not in any very consistent way.

About the only sexual traits that are fully gender-reversed in gay people are those that are almost part of the definition of homosexuality. The fact that gay men are sexually attracted to men carries with it a preference for masculinity—both physical and psychological—in their sex partners. In fact, femininity in looks or manner is strongly rejected by many gay men, according to a study of personal ads and questionnaire data by Bailey's group.[54] Some gay men fantasize about or actually seek sexual relationships with straight men, presumably because straight men are perceived as particularly masculine. Even among the majority who seek gay partners, it's fairly common for gay men who place personals to mention "straight-acting" as a desirable attribute in the sought-after partner or as a selling point in themselves—however politically incorrect that may seem. Conversely, Bailey's group found that lesbians prefer feminine- over masculine-looking women as partners, although they do not reject masculine-*acting* women. Of course these generalizations mask considerable variability in what individual lesbians and gay men find attractive in their partners, both within present-day gay communities and across the course of history.[55]

With regard to jealousy, gay men are gender-atypical. Like heterosexual women, they are more concerned about emotional infidelity than sexual (physical) infidelity, according to a large-scale study by psychologists David Frederick and Melissa Fales.[56] The same is true for bisexual men. Lesbians and bisexual women, on the other hand, are gender-typical: Their patterns of jealousy resemble those of heterosexual women. Thus straight men are exceptional in terms of their great concern with sexual infidelity.

In some other aspects of their sexuality, gay men are fairly like straight men and lesbians are fairly like straight women. Lesbians have the same low interest in uncommitted sex and multiple partners as do straight women, for example, whereas gay men have the same high interest as straight men.[57]

In terms of their actual behavior, gay men have even more sex partners than straight men do, though the numbers have varied greatly over time, even within a single country such as the United States.[58] This behavioral difference between gay and straight men probably has a very practical explanation: Men who seek sex with men are not limited by women's reluctance to engage in uncommitted sexual encounters.

Another trait in which gay people resemble their same-sex peers is the emphasis they place on their partners' physical attractiveness. Gay men rate physical attractiveness to be as important as straight men do, while lesbians rate it to be as unimportant as straight women do.[59]

Gay men are at least as likely as straight men to be interested and involved in unusual sexual practices, such as fetishism and sadomasochism (S/M). In fact, they may well be more likely than straight men to engage in S/M practices, especially the more extreme or unusual practices.[60] Again, the willingness of their (male) partners may be a factor here. Information on women's participation in S/M is limited, but one survey of several hundred lesbians and bisexual women found that 40% had engaged in at least one S/M or related practice, and 25% had engaged in multiple such practices; this seems higher than would be expected in the general female population.[61] It's possible that the experience of having a minority sexual orientation encourages both gay men and women to explore unconventional sexual practices.

Other Personality Traits

Gay people tend to be gender-atypical in some gendered personality traits other than their basic sense of masculinity or femininity. At least three studies[62] have reported that gay men score higher than straight men on tests of empathy—a trait that favors females—but one study found no difference.[63] Gay and bisexual men also score higher on tests of aesthetic interest, another female-favoring trait.[64] Lesbian and bisexual women score much higher than straight women on tests of technological interest and systemizing, which are male-favoring traits.[65]

Several studies have reported that gay men are less physically aggressive than heterosexual men,[66] and one of these found that lesbians are more physically aggressive than heterosexual women.[67] In one study, Doug VanderLaan and Paul Vasey investigated sexual coercion in gay and straight individuals. They found that gay or bisexual men were less likely than straight men to have committed acts of physical sexual coercion. They did not find any difference between straight and lesbian or bisexual women in this respect.[68]

Gay people also tend to be gender-shifted in instrumentality and expressiveness.[69] (As mentioned above, these are sets of male-favoring and female-favoring traits, respectively.) The basic sex differences in these traits are smaller than for masculinity–femininity, and the differences related to sexual orientation are fairly small too—they are definitely shifts and not inversions. In addition, lesbians and gay men are much more variable in these traits than are their straight counterparts, suggesting that it might be fruitful to study subpopulations of gays and lesbians who are and are not gender-shifted in these characteristics.

Overview

The mind of the "average" gay individual is a patchwork of gendered traits—some indistinguishable from those of same-sex peers, some shifted partway toward the other sex, and others typical of the other sex. All in all, though, what's striking is the large number of traits in which gay people's minds are at least partway shifted in a gender-atypical direction. In other words, the stereotype about "feminine" gay men and "masculine" lesbians *is* a stereotype, because it is an exaggeration and because it generalizes across diverse populations of gay men and of lesbians, but it nonetheless contains a substantial kernel of truth.

Most people, gay or straight, accept that there is some truth to the stereotype, but they may have a range of explanations for it. One idea heard from time to time is that gay people develop or act out cross-gendered characteristics as a reaction to the realization that they are gay. For example, a gay man might go through a thought process (not necessarily conscious) of the following kind: "I'm attracted to men, so I must be a woman, so I should act like a woman." Alternatively, a gay person might be pressured into a cross-gendered personality by the force of social labeling.

It's possible that these factors do operate to some limited degree, but they are woefully inadequate as an explanation for the findings of this chapter and the foregoing one. For one thing, gay people are already quite gender-nonconformist during childhood—perhaps more so than when they reach adulthood. Yet most people are still unaware of their sexual orientation in childhood. Given this timetable, it would be much more logical to argue that gay people are gay as a consequence of their gender nonconformity than the reverse. This in fact is the logic behind Daryl Bem's "exotic becomes erotic" theory (see Chapter 4), and although I don't believe that that theory is likely to be correct, it at least has things arranged in a believable temporal order.

Another reason for doubting that the awareness of homosexuality (by oneself or others) is what induces gender-nonconformist traits is the nature of the traits themselves. Some of them, especially in the cognitive area, are things about which most people know little and care less. Few people have preconceived ideas about how men and women should perform on arcane tasks such as mental rotation or object-location memory, and for the most part it's not obvious how parental pressure or any other forms of socialization would cause gay people to develop attributes or skills in these areas that differentiate them from straight people.

Sometimes, to be sure, socialization does come to mind as a possible causal factor. Gay men's relatively poor targeting skills, for example, might be explained by saying that they failed to participate in childhood sports that hone those skills. However, when the researchers in the study that showed poor targeting in gay men "factored out" the effect of sports experience using statistical procedures, the gay/straight difference persisted.[70]

Thus in general, the researchers who have carried out the studies described above have interpreted their findings in terms of a biological difference between gay and straight people, most likely related to levels of testosterone during early brain development, rather than in terms of environmental factors operating during childhood or adult life. The association between sexual orientation and a "package" of gendered traits arises, according to this idea, because several brain systems that mediate such traits develop in the same developmental time period and are all sensitive to circulating testosterone levels. The parallels with research on nonhuman animals as well as with the observations on CAH girls support this interpretation.

In the following two chapters, I will look more closely at two biological factors, sex hormones and genes, to see whether the evidence supports a role for them in the development of sexual orientation.

6

The Role of Sex Hormones

The idea that sex hormones influence sexual orientation goes back to the experiments of the Austrian endocrinologist Eugen Steinach (1861–1944). During the first decade of the 20th century Steinach demonstrated that secretions from the testes and ovaries influence sexual behavior in laboratory animals. He later claimed to have discovered that the testicular secretions of gay men were abnormal, and he even reported that transplantation of testicular tissue from heterosexual men into gay men converted those men to heterosexuality—an assertion that turned out to be wrong.[1]

Most attention has been paid to those sex hormones that, chemically speaking, are *steroids*. These include testosterone, estrogen, progesterone, and related substances. They are therefore known collectively as sex steroids. Initially, research on sex steroids and sexual orientation focused on the hypothesis that the nature and quantities of those hormones differed in gay and straight adults; later, attention shifted to the idea that prenatal hormones had a more important influence on orientation. For much of the 20th century, these hypotheses were used as the rationale for attempts to convert gay people to heterosexuality through hormonal means or for proposed interventions to prevent fetuses from becoming gay adults.

Few if any scientists working in this area today think in terms of pathology, cures, or prevention. Still, the idea that hormones hold the key to understanding sexual orientation is, if anything, even more widely held today than it was in the past. In part, this reflects the increasingly obvious weaknesses of competing theories, especially psychodynamic ones, as discussed in Chapter 2. In addition, the emphasis on hormones has come about as a result of new research that points more strongly to their importance than ever before. In this chapter I review that research.

Hormone Levels in Gay and Straight Adults

In 1984 neuroendocrinologist Heino Meyer-Bahlburg of Columbia University reviewed the studies published up to that time that compared blood testosterone

levels in gay and straight adults.[2] He concluded that there is no consistent difference in testosterone levels between gay and straight men. The data suggested
that most lesbians have testosterone levels in the same range as straight women,
but that up to 30% of lesbians may have testosterone levels that are elevated
(though still below the male range).

Very little research has been done in this area since the time of Meyer-
Bahlburg's review. There seems to be a consensus that gay and straight men
have similar testosterone levels and that further research on that topic is not
warranted. With regard to women, two studies suggest that self-identified
butch (masculine or dominant) lesbians may have relatively high testosterone
levels or that butch lesbians in partnerships with *femme* (feminine) lesbians
have higher testosterone levels than their partners.[3] By itself this doesn't
mean that there's some fundamental endocrinological difference between
butch and femme lesbians, because testosterone levels are influenced by a
variety of circumstances, such as relationship status, sexual activity, social
dominance, stress, phase of the menstrual cycle, and time of day.[4] I will revisit
the question of whether there are biologically different types of gay people in
Chapter 11.

Why Focus on Prenatal Sex Hormones?

The hypothesis that prenatal sex steroid levels influence people's sexual orientation comes from three main sets of observations. First, the experiments
conducted using nonhuman animals described in Chapter 3 indicate that testosterone levels during a critical period before and around the time of birth
influence an animal's preference for male or female sex partners after puberty.
It's reasonable to suspect that a similar developmental mechanism might operate in us. The critical period, if it exists in humans, would probably be entirely
before birth, given that humans are born at a much later stage of brain matura-
tion than most laboratory animals.

Second, observations in humans suggest that gendered traits other than
sexual orientation are influenced by prenatal hormones. For example, the
observations on girls and women with congenital adrenal hyperplasia (CAH;
Chapters 4 and 5) support this point of view.

Third, the link between homosexuality and a variety of other gender-atypical
traits in childhood and adulthood, discussed in Chapters 4 and 5, suggests that
sexual orientation might be part of a gender "package" that has some common
developmental roots. Thus if prenatal hormones influence those other gendered
traits, it's reasonable to ask whether they influence sexual orientation too.

Together, these three sets of observations provide the impetus for a hypothesis about a causal connection between prenatal testosterone and adult

sexual orientation. However, they do not by themselves prove that any relationship exists between those two factors, let alone that the relationship is causal. We need to consider whether there is more-direct evidence.

Hormone Levels During Development

There are three main periods during which testosterone levels are markedly elevated in males.[5] The first period begins about 7 weeks after conception, peaks at weeks 12–18, and tails off at around 24 weeks. During the early part of this period, testosterone drives the development of the male genitals and reproductive system; during the latter part, it influences development both of the genitals and of the brain.

The second period of raised testosterone begins at or shortly before birth and tails off after a few weeks.[6] The function of this second period—sometimes described as a "mini-puberty"—is not well understood, but it appears to play a role in the maintenance of male genital development.[7] In addition, there is evidence that natural variations in testosterone levels during mini-puberty influence gendered behavior in both boys and girls, independent of the prenatal effects of the same hormone.[8]

The third period of elevated testosterone begins at real puberty and is lifelong, though testosterone levels decline gradually with aging. During this period testosterone and its metabolites induce and sustain most of the anatomical and behavioral changes associated with male puberty.

On average, females have lower testosterone levels than males at all times, but there is overlap between the sexes during some portions of fetal life as well as during the neonatal mini-puberty.[9] Although low, the levels of testosterone and other androgens in female fetuses (where they are secreted by the adrenal glands) are thought to play a role in the development of the female genitals, because some women who are completely insensitive to androgens (see below) have underdeveloped clitorises and labia minora.[10]

Females experience a transient rise in estrogen during the neonatal period. Although estrogen then falls to very low levels in girls and remains low until puberty, these levels are still about eightfold higher than they are in boys. This childhood sex difference could be relevant to some aspects of development, especially of the bones (see Chapter 9).[11]

Although testosterone levels rise in girls at puberty (along with the levels of estrogen and progesterone secreted by the ovaries) and fluctuate with the menstrual cycle, they remain well below male levels. Testosterone influences sexual feelings and other gendered traits in women. The question of the relative contributions of testosterone and estrogen to sexual feelings in women is not completely settled. Most likely, both hormones play a role.

Congenital Adrenal Hyperplasia

I've already mentioned studies of females affected by CAH as evidence that elevated prenatal levels of testosterone and other androgens are capable of shifting a variety of gendered traits in a masculine direction. What about sexual orientation? No less than 19 studies have investigated the sexual orientation of CAH women, and most (especially those that have compared CAH women with matched control groups such as their unaffected sisters) have found these women to be very significantly shifted, on average, in the homosexual direction.[12]

Congenital adrenal hyperplasia comes in several forms that vary in severity; the most severe ("salt-wasting") form is associated with the most marked shift in sexual orientation (see Figure 6.1), while the mildest ("non-classical") form

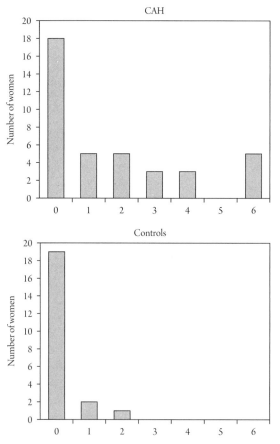

Figure 6.1 Congenital adrenal hyperplasia (CAH) and sexual orientation. The graphs show the numbers of individuals with different Kinsey ratings (0 = exclusively heterosexual; 6 = exclusively homosexual) in 39 women with the severest form of CAH (top) and in a control group consisting of 22 unaffected sisters or female cousins of CAH women (bottom). Data from Meyer-Bahlburg et al. (2008).

is associated with only a modest—but still significant—shift. This difference suggests that those affected female fetuses with the greatest exposure to androgens are the most likely to experience same-sex desire in adulthood. Not surprisingly, there is an association between childhood gendered traits and adult sexual orientation: CAH women who showed the most gender-atypical play behavior during childhood are the most likely to report sexual attraction to women in adulthood.[13]

Still, even the most severely affected group of CAH women—those with the salt-wasting condition—show only a moderate (though statistically very significant) shift of sexual orientation. In fact, while some of the affected women are out-and-out lesbian (6 on the Kinsey scale), a greater number are completely heterosexual, as shown in Figure 6.1. This finding could be interpreted to mean that prenatal testosterone levels by themselves do not dictate sexual orientation but merely influence it. It's also possible, however, that the levels or timing of testosterone exposure in many female CAH fetuses do not match the levels or timing of exposure that typically characterize male development. Thus the observation that there is *any* shift in the sexual orientation of CAH women is probably more meaningful than the fact that the shift is incomplete.

It would be useful to have the converse "experiment of nature," namely, a genetic condition that exposed *male* fetuses to unusually *low* levels of testosterone. The closest we have to that is a condition called *androgen insensitivity syndrome*, in which the gene coding for the androgen receptor—the molecule that senses the presence of testosterone and other androgens—is nonfunctional. This condition causes XY fetuses that would otherwise have become normal males to develop with the outward appearance of females (albeit sometimes with underdeveloped genitalia, as noted above), because their bodies simply don't respond to the testosterone being secreted by their testes. Children with androgen insensitivity syndrome are reared as girls, and they identify as girls. In adulthood they are psychosexually similar to other women; that is, the great majority are sexually attracted to men and are feminine in other gendered traits.[14] This finding is certainly consistent with the idea that testosterone is the key biological player in the development of sexual orientation and gender, but it does not distinguish between the roles played by biological and socialization factors, given that these individuals look like females and are raised as such.

Finger Length Studies

Are the findings on CAH, androgen insensitivity syndrome, and other unusual conditions relevant to healthy people? To approach this question, researchers have looked for anatomical or functional "markers" that might give some indication of the extent to which an individual was exposed to androgens during

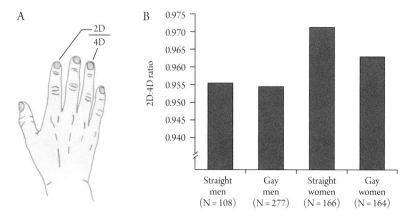

Figure 6.2 Finger length ratios and sexual orientation. (A) The 2D:4D ratio is the length of the index finger divided by the length of the ring finger. (B) Average 2D:4D ratios for straight and gay men and women. Data from T. J. Williams et al. (2000).

fetal life. If these markers do in fact provide such information, then comparing the markers in gay and straight people would help establish whether prenatal androgen levels are related to sexual orientation in the general population.

One potential marker that has triggered a lot of interest is finger length—not the absolute length of the fingers, but the ratios of the lengths of different fingers (see Figure 6.2).[15] The most informative finger appears to be the index finger (second digit). This finger, when measured in relationship to other fingers, tends to be slightly shorter in males than in females. The usual way that the measurement is done is simply to divide the length of the index finger by the length of the ring finger (fourth digit), giving what is called the *2D:4D ratio*.* The lower average 2D:4D ratio in males than females is more marked and consistent for the fingers of the right hand than for those of the left hand.[16] The sex difference in 2D:4D ratios exists prenatally but increases during postnatal life.[17]

Besides the basic sex difference, 2D:4D ratios have been linked to a variety of gendered traits *within* each sex, such that individuals with low ratios tend to be more male-typical and those with higher ratios more female-typical. For example, men engage in more risky behaviors, on average, than women, and men with low 2D:4D ratios tend to engage in more risky behaviors than men with higher ratios.[18] Similarly, the male-favoring task of mental rotation is associated with low 2D:4D ratios among men as well as among women.[19] Still, findings on the relationship between finger length ratios and gendered traits have not been entirely consistent.

---

* Sometimes the second digit is compared with the fifth digit or with a combination of digits 3, 4, and 5.

Several lines of evidence support the notion that the 2D:4D ratio is influenced by prenatal androgens:

- High testosterone levels in fetal amniotic fluid correlate with low (more male-like) 2D:4D ratios at two years of age, independent of the child's sex.[20]
- Women with CAH, who were exposed to unusually high androgen levels before birth, have lower 2D:4D ratios than unaffected women.[21] This effect of CAH may be stronger in the right than the left hand.[22]
- Women with polycystic ovary syndrome—another condition that is thought to be associated with high prenatal testosterone levels—have lower 2D:4D ratios in the right hand than unaffected women.[23]
- Women who were members of an opposite-sex twin pair, and who therefore may have been exposed to testosterone from their brothers during fetal life, have lower 2D:4D ratios than women who were members of same-sex twin pairs.[24]
- Administering testosterone to pregnant rats lowers the 2D:4D ratios of their offspring when measured in adulthood.[25]

So are there differences between gay and straight people in their finger length ratios? The answer appears to be yes, although there is not unanimous agreement among studies. Let's look at the findings for women first. Out of 10 studies that have compared 2D:4D ratios between lesbians and straight women, six reported that lesbians have lower (more male-like) ratios.[26] One Internet-based study found a *trend*[†] in the same direction, but only for White women.[27] Two studies found no difference,[28] and one Finnish study found the reverse effect: a combined sample of bisexual and lesbian women had *higher* 2D:4D ratios than heterosexual women.[29] Nevertheless, a meta-analysis of all studies supported the majority finding, that 2D:4D ratios are on average lower in lesbians than in straight women.[30]

The data for men are less clear. Out of 13 studies that have compared 2D:4D ratios in gay and straight men, six have reported that gay men have higher (more female-like) ratios than straight men,[31] four reported that they have *lower* ratios,[32] and three found no difference.[33] This conflict in results is certainly frustrating—it tempts us to throw up our hands and reject the idea that there is any real difference in gay and straight men's finger length ratios. However, one of the studies that reported that gay men's ratios are higher (shifted in the female direction) than straight men's was based on an Internet survey that had more subjects than all the other studies combined.[34] This study

[†] In statistics, a trend is an average difference between groups that fails to satisfy a minimum criterion for statistical significance.

found the shift only when comparing White gay and straight men, not Black or Chinese men. Because of the size of this study, it does seem likely that there is a small but real shift in the average 2D:4D ratios of White gay men in the direction of female-typical values. (Why there should be a racial difference of this kind is not understood.) The same meta-analysis that supported a difference in 2D:4D ratios related to sexual orientation in women failed to do so for men.[35] However, it excluded the Internet-based study just mentioned on the grounds that the measurements were made by the subjects rather than by the researchers.

One way to reduce the "noise" in the 2D:4D data (such as variations due to race) is to focus on monozygotic ("identical") twin pairs who are discordant for sexual orientation—that is, pairs in which one twin is straight and the other is gay or bisexual. In the two such studies that have been done, both male and female twins who were gay or bisexual had 2D:4D ratios that were shifted toward values typical for the other sex; this was not true of their straight co-twins.[36] Monozygotic twins share the same genome; thus besides supporting a relationship between finger length ratios and sexual orientation in both sexes, these studies suggest that nongenetic factors influence prenatal androgen levels.

Observations on finger length ratios not only support the idea that prenatal androgens influence sexual orientation; they also strengthen the notion that homosexuality is part of a package of gender-atypical traits that share a developmental history. That's because a variety of other gendered cognitive and personality traits have likewise been reported to vary with 2D:4D ratios, and in the expected direction—high ratios being associated with more-female-like scores and low ratios with more-male-like scores.[37] Still, some of the reported associations are weak or inconsistent.[38] Finger length ratios certainly offer a window into people's hormonal history, but the subtlety of the basic sex difference means that detecting differences *within* one sex—between gay and straight men, for example—requires large and carefully designed studies that take ethnicity and other variables into account.[39]

The Inner Ear

We don't usually think of men and women as differing in their sense of hearing, but in fact there are subtle differences between the sexes in auditory function.[40] Women are more sensitive than men (on average) to very quiet sounds, for example, whereas men are better than women at localizing the source of a sound.

Auditory physiologist Dennis McFadden, now retired from the University of Texas at Austin, made close studies of the *cochlea*, the auditory sense organ in the inner ear. The cochlea, as it turns out, doesn't just sense sounds; it also generates sounds. Although these sounds are very weak, they can be picked up by a sensitive microphone placed inside the ear canal (Figure 6.3A). The sounds are called *otoacoustic emissions* (OAEs); they can either occur spontaneously or be evoked in the laboratory by external sounds such as clicks. Any given spontaneous OAE has a certain *frequency* (pitch), and any particular individual

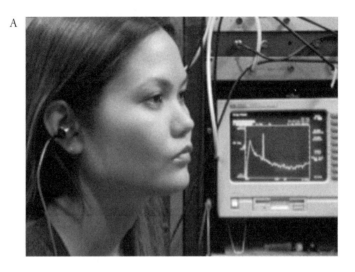

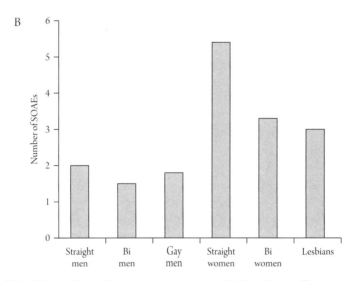

Figure 6.3 (A) Recording of otoacoustic emissions (OAEs). The oscilloscope trace shows the level of sound recorded from the subject's right ear across the entire range of audible frequencies. This subject has one spontaneous OAE (the sharp spike). Photograph courtesy of Dennis McFadden. (B) Average numbers of spontaneous OAEs recorded from the right ear for men and women of different sexual orientations. Lesbians and bisexual women have fewer spontaneous OAEs than straight women. Data from McFadden and Pasanen (1999).

generates a certain number of spontaneous OAEs, each at a different frequency. An individual's spontaneous OAEs may range in number from zero to a dozen or so. The number of spontaneous OAEs remains more or less constant for a given individual from birth until death, unless the ear becomes damaged.

Women, on average, generate more and louder spontaneous OAEs and louder click-evoked OAEs than men do,[41] although one study failed to find a sex difference in click-evoked OAEs.[42] About half of all men generate no spontaneous OAEs at all. The sex difference exists at birth[43] and has also been found in nonhuman animals.[44] Thus it is not likely to be caused by cultural factors such as a difference between boys' and girls' exposure to harmful noise levels.

Three lines of evidence suggest that the sex differences in OAEs result from the greater exposure of males to androgens during prenatal life. First, exposing female sheep fetuses to higher-than-usual levels of testosterone causes their click-evoked OAEs in adulthood to be weaker—that is, the testosterone exposure shifts the female pattern toward the male pattern.[45] Second, women who are members of opposite-sex twin pairs, and who therefore may have been exposed to higher-than-usual levels of testosterone during fetal life, have spontaneous and click-evoked OAEs that are more male-like than those of other women.[46] Third, women with CAH have a male-like pattern of spontaneous OAEs, at least in the right ear.[47]

It has been reported that hormone levels can influence OAEs to some degree in adult men and women.[48] Still, the fact that the basic sex difference exists at birth means that it is established prenatally.

McFadden and his colleague Edward Pasanen measured both spontaneous and click-evoked OAEs in straight, bisexual, and gay men and women (Figure 6.3B).[49] They found that the OAEs of lesbians and bisexual women were weaker and fewer than those of straight women; in other words, their OAE patterns were shifted in the male direction. McFadden and Pasanen interpreted these findings as evidence that non-heterosexual women, on average, experience higher levels of androgens during prenatal life than do their heterosexual peers.

McFadden and Pasanen found no significant difference in OAE patterns among straight, bisexual, and gay men. This negative finding does not constitute substantial evidence against the idea that prenatal testosterone levels influence male sexual orientation, however, for reasons I will discuss later. What's more, according to a Dutch–Belgian group, boys with gender identity disorder (i.e., very feminine boys, many of whom are likely to become gay men) do have stronger, more-female-typical OAEs than conventional boys.[50]

One disadvantage of using OAEs as a marker for prenatal hormonal exposure is that measuring them accurately requires considerable expertise as well as specialized equipment. That's in marked contrast to the use of digit ratios. Anyone with a ruler and five minutes' training can carry out a digit ratio study, and as a result there are plenty of published studies on the topic by different research groups—even though digit ratios are less-than-ideal markers, on account of the rather small sex differences they exhibit. But other than McFadden's lab, not a single research group has compared OAEs in gay and straight adults. Thus the topic remains somewhat on the fringes; it deserves to be explored more fully.

Central Auditory System

The cochlea represents the first stage in the processing of auditory signals; further processing occurs in the brainstem and in the auditory regions of the cerebral cortex. McFadden and Craig Champlin have studied central auditory function by means of electrical recordings from the scalps of subjects who are listening to clicks or other sounds.[51] These recordings, called *auditory evoked potentials*, are essentially a kind of electroencephalograph, or EEG. McFadden and Champlin reported that some of these evoked potentials show sex differences and that lesbians and bisexual women exhibit evoked potentials that are intermediate between those typical of straight women and straight men. This finding invites the same interpretation as for the cochlear data, namely, that the brains of bisexual and lesbian women are exposed to greater levels of testosterone before birth than are the brains of straight women.

With regard to men, McFadden and Champlin obtained unexpected results: Some of the patterns of evoked potentials in gay and bisexual men were shifted *away from* female values. They might be described as "hypermasculinized" rather than "feminized." In terms of the simplest hormonal model, such findings would suggest that gay and bisexual men were exposed to *higher* prenatal testosterone levels than were straight men, contrary to what the majority of data suggest. Other explanations are possible, however, and I will put off discussion of this finding until later in the chapter. Another note of caution: A more recent study, of which McFadden was a coauthor, failed to verify the originally reported sex differences in auditory evoked potentials, for reasons unknown.[52] That report muddies the interpretation of the findings in non-heterosexual subjects.

Another auditory study was carried out by Qazi Rahman and his colleagues.[53] Rahman's group focused on the *eye-blink auditory startle response*, a phenomenon that may be even more esoteric than OAEs. The basic phenomenon is that people blink when startled by a sudden loud sound. There is no obvious sex difference in this startle response. Men's startle response is greatly attenuated, however, if the loud sound is preceded by a much softer sound (a "prepulse"—the phenomenon is called *prepulse inhibition*). Women's startle response is much less affected by a prepulse.[54] When they compared straight and gay men and women, Rahman's group obtained results comparable to McFadden's findings on the cochlea; that is, lesbians showed stronger (more male-like) prepulse inhibition than did straight women. There was also a trend for gay men's responses to show weaker (more female-like) prepulse inhibition than straight men's responses.

In summary, then, three sets of auditory system findings (on OAEs, auditory startle responses, and perhaps auditory evoked potentials) are reasonably consistent in showing that the response patterns of non-heterosexual women are shifted in a male-typical direction. The findings in males show little or no difference related to sexual orientation, or may actually be in the opposite direction to what we might have predicted.

Action of Sex Hormones on the Developing Brain

After testosterone enters the fetal brain, some of it is converted to estrogen. As mentioned in Chapter 3, this conversion is performed by the enzyme aromatase. Thus both testosterone itself and the estrogen produced from it are candidates to drive brain development in a male-typical direction. As also discussed in Chapter 3, estrogen appears to be the key player in some animals, but in humans testosterone may be sufficient for brain masculinization, because men with a genetic mutation that knocks out aromatase nevertheless go through male-typical psychosexual development.[55]

The presence of testosterone and estrogen is sensed by *receptor* molecules. Earlier in the chapter I mentioned the androgen receptor, the absence of which leads to female-like development and, usually, sexual attraction to males. The brain also contains estrogen receptors.

Some of these androgen and estrogen receptors are present on the outer cell membranes of neurons. These receptors are responsible for rapid actions of sex hormones—within seconds in some cases. Other receptors, present inside neurons, are responsible for slower actions of sex hormones—over hours or days. It's these latter receptors that seem to be involved in the long-term effects that we are interested in here. I'll briefly describe their mode of action.

After a sex steroid molecule binds to a receptor, the steroid–receptor complex interacts with the DNA in the cell's nucleus. Certain genes carry specific DNA sequences that can bind to the steroid–receptor complex, thereby activating the genes, while other genes do not. Thus androgens activate their own particular suite of genes, and estrogens their own suite. Further complicating the matter is the existence of groups of proteins called *coactivators* and *corepressors*, which are capable of enhancing or inhibiting hormone action, respectively.[56]

Studies of one particular gene offer an interesting insight into how sex steroids exert their effects. This gene codes for a growth factor called *NELL2*. In the developing SDN-POA of the rat's hypothalamus, NELL2 is present in the same neurons that contain estrogen receptors—probably because the gene for NELL2 is one of the suite of genes that are activated by the estrogen receptor. A group of South Korean researchers, led by J. K. Jeong, wanted to know what would happen if the NELL2 gene were silenced during development.[57] They therefore injected into the hypothalamus of newborn male rat pups an "antisense DNA"—a stretch of DNA designed to neutralize the messenger RNA that normally carries the genetic instruction to synthesize NELL2. It turned out that with the NELL2 gene disabled, the male rats' SDN-POA developed to a smaller size than in untreated males—though not as small as in females. It appears that NELL2 normally participates in keeping SDN-POA neurons alive, so without it many cells died. NELL2 is probably just one of several growth factors that are involved in the sexual differentiation of the hypothalamus and other parts of the brain.

Sex steroids don't just affect how many neurons in SDN-POA survive; they also affect the synaptic connections established by those neurons. In male rats, SDN-POA neurons receive twice as many of a certain class of excitatory synapse as they do in females, and this high synaptic density is crucial for the establishment of male-typical sex behavior.[58] The high levels of testosterone in male fetuses during brain development are ultimately responsible for this high synaptic density, but the process involves a series of intermediate steps. Testosterone is converted in the rat's brain to estrogen, which in turn activates certain genes that raise the levels of a signaling molecule known as prostaglandin E_2, or PE_2. This molecule in turn promotes synapse formation by the neurons in SDN-POA. Simply injecting PE_2 into the hypothalamus of female rat pups raises the SDN-POA synaptic density to the level of males, even in the complete absence of sex steroids. Conversely, blocking PE_2 in male rat pups keeps the synaptic density low, even when sex steroids are present. In other words, PE_2 is a vital intermediate in this developmental pathway. The role of PE_2 has largely been elucidated by a group at the University of Maryland School of Medicine led by Margaret McCarthy.[59]

Yet another interesting effect of steroids involves the neurotransmitter *gamma-aminobutyric acid*, or GABA. In adults, GABA is the brain's principal inhibitory transmitter, but during early fetal development it has an excitatory action, and this excitation has a strong influence on the survival of neurons and the establishment of synaptic connections.[60] Testosterone delays the switch from excitation to inhibition. Thus there is a period during development (around the time of birth in rats, probably prenatally in humans) when GABA has opposite effects on testosterone-sensitive hypothalamic neurons in the two sexes: It is still excitatory in males (because they have been exposed to testosterone) but has already switched to an inhibitory function in females. This puts GABA in the position of being able to drive development in different directions in the two sexes, and it seems to actually do so: Reducing GABA levels in newborn rats weakens the development of both male-typical sexual behavior in males and female-typical sexual behavior in females.[61]

Finally, there is evidence that epigenetic processes (processes involving chemical changes to DNA or associated proteins but not to the DNA sequence itself) are involved in the sexual differentiation of the brain. I'll postpone discussing this topic until the next chapter.

The main point of this excursion into the world of brain molecules is that a prenatal hormonal theory of sexual orientation potentially involves any of a host of molecular processes. First and foremost, there could be differences between pre-gay and pre-straight fetuses in the levels of circulating testosterone during the critical period for the organization of brain circuits underlying sexual orientation. But alternatively or additionally, there could be differences in the activity of the converting enzyme aromatase or in the function or distribution of androgen or estrogen receptors—any of which might cause testosterone to have a greater or lesser effect on brain development. Coactivators or corepressors might differ between pre-gay and pre-straight fetuses. Or there might be differences in the suites of genes that are responsive to androgens and estrogens, such as the NELL2 gene or the genes responsible for the synthesis of PE_2. There could also be differences in the GABA mechanisms just described. And there are plenty of other potential players that I haven't even mentioned. Thus a prenatal hormonal theory, broadly defined, could involve other factors besides actual differences in hormone levels, and different factors might be operative in different individuals.

Continuing this line of thought, it is possible to understand how the findings concerning prenatal hormones and sexual orientation may sometimes be inconsistent. Sexual orientation and other sex-differentiated traits (gendered mental traits, finger length ratios, OAEs, and so forth) may be developmental fellow travelers, but they don't march in lockstep. This could be so for at least three kinds of reasons:

- *Timing effects.* The critical periods for sexual orientation and other traits may be exactly synchronized, may partially overlap in time, or may not overlap at all.
- *Localization effects.* Different regions of the brain and body may respond to hormones in the same way or in different ways.
- *Range effects.* The range of testosterone levels that influences sexual orientation could differ from the range that influences some other traits. To give a specific example, range effects could explain why OAEs differ between lesbian or bisexual women and straight women but not between gay and

straight men. We would just have to imagine that gay men were exposed to prenatal testosterone levels that were far enough below typical male levels to affect their sexual orientation, but not low enough to give them female-typical OAEs. Lesbian and bisexual women, on the other hand, might have been exposed to testosterone levels high enough to affect both their sexual orientation and their OAEs.

Possible Causes of Variability in Prenatal Androgen Levels

If variations in prenatal androgen levels do influence sexual orientation, how do these variations arise? One possibility is that they are caused by genetic differences between individuals. I've already described one clear-cut example of such a genetic effect—CAH. Women whose sexual orientation has been shifted in the homosexual direction on account of CAH owe this shift to a specific gene that they inherited—the gene that caused them to have CAH and thus to be exposed to unusually high androgen levels before birth. Genes may also contribute to variability in androgen levels among healthy individuals; I will discuss evidence bearing on the role of genes in the next chapter.

Prenatal androgen levels may also vary on account of nongenetic factors, including random variability. As discussed in Chapter 3, a good example of such variability from animal research is the uterine proximity effect in rodents—a female fetus that by chance is located between two males is exposed to testosterone derived from those males and consequently experiences some behavioral masculinization in adulthood. Whether this particular effect influences sexual orientation in humans (in the few women who are members of opposite-sex twin pairs) is not clear. However, random variations in hormone levels can no doubt arise in many other ways during development. I will discuss this issue further in later chapters.

Environmental factors also might affect prenatal androgen levels sufficiently to influence sexual orientation in adulthood. One candidate for such an environmental factor is stress. As I mentioned in Chapter 3, there is evidence that placing a pregnant rat or mouse under repeated stress (by immobilization, exposure to bright lights, and the like) can alter the sexual behavior and partner preference of males born of that pregnancy. This happens because stress hormones secreted by the mother reduce the levels of circulating testosterone in the male fetuses.[62]

Intriguingly, it has been reported that some demasculinizing effects of prenatal stress are also seen in the male offspring of prenatally stressed mice—more precisely, in mice whose paternal grandmothers experienced stress during pregnancy.[63] This appears to be an example of a transgenerational epigenetic effect: Stress on a pregnant female leads directly or indirectly to epigenetic changes in the genomes of their male offspring's sperm—changes that in turn affect sexual differentiation of the brains of males in the next generation.

In the early 1980s, Günter Dörner proposed that prenatal stress was an important cause of homosexuality in men.[64] Dörner and his colleagues reported that the rate of male homosexuality was unusually high among men born in Germany during World War II, when the population was exposed to many kinds of stress. They also found that most gay men (and, to a lesser extent, bisexual men) reported that their mothers had been exposed to stressful events during pregnancy, whereas straight men seldom reported such events. These events included air raids, the death of the father, and the fact that the pregnancy was unwanted. On the basis of Dörner's results it looked as if prenatal stress was the major cause of male homosexuality.

Subsequent research has not substantiated Dörner's hypothesis. A more careful analysis revealed no effect of World War II on the prevalence of male homosexuality in the German population.[65] Likewise, a more recent study found no effect of the Dutch famine of 1944–1945 on the sexual orientation of men (or women) who were fetuses at the time of the famine.[66] (However, the very low rate of exclusive homosexuality reported by men in that study—only 1 out of 374 men overall—raises some doubt about the researchers' ability to correctly assess their subjects' sexual orientations.)

Two US research groups have investigated the incidence and severity of stressful events experienced by women during pregnancies that gave rise to gay men. These groups improved on Dörner's methodology by interviewing the mothers themselves rather than relying on the men's reports. One study, by Michael Bailey's group, found no tendency for mothers to report greater stress during pregnancies that gave rise to gay men than during pregnancies that gave rise to straight men.[67] The other study, by Lee Ellis of Minot State University and his colleagues, likewise found no increase in reported stressful events during pregnancies that gave rise to gay men.[68] The study did find an apparently significant increase in severely stressful events during a three-month period 9–12 months *before* the pregnancies that gave rise to gay men. This unexpected finding could well be a fluke that resulted from subjecting the data to too many statistical tests. It could also reflect the fact that gay men are more likely to have older brothers than are straight men (see Chapter 10): Those older brothers could have been a source of increased stress for their mothers. All in all, the idea that stress is a significant cause of homosexuality in men is not supported by data.

Curiously, Bailey's group did find a slight but statistically significant effect in *women:* Mothers of lesbian or bisexual women reported experiencing a somewhat greater number of stressful events during the pregnancies that gave rise to those daughters than during pregnancies that gave rise to heterosexual daughters. Because this effect was not predicted by the animal experiments and was quite weak, it is possible that it was a fluke or was caused by some irrelevant factor, such as mothers' looking for events that might have caused their daughters' homosexuality.

Considering all the studies mentioned in this chapter, it seems reasonably well established that prenatal androgen levels have a significant influence on sexual orientation in both men and women, although the effect may be stronger in women than in men. Applying this conclusion to a more general theory of sexual orientation requires consideration of several other factors, starting with genes—the topic of the next chapter.

The Role of Genes

Boston University psychiatrist Richard Pillard is gay. Not only that; he has a gay brother, a lesbian sister, and a bisexual daughter. And his father—as Pillard found out when he read his father's diaries after his death—was in a sexual relationship with another man early in his adult life.[1] This personal history was Pillard's motivation to investigate whether homosexuality generally runs in families, a line of research he began in the early 1980s.

There could be a variety of reasons why gay people cluster in certain families. If Freud was right that a close-binding mother or hostile father makes a boy gay, then two or more boys in the same family could easily be subjected to the same influence and thus both end up gay. Alternatively, an older sibling might act as a role model, leading a younger sibling down a shared path toward homosexuality. In fact, pretty much any environmental factor could cause clustering among siblings, so long as it operates before the age at which siblings go their separate ways. Another possibility, however—and the one that we're concerned with in this chapter—is that the clustering is caused by genes that run in certain families but not in others. In other words, it could be that homosexuality is heritable.

Sibling Studies

Reports supportive of the idea that homosexuality clusters in families actually go back many decades.[2] Pillard and his colleagues, however, performed more-systematic studies. They recruited gay and straight individuals (*index subjects*) who had siblings and then ascertained the sexual orientations of the siblings, either from the statements of the index subjects or (whenever possible) from interviews with the siblings themselves.[3]

From these studies it became apparent that gay men and women have more gay siblings than do straight men or women. In Pillard's early data, about 22% of the brothers of gay men were gay or bisexual, compared with about 4% of the brothers of straight men. Similarly, about 25% of the sisters of lesbians were lesbian or bisexual, compared with about 11% of the sisters of straight women.

Subsequent studies by Pillard and others have confirmed the clustering among siblings, although the degree of clustering has generally been less than Pillard's early studies suggested.[4] Typically, about 7–16% of the same-sex siblings of gay people are found to be gay. It may be that the early studies recruited somewhat atypical samples or used broader criteria for deciding whether a sibling was gay.

An important question that hasn't been fully resolved is whether this clustering crosses the sex lines: Are the sisters of gay men more than usually likely to be lesbian, and are the brothers of lesbians more than usually likely to be gay? Pillard's personal history illustrates the clustering of male and female homosexuality in a single family, but that could have been an unusual coincidence. One study, based on data collected in the 1970s, found that opposite-sex siblings of gay index subjects were as likely to be gay as are same-sex siblings,[5] but other studies, based on more-recent data, have failed to detect any increased rate of homosexuality among opposite-sex siblings of gay people[6] or have reported rates that are increased but less so than for same-sex siblings.[7] Most likely, there is some cross-sex clustering, but not nearly as much as there is same-sex clustering.

When two brothers are gay, they tend to resemble each other in other traits related to their sexual orientation. Most notably, they are similar in their childhood characteristics: If one brother was a markedly feminine or unmasculine boy, then the same was usually true for his brother; if one brother was conventionally masculine, then the other was usually masculine too.[8] This suggests that family clustering relates not just to homosexuality in general but also to different *kinds* of homosexuality.

Is the Family Clustering Caused by Genes?

Several methods are available to tease apart the two potential main causes of family clustering: shared genes and shared environment. First, if genes are responsible, then one would expect to find increased rates of homosexuality even among relatives who were not brought up in the same family environment as gay index subjects; these could include parents, children, aunts, uncles, and cousins, as well as siblings who were separated from the index subjects soon after birth. Conversely, unrelated children who were adopted into a family should not show any increased likelihood of growing up to be gay, no matter how many other children in the family do so.

A number of studies have reported increased rates of homosexuality or bisexuality among non-sibling relatives of gay or bisexual people. These include the daughters, nieces, and female cousins of lesbian or bisexual women[9] and the uncles, male cousins, and possibly the sons of gay men.[10] As with siblings, the increase in homosexuality applies predominantly to same-sex rather than opposite-sex relatives. These findings suggest that genes are at least partly responsible the clustering of homosexuality in certain families and that different genes may predispose men and women to homosexuality.

Twin Studies

Twins are the workhorses of human behavioral genetics. They offer a fairly straightforward means to distinguish between genetic and nongenetic influences on psychological traits. They can also help distinguish between different kinds of nongenetic influences.

Twin studies compare the trait of interest—here, homosexuality—in two kinds of twins. Monozygotic ("identical") twins are the products of a single fertilized egg that split in two early in development, so they have nearly all their genes in common. (Not even monozygotic twins have precisely identical genomes, however.[11]) Dizygotic ("fraternal") twins develop from two different eggs fertilized by two different sperm, and they therefore have the same genetic relatedness as regular siblings, which is to say they share about half of their genes.

In traditional twin studies of homosexuality, index subjects are recruited who are gay and are members of same-sex twin pairs. The researchers then ascertain the sexual orientation of the other member of each pair (the co-twin), either by asking the index subject or, better, by interviewing the co-twin directly. The percentage of the co-twins who are also found to be gay is called the *concordance rate*. To the extent that homosexuality is heritable, the concordance rate will be higher for monozygotic twin pairs than for same-sex dizygotic pairs. If homosexuality were determined completely by genes, then the concordance rate for monozygotic twins would be 100%, while the concordance rate for dizygotic twins would be 50% or less.

The data from twin studies, along with an estimate of the base rate of homosexuality in the population, can be used to estimate the strength with which three factors affect sexual orientation:

- *Genes*. A genetic influence causes the concordance rate for monozygotic twins to exceed that for dizygotic twins, as just mentioned. The fraction of the total variability in a trait in a population that can be ascribed to genes is called the trait's *heritability*.
- *Shared environment*. This includes any nongenetic influences that promote homosexuality in both members of twin pairs; it typically would mean

influences that children experience while they live together, such as similar parental treatment of both twins or epigenetic (see below) or nongenetic factors that affect both twins in the womb. If shared environment is the dominant factor influencing sexual orientation, concordance rates will be high and roughly equal for monozygotic and dizygotic twin pairs.

• *Unshared environment.* This is a catch-all term for any nongenetic influences that promote homosexuality in one twin but not the other. The word "environment" is a bit misleading in this context: It includes biological sources of variability unique to individuals (such as variations in prenatal hormonal levels that are not controlled by genes) as well as the different life experiences that individuals are exposed to (which could include differential treatment by parents, sexual molestation of one twin but not the other, encountering certain role models or sex partners in adolescence and adulthood, and so on). Any random measurement error (caused by untruthful responses, for example) also raises the estimate of this factor. If the unshared environment is the dominant factor influencing sexual orientation, the concordance rates will be low and roughly equal for monozygotic and dizygotic twin pairs.

In twin studies published in the early 1990s by Michael Bailey, Pillard, and others, concordance rates for homosexuality in monozygotic twins (both male and female) were around 50%, whereas concordance rates for dizygotic twins were much lower.[12] Another study from the same period, led by Fred Whitam of Arizona State University, found an even higher concordance rate for monozygotic male twins (65%, compared with 29% for dizygotic twins).[13]

The Bailey–Pillard studies yielded estimates of heritability of roughly 50% in both sexes (though with a considerable range of uncertainty). Unshared environment contributed about as much as genes, whereas shared environment contributed little or nothing. These findings suggested not only that genes have a strong influence on sexual orientation but also that parental treatment of children (insofar as it is similar for both members of a twin pair) plays little or no role.

These early studies relied on recruiting gay twins through advertisements and so may have suffered from distortions. For example, if gay individuals with monozygotic co-twins were especially likely to volunteer if they knew that their co-twins were also gay, while dizygotic twins were less susceptible to such a bias, this would have artificially inflated the observed concordance rates for monozygotic twins, giving rise to exaggerated estimates of heritability.

To get away from this kind of problem, more-recent studies have recruited pairs of twins from large preexisting lists or registries of twins that were created without reference to sexual orientation. Studies based on this approach have been conducted in several countries. An Australian study came up with heritabilities of 30% for men and 50–60% for women.[14] A Swedish study found heritabilities of 34–39% for men and only 18–19% for women.[15] A Finnish study (the Alanko study already discussed in Chapter 4) found 45% for men and 50% for women.[16] One US study found 0% for men and 48% for women;[17] another treated men and women together and found a heritability of 28–65%.[18] All the studies found little or no effect of shared environment but a substantial effect of the unshared environment.

The large quantitative differences among the studies are disconcerting, but they are probably not worth trying to dissect in detail. For one thing, the differences may not be significant, given that these studies tend to have fairly low statistical power. (Although the studies may recruit up to a few thousand twin pairs, most pairs are uninformative because neither member is gay.) Differences may also result from the criteria employed for selecting subjects or for defining homosexuality: The Swedish study relied solely on the numbers of same-sex partners individuals had had, for example, whereas the Australian study asked about a whole range of issues related to sexual orientation. Finally, it should be borne in mind that measures of heritability can differ between populations even when there is no difference in the prevalence of the relevant genes. That's because the strength of nongenetic effects may vary, leaving genes in greater or lesser control of the trait in question.

In some of the twin studies, participants were asked about their childhood gender characteristics.[19] It turns out that monozygotic twins who are both gay are also very similar to each other in how gender-nonconformist they were during childhood. From the data in these studies it appears that childhood gender nonconformity, like homosexuality, is substantially heritable. In fact, a Dutch twin study that focused on childhood gender nonconformity without regard to adult sexual orientation obtained an estimated heritability of 70%, which is remarkably high.[20] According to the Finnish registry study, it appears that a shared set of genes is partially responsible both for childhood gender nonconformity and adult homosexuality.[21]

Monozygotic twins reared separately from birth offer an especially useful paradigm for studying the origin of psychological traits. If such twin pairs share traits on more than a chance basis, those traits are likely to be influenced by genes or by the shared intrauterine environment, not by the postnatal environment. Unfortunately, it is very difficult to find separately reared monozygotic twin pairs in whom at least one member is gay or bisexual. The research group of Thomas Bouchard Jr. at the University of Minnesota identified six such pairs, two male and four female.[22] Both members of one male pair were unambiguously gay—in fact, they didn't know of each other's existence until one of them was mistaken for his brother at a gay bar, after which they met each other and became lovers. (This could be considered an extreme example of what is popularly called "genetic sexual attraction"—the strong sexual attraction that can arise between biologically related persons who were raised apart.) The other pair consisted of a man who identified as gay (though he had had relationships with women earlier in his life) and a man who identified as straight (though he had had a homosexual relationship earlier in his life). This pair might be considered concordant for some degree of bisexuality. Whitam and colleagues reported another male monozygotic twin pair concordant for homosexuality.[23] These three examples, though hardly enough to build a statistical case, do support the idea that male homosexuality is strongly influenced by genes or the prenatal environment.

The four female pairs studied by the Bouchard group were all *discordant* for sexual orientation: One member of each pair was lesbian or bisexual and the other heterosexual. Thus the study offered no support at all for the idea that female homosexuality is heritable, although the small number of cases prevented any strong conclusion on this score.

Twin studies can suffer from various potential shortcomings. The diagnosis of each pair as monozygotic or dizygotic is not always done correctly, especially when it is based on appearance (as was the case in most of the studies just discussed) rather than molecular tests.[24] Recruitment biases can exist, as I've mentioned. And the causes of homosexuality in twins may not always be the same as in singletons.[25] Nevertheless, looking at the twin studies as a whole it seems reasonable to draw the following conclusions: Homosexuality is significantly heritable in both sexes, and the unshared environment is also important in determining sexual orientation; the shared environment, however, plays little or no role.

Molecular Genetics

Candidate-Gene Studies

The results of the family and twin studies have motivated attempts to find actual genes that might predispose to homosexuality in men or women—so-called gay genes.* One approach that has been taken is simply to guess that a specific, "candidate" gene might be involved and then to compare this gene in gay and straight people.

In the early 1990s molecular geneticists Dean Hamer, Jeremy Nathans (of the Johns Hopkins University), and their colleagues tried this approach with the gene that codes for the androgen receptor, a key player in the interaction between testosterone and the brain.[26] Obviously, gay men don't completely lack

---

* I use the phrase "gay gene" as shorthand for a hypothetical gene that, possibly in conjunction with other genes or nongenetic factors, increases the probability that its possessor will become homosexual.

this gene, because if they did they would have androgen insensitivity syndrome and would have the outward appearance of females (see Chapter 6). However, a range of variations in the DNA sequence of this gene are known or suspected to affect the activity of the androgen receptor in a variety of ways. Hamer and Nathans looked for consistent differences in the gene between gay and straight men but drew a blank. More recently a group in Hamer's lab, led by Michael DuPree, focused on the gene that codes for aromatase, the enzyme that converts testosterone to estrogen.[27] Again, they found no evidence that variations in this gene influence men's sexual orientation.

In 2012 a Chinese group published a study in which they focused on a gene named *sonic hedgehog*.[28] This is an important developmental gene that helps set up our basic body plan. The researchers reported that a certain mutation within the gene was more common in gay than in straight men, but the difference was not particularly large.

Genome Scans

Another approach to finding gay genes is to search large sections of the genome or the entire genome without any preconceived ideas as to which genes might be involved. The first study of this kind was published by Hamer's group in 1993.[29] Hamer and his colleagues first recruited a sample of gay men and asked about the sexual orientations of their relatives. The researchers found increased rates of male homosexuality among the brothers, uncles, and male cousins of the index cases, in line with what I've mentioned above. However, of the two kinds of uncles (maternal and paternal), only maternal uncles had significantly increased rates of being gay, and among the four kinds of male first cousins (sons of maternal aunts, sons of maternal uncles, sons of paternal aunts, and sons of paternal uncles), only the sons of maternal aunts had significantly increased rates. In other words, only men connected to the index cases through the female line had an increased likelihood of being gay.

This pattern suggests that there might be maternal inheritance of genes predisposing to male homosexuality. Reinforcing this conclusion, Hamer presented several family trees in which multiple gay men were found; in each tree, all the gay men could be connected to each other through females. (Figure 7.1 shows an example.) Such a pattern of inheritance usually points to genes on the X chromosome, because this is the only chromosome that men inherit exclusively from their mothers. Hamer therefore focused his molecular studies on the X chromosome.

I should say right away that data from subsequent studies have not uniformly confirmed a higher rate of male homosexuality among maternal-line than paternal-line relatives of gay men: Some studies have,[30] while others have not.[31] A study led by Gene Schwartz of Northwestern University, for example,

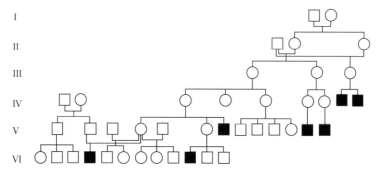

Figure 7.1 Six-generation family tree including seven gay men (black squares) in the three youngest generations. Squares indicate men, circles indicate women. The tree is consistent with the existence of a gay gene that was passed down from the woman in generation I, via female descendants, to each of the gay men. From Hamer et al. (1993).

found the same elevated rate of homosexuality among all four kinds of first cousins.[32] I will return to this issue later in the chapter.

From the index subjects and their relatives in the X chromosome study, Hamer and colleagues recruited 40 pairs of brothers who were both gay. Recall that women possess two X chromosomes and men just one. Thus if the brothers in each pair were gay on account of a gene on the X chromosome (an *X-linked* gene), then they should both have inherited the same genetic material from the same maternal X chromosome—the one that carried the putative gay gene. Because of the phenomenon called *crossing over*, in which the two maternal X chromosomes exchange segments during the development of the ovum, only the region of the X chromosome near the gay gene would have been co-inherited by the brothers at an above-chance rate. Hamer's group therefore examined 22 DNA markers—sites where DNA sequences are known to vary among individuals in the population—that are scattered along the length of the X chromosome. This is called a *linkage study*.

In Hamer's data, the pairs of brothers shared the same markers at an above-chance rate in just one part of the X chromosome, a region named Xq28, which lies near the tip of the long arm of the chromosome. Straight brothers of these gay siblings did not share the same markers. Hamer and colleagues interpreted these results to mean that a gene or genes predisposing to homosexuality lay in region Xq28.

Subsequent to Hamer's study, several other linkage studies were published, with negative or only weakly positive findings.[33] More recently, however, a research group at Northwestern University published the findings of an independent and much larger linkage study.[34] This study confirmed Hamer's finding concerning Xq28. In addition, it found evidence for a gene or genes influencing male sexual orientation on a different chromosome, chromosome 8. There was no evidence in this study for any gay genes on chromosome 7, on which *sonic hedgehog* is located.

The linkage studies don't have enough precision to identify specific genes, but they narrow the search to perhaps a couple of dozen genes that might be relevant to sexual orientation. To mention just one of these, there's a gene at Xq28 named *Cnga2*, which is involved in olfactory communication: When this gene is knocked out in mice, the animals' sexual behavior is greatly impaired.[35] They don't become "gay mice," though.

Neither of the two linkages identified in these studies explains more than a small fraction of the total genetic influence on men's sexual orientation, if we are to believe the estimates of heritability that have been derived from family and twin studies. Thus there are probably genes at other locations, as yet unidentified, that also play a role. In general, it has proved difficult to identify single genes that explain a large portion of the variation in any behavioral trait researchers have investigated—even for traits, such as intelligence, that are known to be highly heritable.[36] Still, it's possible that single genes do sometimes have powerful effects. The family trees presented by Hamer and colleagues, for example, suggest that the presence or absence of a particular X-linked gene has an almost decisive influence on who is gay and who is straight in those particular kinship groups.

Unlike linkage studies like those just described, *genome-wide association studies* dispense with the need to find pairs of gay brothers. Association studies make use of the fact that there are over a million locations within the genome where people may have slightly different DNA sequences. These differences, affecting just a one DNA nucleotide or "letter," are called *single-nucleotide polymorphisms,* or SNPs (pronounced "snips"). If a certain gene is reliably different between gay and straight individuals, then SNPs at the location of that gene may also be reliably different.

The company 23andMe, which offers personalized genetic information to the general public, has collected and analyzed DNA samples from hundreds of thousands of men and women. Using this database, researchers at the company compared SNPs between gay and straight men as well as between lesbian and straight women.[37] In women they recorded no significant "hits," that is, SNPs that were statistically different for lesbians and straight women. They recorded no significant hits in men either, but the SNP that came closest to statistical significance was found at the same location on chromosome 8 where the Northwestern group's linkage study had its most significant hit. Thus the 23andMe study strengthens the evidence that there is indeed a gay male gene at that location.

As the cost of DNA sequencing falls, it is becoming affordable to dispense with SNPs and simply sequence the entire genomes of individuals with and without a certain trait. No such study has yet compared the genomes of gay and straight people, however.

Epigenetic Effects

Epigenetic effects are biological effects brought about by chemical modifications to DNA or to the proteins associated with DNA—modifications that don't involve changes to the DNA sequence itself. A common change is the addition of a methyl group ($-CH_3$) to cytosine, which is one of the four DNA nucleotides. Genes that have many methylated cytosines are less active and may be switched off completely. When a cell divides, the methylation pattern of its DNA is passed on to its daughters. The stability of these epigenetic "marks" probably helps ensure that different tissues maintain their specific characteristics over a lifetime. Epigenetic processes play a complex role in the sexual differentiation of the brain and behavior, although the evidence for this comes mainly from experiments on mice and other nonhuman animals.[38]

The activity of the enzymes that methylate DNA is controlled partly by genes and partly by nongenetic factors. For example, monozygotic twins at birth have DNA methylation patterns that differ from each other (demonstrating a nongenetic influence), but they are more similar to each other than is the case for dizygotic twins (demonstrating a genetic influence).[39]

Nongenetic factors fall within the category of unshared environment (see above). It may seem strange that newborn twins could have been exposed to different environments when they developed at the same time in the same uterus. However, differences in such things as blood supply can lead to different methylation patterns. In addition, the unshared environment includes purely random variations that are unique to individuals, and this kind of randomness seems be an important developmental factor not just in twins but in everyone.[40]

How does this relate to the development of sexual orientation? As mentioned above, twin studies show that genes contribute no more than about half of the total causation of homosexuality in men and perhaps less than that in women, so there is plenty of space for epigenetic mechanisms to play a causal role too. And as there is a long time lag between the events presumed to cause homosexuality and the actual expression of that trait (i.e., from prenatal life until puberty), epigenetic mechanisms are possible candidates for maintaining a corresponding "silent signal" over the intervening years.[41]

In the previous chapter I mentioned the work of Margaret McCarthy's group at the University of Maryland School of Medicine demonstrating the role of prostaglandin E_2 (PE_2) as an intermediate step between rising steroid hormone levels in the developing hypothalamus and the masculinization of synaptic anatomy and sexual behavior. More recently the same group has discovered a crucial role for epigenetic processes in this developmental sequence.[42] In a rodent model, estrogen (derived from testosterone) inhibits the enzymes that methylate DNA during the critical period of development. Thus in males the suppressive effect of methylation is weaker than in females, and as a consequence masculinizing genes (perhaps including those responsible for the synthesis of PE_2) are permitted full sway. In females, on the other hand, the much greater prevalence of methylation represses the masculinizing genes and so the hypothalamus follows the female developmental pathway. If methylation is blocked in males (by drugs or by genetic manipulation), the male rodents develop female-like synaptic patterns in the medial preoptic area of the hypothalamus, and their sexual behavior in adulthood is feminized (including preferring to associate with other males). We don't yet know, however, whether differences in these epigenetic processes can account for different sexual orientations in humans.

In a study that was presented at a conference in 2015 but has not yet been published, a large research group with Tuck Ngun of UCLA as first author described an analysis of DNA methylation patterns in male monozygotic twin pairs.[43] The pairs were discordant for sexual orientation—one gay and one straight. The researchers found consistent differences between the gay and straight twins at five locations in the genome. Using information about methylation at just these five sites, they were able to devise an algorithm that predicted the sexual orientations of a new set of discordant twins with 67% accuracy. Note, however, that random guesswork would have yielded about 50% accuracy, so the algorithm's performance was in a sense closer to guesswork than it was to perfect prediction. It remains to be seen whether these findings hold up in other studies. If they do, it will be interesting to know how these key epigenetic markers come to differ in gay and straight twins, and what effect the different methylation patterns have on gene expression.

Genes and Sexuality in Fruit Flies

In a state of nature the male fruit fly, *Drosophila melanogaster*, is resolutely heterosexual. In the early 1960s, however, Indian geneticist Kulbir Gill, working at Yale University, created a mutant strain of fruit flies in which males courted males and females with equal enthusiasm.[44] When these flies were put together in all-male groups they formed long, moving chains resembling conga lines, with each male attempting (unsuccessfully) to mate with the male in front of it. The change from a heterosexual to a bisexual orientation was caused by a single mutation affecting a gene that Gill named *fruity*, given the standard three-letter abbreviation *fru*. The full name was a crude joke at the expense of gay people, and it was later changed to the less obnoxious *fruitless*.

The *fru* gene was isolated and sequenced in 1996 by a group working at Stanford University[45] and by a Japanese group led by Daisuke Yamamoto.[46] Both male and female flies possess the *fru* gene, but the product of the gene (the messenger RNA) is processed differently in the two sexes.[47] In males the product of the non-mutant *fru* gene activates a cascade of lower-order genes in the brain, enabling male-typical sexual behavior and suppressing female-typical behavior. If female *Drosophila* are engineered to process *fru* in the male fashion, they remain anatomically female, but they court other females rather than males, as shown in Figure 7.2.

Rather as testosterone does in the developing brains of male mammals, the *fru* product promotes the survival of certain clusters of neurons in male fruit flies so that these clusters end up sexually dimorphic, containing more cells in males than in females.[48] The main difference is that testosterone in mammals is a hormonal signal that enters the brain and masculinizes it, whereas the *fru* product in *Drosophila* operates within brain cells themselves if the chromosomal sex of those cells is male.

Yamamoto's group used molecular-genetic trickery to insert just one of these male-specific neuronal clusters, named P1, into the brains of female flies.

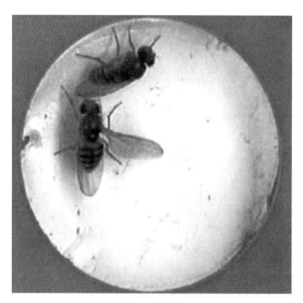

Figure 7.2 Homosexual courtship in fruit flies. The lower of these two flies is a female that was genetically engineered to process the product of the *fru* gene in a male fashion. She is courting another female by "singing" to her with the vibrations of her right wing. Photo courtesy of Barry Dickson.

Even though the rest of the brain, and the body, of these flies were female, they displayed male-typical sexual behavior, including courtship of females.[49] This was a striking demonstration of the relevance of sexual dimorphism in the brain to sex differences in partner choice.

Many mutations or other genetic manipulations are now known that can induce homosexual behavior in fruit flies.[50] In addition, two neurotransmitters, *glutamate* and *dopamine*, are known to play a role. Suppressing glutamate neurotransmission in male flies causes them to court other males.[51] Raising dopamine levels in male flies has the same effect.[52]

Finally, *lowering* dopamine levels in male flies causes *other* males to court them.[53] This is thought to happen because, without sufficient dopamine, males produce less than usual of a chemical that is aversive to males—a kind of "no males need apply" *sex pheromone*. A similar effect has been observed in flies that are entirely male except that the pheromone-secreting tissue has been genetically engineered to be female. Like the low-dopamine flies, these male flies court females but are courted by males.[54] These observations serve as a reminder that sexual attraction involves two participants, an attractor and an attractee, and characteristics of either can induce or suppress homosexual behavior.

No one considers it likely that the detailed findings in *Drosophila* apply to humans—the two species differ too much in genetics, development, and brain organization. Still, there may be some useful lessons to be learned about humans from fruit flies. First, there is simply the fact that it is proving possible to understand the basis of sexual partner preference in flies at the level of specific genes, molecules, and brain cells and the interactions among them. This offers hope that it will eventually be possible to do the same for our own species.

A second lesson from *Drosophila* is that the lower-level neural circuits that mediate courtship of males and females exist in all flies; what differ between flies are the higher-level control centers that activate one circuit and inhibit the other. There is reason to believe that the same might be true in mammals, including humans, as I will discuss in the next chapter.

Finally, although the sexual differentiation of the mammalian brain is largely controlled by circulating hormones, some influence is also exerted by the intrinsic chromosomal sex of the brain itself, as happens in *Drosophila*. I already touched on this issue in Chapter 3. The evidence for this influence comes from a variety of studies, including ones where researchers used genetic-engineering technologies to manipulate the intrinsic brain sex of mice independently of the sex of the gonads.[55] There is no direct evidence as yet that these hormone-independent processes influence partner preference in either mice or humans, but Sven Bocklandt and Eric Vilain of UCLA have discussed how such processes might do so.[56]

Genes, Homosexuality, and Evolution

The idea that genes predispose certain people to homosexuality is paradoxical. We might expect such genes to reduce their possessors' *reproductive success*[†] and thus to be eliminated from the gene pool by natural selection. Doesn't this problem throw doubt on the very existence of gay genes?

Actually, plenty of genes exist that lower reproductive success. I've already mentioned a couple: the gene that causes androgen insensitivity, which renders its possessor infertile, and the genes that cause congenital adrenal hyperplasia, which (untreated) can kill their possessors long before they are old enough to have children.

A number of factors may help save such a gene from extinction. If it is a *recessive gene* it will harm its possessor's reproduction only when the possessor has inherited copies of the gene from both parents (the so-called *homozygous state*), and not when the possessor has inherited a copy from just one parent (the *heterozygous state*). The homozygous state isn't common, so natural selection acts only slowly to eliminate harmful recessive genes. New mutations that cause the same trait may occur fast enough to compensate for the gradual elimination of the gene. In the case of androgen insensitivity syndrome (which is caused by X-linked recessive genes, so XX female heterozygous carriers are healthy), about a third of all cases of the disorder are caused by new mutations.[57]

In some cases, "harmful" genes are actually beneficial when they occur in the heterozygous state. This is known as *heterozygous advantage* or (more technically) overdominance. The classic example is the gene that causes *sickle cell anemia*: Persons with two copies of the gene develop the disease, but persons with one copy (the heterozygous state) enjoy partial resistance to malaria. Therefore, in malaria-prone regions, the heterozygous state confers an advantage, and the sickle-cell gene persists.

In real life, genes may have multiple effects, and they may interact with one another and with the environment in complex ways that make it hard to predict their net effects on reproductive success. Still, that uncertainty hasn't prevented people from coming up with hypotheses about how gay genes are able to stay afloat in the gene pool, and even looking for evidence in support of those hypotheses.

One idea is this: Maybe being gay doesn't have as severe an impact on reproductive success as we imagine.[58] After all, many famous gay people, such as Oscar Wilde, have been parents. Perhaps traditional societies forced everyone

---

[†] "Reproductive success" is a standard term meaning the total number of an individual's offspring that survive to maturity. I don't mean to imply that there is anything particularly meritorious about having large numbers of children.

to marry and have all the children they were capable of, regardless of their sexual orientation. In that situation, genes predisposing to homosexuality would not be weeded out.

This idea doesn't hold water, however—for men, at least. Whatever the situation in traditional societies, gay men in contemporary Western cultures are far less likely to have children than are their straight peers. In a US random-sample survey conducted in 1994, for example, only 27% of men who identified as gay or homosexual said they were fathers, compared with 60% of other men.[59] A more recent Italian study found that gay men have only one-fifth the number of children that straight men have,[60] and a British study (which focused on White men) found an even larger difference.[61] The *fa'afafine* (androphilic men) of Independent Samoa, about whom we will say more later in this chapter, usually have no biological children at all.[62] These huge disparities should eliminate any gene for male homosexuality in the blink of an evolutionary eye. The 1994 US study found only a small difference in motherhood between lesbians and other women (67% versus 72% said they had children, respectively), but even that difference, if consistently maintained, should eliminate genes for female homosexuality quite quickly.

About the only way that the existence of gay genes could be compatible with the lower reproductive success of gay people is if there is a compensatory increase in the numbers or reproductive success of heterosexual *relatives* of gay people: individuals who, because of their relatedness to the gay person, have some likelihood of also carrying the gay genes. The transmittal of these "extra" copies of the genes to the next generation could balance the loss of copies caused by the lowered reproduction of gay people themselves, thus maintaining gay genes in a state of equilibrium through the generations. This explanation of course would require that not every person carrying a gay gene is actually gay.

Gay men do indeed have more relatives than straight men. In the British study just mentioned, which was led by psychiatrist Michael King, the combined total number of siblings, aunts, uncles, and cousins (i.e., relatives belonging to generations that were likely to be complete at the time of the survey) averaged 19.8 for the gay men and 16.9 for the straight men; in other words, the gay men had nearly three extra relatives.[63] Gay men also had more nephews and nieces than straight men, but that generation was probably incomplete at the time of the survey, so the numbers were more difficult to interpret.

Kin Selection

What causes gay men to have extra relatives? One possibility is that gay men (and possibly lesbians too) actually help their relatives reproduce. For example, gay people might give their siblings money or assist them with child care, thus enabling them to have extra children. There are nonhuman species in which some individuals do not have offspring but dedicate themselves to the reproductive success of their close relatives. The best-known examples are the social insects such as ants and bees, in which sterile female workers help the queen reproduce.

This "kin selection" model, which was first applied to homosexuality by sociobiologist E. O. Wilson,[64] does not work well to explain the persistence of gay genes in humans. Admittedly, one set of studies seems to support it: Paul Vasey and Doug VanderLaan have reported that the homosexual men in Samoa known locally as *fa'afafine* are significantly more willing to assist their siblings with childrearing duties than are straight men.[65] This helpfulness is not directed to the children of non-kin, and it is not explained simply by the men's general femininity, so in those respects it fits well with the kin selection model. However, it is unclear that *fa'afafines* provide *enough* assistance to their kin to meet the model's requirements. For the *fa'afafines'* behavior to satisfy kin selection theory, they must, on average, help their siblings to have at least *two* extra surviving offspring for every *one* offspring that they give up on themselves. That is a difficult condition to fulfill.

Comparable studies in the United States and the United Kingdom have found no evidence in favor of a kin selection model.[66] What's more, gay people devote considerable resources to their own (reproductively inefficient) sex lives, but this behavior has little value in terms of a kin selection model. And however benevolent gay people's feelings towards their relatives might be, this benevolence could hardly increase the number of their relatives in the generation *before* their own, yet there are in fact extra relatives in that generation, according to the King study.[67]

The "Fertile Female" Hypothesis

A more likely explanation for why gay people belong to larger extended families than straight people is that gay genes act directly within some of the relatives of gay people to increase their reproductive success. There are at least two models for how this might work. Both require that gay genes have other effects besides conferring a predisposition to homosexuality.

In one model, gay genes promote the reproductive success of the opposite-sex relatives of gay people. Because the relevant research has been done on the relatives of gay men, this model is often called the "fertile female" hypothesis.[68] In the simplest version of this hypothesis, the male gay gene is not really a gene for homosexuality per se but rather a gene for sexual attraction to males (androphilia). If so, those female relatives of gay men who inherited the gene might be, as it were, "hyper-heterosexual." That is, they would have the regular tendency to experience sexual attraction to males that most women share, plus an extra dose conferred by the androphilic gene that runs in their families. As a result, they might engage in more sex with men and thus become pregnant more often. Alternatively, the male gay gene might make women who carry it look or act more feminine than other women, thus increasing their attractiveness to men.

To the extent that this *sexually antagonistic model* is correct, the larger average size of gay men's extended families should result from the greater fecundity (number of children) of their female relatives rather than of their male relatives. Although the King study mentioned above did not observe this effect, an Italian research group led by Andrea Camperio-Ciani of the University of Padua has reported a difference of this kind in three studies.[69] What's more, the females with extra children were found only on the maternal side of the gay men's families. This pattern supports the notion that at least one gene promoting male homosexuality is located on the X chromosome. That's because, as discussed above, men inherit their X chromosome from their mothers, not from their fathers, so there's no increased likelihood that paternal relatives will carry an X-linked gay gene. In other words, the Italian studies support the molecular-genetic findings indicating the existence of a gay gene on the X chromosome.

Thus the fertile female hypothesis for the maintenance of genes promoting male homosexuality has some observational support. What's more, detailed mathematical modeling has shown that with certain assumptions (i.e., that two genes influence male sexual orientation and that at least one of them is located on the X chromosome), the sexually antagonistic model explains why male homosexuality persists at a constant low frequency in the population without either dying out or increasing in frequency.[70]

Incidentally, the fertile female hypothesis offers a possible explanation for the high prevalence of male homosexuality in domestic sheep, as described in Chapter 3. Sheep farmers select the most-fertile ewes for breeding,[71] so any genes that promote both fertility in ewes and homosexuality in rams would likely persist. In one experimental study, however, selecting ewes for high fertility did not increase the percentage of the male offspring who showed homosexual behavior.[72]

A variation on the fertile female hypothesis has been put forward by a French group led by Julien Barthes.[73] As already mentioned in Chapter 1, these researchers reported evidence that male homosexuality (in the sense of a durable preference for male sex partners) is found primarily in socially stratified societies—that is, societies with hierarchical classes. In such societies, they say, women who marry into a higher class enjoy greater reproductive success. A male gay gene might confer signs of high fertility when present in women, thus making them more attractive to higher-class men and increasing their chances of "marrying up." As with the basic fertile female hypothesis outlined above, the reproductive benefit of the gene in women could outweigh its reproductive cost in their gay male relatives. The validity of these ideas has been the subject of some debate.[74]

Beneficial Effects on Same-Sex Relatives

I've just described a mechanism whereby a gene predisposing to homosexuality in one sex would increase the reproductive success of heterosexual persons of the other sex. There are other possible mechanisms, however, in which a gene promoting homosexuality in one sex would increase the reproductive success of heterosexual persons of the *same* sex, or of both sexes. The most detailed model of this kind was developed by economist Edward Miller of the University of New Orleans.[75] As with the other models, this one was directed primarily at explaining male homosexuality, though it could be applied to both sexes.

Miller started from the assumption (for which I have described evidence earlier in this book) that male homosexuality is not an isolated trait but rather is part of a package of gender-variant traits. Miller proposed that several "feminizing" genes control these traits. If a man inherits a few of these genes, he will have some feminine characteristics, which might include increased empathy and kindness, decreased aggressiveness, and the like. These traits, Miller suggests, will increase his attractiveness to women, giving him more sexual access to them and thus making him likely to have more offspring. If a man inherits *all* of these genes, however, he will be feminized to the point of homosexuality, and his reproductive success will drop markedly. These two possibilities lead to an equilibrium state that maintains a certain constant percentage of gay men in the population. Because each feminizing gene is present in many more straight men than gay men, it only has to raise each straight man's reproductive success by a small amount to compensate for the lowered reproductive success of gay men.

This model generates three important predictions. First, straight men who exhibit certain feminine traits should experience greater reproductive success than straight men who lack such traits. Second, straight men who have gay relatives should be more likely to exhibit feminine traits than straight men who lack gay relatives. And third, straight men with gay relatives should experience greater reproductive success than heterosexual men who lack gay relatives.

Miller did not test these predictions, but a group led by Brendan Zietsch of the Queensland Institute of Medical Research and including Michael Bailey made an initial attempt to do so, using nearly 5000 male and female subjects from the Australian twin registry mentioned earlier.[76] The subjects filled out questionnaires about their masculinity or femininity, their sexual orientation, and the number of opposite-sex sex partners they had had over their lifetime. (The researchers used the number of sex partners in preference to fecundity—the total number of offspring—on the assumption that modern culture has divorced fecundity from the psychological traits that used to regulate it.)

Zietsch's group found, first, that femininity in men and masculinity in women were associated with an increasing likelihood of being gay. This was fully expected, of course. However, among *straight* men, femininity was associated with a larger number of female sex partners, and among straight women, masculinity was associated with a larger number of male sex partners. Thus in accordance with Miller's model, gender-atypical traits do seem to promote reproductive success in both straight men and straight women.

Second, by analysis of concordance rates in monozygotic and dizygotic twin pairs, the researchers were able to show that overlapping genetic factors were partly responsible for the correlation between gender identity and sexual orientation and (in straight men and women) between atypical gender identity and number of sex partners. This is also consistent with Miller's model.

Finally, the researchers found that heterosexual individuals with gay twins had more opposite-sex sex partners than did heterosexual individuals without gay twins, although the difference reached statistical significance only for females. This suggests that, among females at least, close same-sex relatives of gay individuals inherit genes that aid their reproductive success by conferring atypical gender characteristics.

In general, it's clear that there are several robust models that can account for the persistence of gay genes. My hunch is that the sexually antagonistic model is the correct one (but my hunches are often wrong).

8

The Brain

All mental traits, including sexual orientation, have some durable representation in the brain. These representations are not merely a matter of neuronal activity patterns; we know this because their influence re-emerges after our thoughts have been diverted into other channels, after we have been asleep or under general anesthesia, and even after our brains have been cooled to a temperature at which all neuronal activity ceases. Therefore these brain representations are structural in a broad sense, a description that could include the numbers, kinds, and arrangements of neurons, synapses, or molecules.

Finding these representations could be difficult. Take our preference for one musical composer over another. This has to have some representation in the brain, but it is likely to be an inconspicuous one. Finding it might be like finding, in a haystack, not a needle but an unmarked stalk of hay. Our hope that the brain representation of sexual orientation is findable rests on the assumption that there is something unusual about this trait—that it involves very basic and specialized neural hardware rather than general-purpose networks.

Even finding a brain representation for a person's sexual orientation—whether straight, bisexual, or gay—wouldn't mean that we understood how it came into being. Figuring that out would require putting together information from many different approaches, some of which I have discussed in previous chapters. I will make only some brief comments on this topic at the end of this chapter and postpone further consideration of it until later in the book. Here I will focus on what has been learned from studying the brains of people of different sexual orientations. Right away I should caution that many of these studies have not yet been confirmed (or disconfirmed) by other researchers.

A Brief Tour of the Brain

The brain has a dauntingly complex organization, but for the present purposes I need only give a quick sketch, focusing on a few structures that may be relevant to our enquiry (Figure 8.1). The brain consists of two general parts,

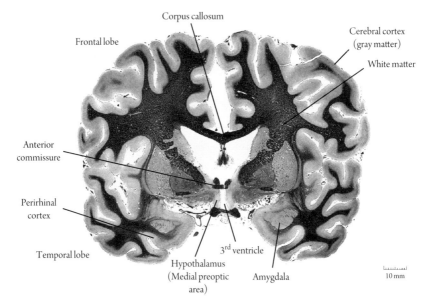

Figure 8.1 Transverse section through the human brain, showing some of the structures mentioned in this chapter. The white matter (fiber tracts) has been stained dark. Image adapted with permission from the Michigan State University Brain Biodiversity Bank, produced with support from the National Science Foundation.

the forebrain, which takes up most of the brain's volume, and the brainstem, which connects the forebrain to the spinal cord. It's the forebrain that interests us here.

The most obvious feature of the forebrain is the cerebral cortex, the wrinkled, layered sheet of *gray matter* (neurons and synapses) that forms most of the outer surface of the left and right cerebral hemispheres. The cerebral cortex is the principal site of cognitive processing. On each side of the brain the cerebral cortex is divided into four major lobes—the frontal, temporal, parietal, and occipital lobes—and these lobes are further divided into anatomically and functionally specialized regions that are designated with numbers or names. Under the cortex is *white matter* (stained black in Figure 8.1), which consists of neuronal fibers connecting cortical regions with each other and with brain regions that are not part of the cortex. The major band of subcortical white matter that interconnects the left and right hemispheres is called the *corpus callosum*; another, much smaller one is called the *anterior commissure*.

Even deeper under the white matter are large groups of nuclei—clusters or masses of neurons that are not organized into layers. I'll mention just three of these groups. The *thalamus* acts as a way station between lower centers and the cerebral cortex, converting sensory signals into a form that the cerebral cortex can process. It also participates in cognitive processes by means of its two-way connections with the cortex.

Below the thalamus is the hypothalamus, which I've already mentioned several times in earlier chapters. The hypothalamus can be seen on the underside of the brain. It is situated on either side of the *third ventricle*, a slit-like space filled with cerebrospinal fluid that lies in the brain's midline. In spite of its rather small size, the hypothalamus participates in a wide variety of "life-preserving" functions, such as feeding and drinking, keeping body temperature in the right range, and reproduction. The hypothalamus also controls the function of the pituitary gland, the master gland of the endocrine system, which sits immediately under the hypothalamus. The hypothalamus is divided into many small nuclei with specialized functions, and these are connected with many other brain regions, including the cerebral cortex.[1]

Another subcortical structure that needs to be mentioned is the *amygdala*, which lies to the side of the hypothalamus at the base of each cerebral hemisphere, within the temporal lobe. Each amygdala is a ball-like mass of neurons about 1 cm in diameter, and like the hypothalamus it consists of several individual nuclei. Although the different nuclei within the amygdala have a variety of connections and functions,[2] one important function of the amygdala is processing emotion—most notably, forming emotional associations sparked by, for example, seeing happy or fearful faces.[3] Parts of the amygdala are involved in sexual functions; these connect richly with hypothalamic nuclei concerned with sexual behavior[4] and differ between the sexes in their synaptic architecture.[5]

Hypothalamic Anatomy and Sexual Orientation

As I already discussed in Chapter 3, a region at the front of the hypothalamus called the medial preoptic area is involved in the regulation of male-typical sexual behaviors, and within this area lies at least one cell group that is larger, on average, in males than in females. In rats this cell group is called the sexually dimorphic nucleus of the preoptic area (SDN-POA), and in humans it is called the third interstitial nucleus of the anterior hypothalamus (INAH3) (Figure 8.2A). It is suspected, but not proven, that the rat SDN-POA and the human INAH3 are homologous structures, meaning that they evolved from the same structure in the common ancestor of rats and humans.[6*]

* In 1985 Dick Swaab's group at the Netherlands Institute for Brain Research reported that a different hypothalamic cell group, INAH1, was larger in men than in women (Swaab & Fliers, 1985). They named this cell group "SDN-POA," described it as "analogous" to the rat SDN-POA, and performed a number of subsequent studies of its structure and development (Swaab & Hofman, 1988; Hofman & Swaab, 1989; Swaab, 1995). They also reported failing to find any difference

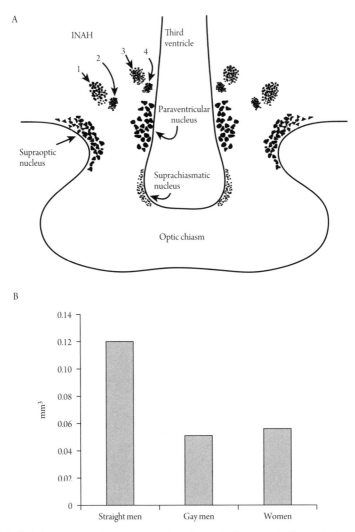

Figure 8.2 (A) Diagram of transverse slice through the anterior hypothalamus (same level as Figure 8.1), showing layout of the interstitial nuclei of the anterior hypothalamus (INAH1–4). (B) Average volumes of INAH3 in straight and gay men and in women. Data from LeVay (1991). (C) Same as (B), but with data from Byne et al. (2001). (D) Average volumes of the equivalent cell group in sheep (oSDN) for heterosexual and homosexual rams and for ewes. Data from Roselli et al. (2004a).

between the size of INAH1 in gay and straight men, and used this result to reject the idea that the hypothalamus of gay men develops in a sex-atypical fashion (Swaab et al., 1992). Since that time, however, three other laboratories have failed to confirm the basic sex difference in INAH1 (Allen et al., 1989; LeVay, 1991; Byne et al., 2001). Thus the reliability of Swaab and Fliers' observation, the merits of any theoretical conclusions based on it, and the appropriateness of the name SDN-POA in reference to INAH1 are open to serious question. The function of INAH1 (now more commonly known as the ventrolateral preoptic nucleus) likely has nothing to do with sex: There is evidence that it is involved in the regulation of sleep (Gaus et al., 2002; Lim et al., 2014).

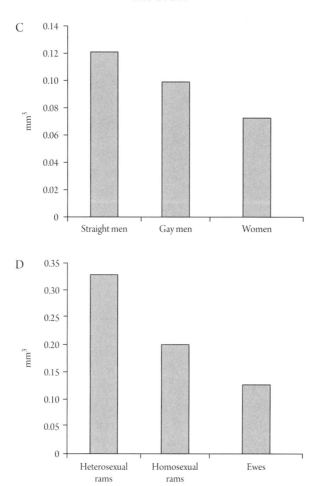

Figure 8.2 (Continued)

In the 1991 study already mentioned at the beginning of this book, I reported that INAH3 was significantly smaller, on average, in gay men than in straight men (Figure 8.2B).[7] In fact there was no significant difference between its size in the gay men and the six women in my sample, although one might have emerged with larger numbers of subjects.

Because my 1991 study was an autopsy study, various questions of interpretation arose, especially because all the gay men in the study, but only about half of the straight men, had died of complications of AIDS. A number of critics have raised the possibility that I was seeing an effect of that disease rather than something related to the men's sexual orientation. I don't think that was the case, for a variety of reasons: There was no difference in the size of INAH3 between the straight men who died of AIDS and those who died of other diseases; there was no obvious pathology in the specimens I studied; other, nearby nuclei (INAH1, INAH2, and INAH4) showed no size differences between the subject groups; and the INAH3 of one gay man who died of non-AIDS causes, which I obtained after publication of the 1991 study, was as small as those of the gay men in the study. Still, autopsy studies do have their limitations; later in the chapter, I will discuss results from brain imaging studies on living, healthy people.

There has been only one attempt to replicate my study, by psychiatrist and neuroscientist William Byne of the Mount Sinai School of Medicine, New York, and several colleagues.[8] Byne's group confirmed that INAH3 was sexually dimorphic and that it did not differ in size between persons who died of complications of AIDS and those who died of other causes. With regard to sexual orientation, they found INAH3 in gay men to be intermediate in size between the average sizes for (presumably) straight men and women (Figure 8.2C). The size difference between the gay and straight men did not quite reach statistical significance by the test that Byne employed, so he described it as a trend.[†]

Byne's group also measured neuronal packing density (the number of neurons per cubic millimeter) in INAH3, and found a "strong trend" for it to be higher in the gay men than in the straight men. Neuronal density is relatively high when the structures that usually occupy the spaces between neurons, such as synapses, are smaller or fewer, allowing the neurons to pack more closely together; Byne suggested that that might be the case in gay men relative to straight men.

Byne's findings were in no way a refutation of the findings of my study, but neither were they a clear-cut confirmation. Further studies are certainly needed. Other studies have strengthened the general conclusions of my own in indirect ways, however. First, very similar findings to those of my human study have been made in sheep (see below). Second, Dick Swaab's group at the Netherlands Institute for Brain Research reported that INAH3 was smaller in male-to-female transexuals than in non-transexual men.[9] Third, activity patterns in this region of the hypothalamus have been reported to differ between gay and straight men (see below).

One other structure in the hypothalamus has been reported to differ in size between gay and straight men. As I mention in the Introduction, Dutch researchers (Swaab's group) reported in 1990 that a cell group called the *suprachiasmatic nucleus* was larger in gay men than in straight men.[10] The suprachiasmatic nucleus is concerned with the regulation of circadian rhythms, not sex.

[†] Byne used a two-tailed *t*-test, which is the appropriate test when there is no advance prediction about the direction of a difference. Given that my study had already reported INAH3 to be smaller in gay men, a one-tailed test might have been appropriate, and it would have yielded a significant difference.

Swaab's report has not been followed up by other groups. If the finding is real, its significance is uncertain.

Other Brain Regions

Several brain regions outside of the hypothalamus have been reported to differ in structure between gay and straight people. Both of the fiber tracts interconnecting the two cerebral hemispheres that were mentioned above, the anterior commissure and the much larger corpus callosum, have been reported to be larger in gay men than straight men—a difference in the opposite direction from what I reported for INAH3.

The anterior commissure study—based on autopsy material—was carried out by Laura Allen and Roger Gorski of UCLA.[11] They had previously reported that the anterior commissure was larger, on average, in women than in men; thus, their report that the anterior commissure was larger in gay than in straight men seemed to provide another example of a brain structure that is shifted in the feminine direction in gay men. When Byne's group attempted to replicate this finding, however, they were unable to find any difference in the size of the anterior commissure, either between gay and straight men or between men and women.[12]

The study on the corpus callosum was carried out more recently, by Sandra Witelson and her colleagues at McMaster University, using magnetic resonance imaging (MRI) in living subjects. The corpus callosum is slightly larger in men than women, on average, but this difference disappears if one compares men and women of equal brain volume. In other words, the difference simply reflects that men's brains tend to be larger than women's.[13] Witelson's group reported that one section of the corpus callosum was significantly larger in gay men than straight men.[14]

A group led by Jorge Ponseti of the University of Kiel, Germany, used MRI to examine the distribution of gray matter and white matter throughout the brains of gay and straight men and women.[15] They found no differences between gay and straight men, but they did find several locations where lesbians had significantly less gray matter than did straight women. The most marked difference was in a region of the left cerebral hemisphere called the *perirhinal cortex*. This region, whose location is shown in Figure 8.1, typically has more gray matter in women than in men, so Ponseti's finding was another example of a sex-atypical structure in gay people—in lesbians, this time. The perirhinal cortex is involved in olfactory processing, spatial processing, and memory encoding; as discussed in Chapter 5, all of these functions differ between men and women in some respects.

Yet another anatomical study was carried out by Ivanka Savic and Per Lindström of the Karolinska Institute in Stockholm, Sweden, using both MRI and positron emission tomography (PET).[16] They studied 90 subjects, including both straight and gay men and women. In the MRI portion of the study, Savic and Lindström compared the volumes of the left and right cerebral hemispheres. In the straight men, the right hemisphere was 2% larger than the left—a modest but highly significant difference. In the straight women, the two hemispheres were the same size. In gay men, the two hemispheres were also the same size; in other words, gay men were sex-atypical in this regard. In the lesbians, the right hemisphere was just slightly larger than the left, perhaps indicating a small shift in the male direction.

The Swedish researchers used the PET scanner to visualize functional connections within the brains of their subjects.[†] The main findings of interest concerned the left and right amygdalas. There were marked differences between straight men and women: In straight men the right amygdala was more richly connected with other brain regions than was the left amygdala, while in straight women the left amygdala was more richly connected. What's more, the main functional connections formed by the amygdala were to different brain regions in the two sexes. In the gay men and women, these characteristics were almost entirely sex-atypical: The findings in gay men resembled those in straight women, and the findings in lesbians resembled those in straight men.

Brain Activity

In Chapter 6 I mentioned two studies that reported on differences in brain activity between individuals of different sexual orientation, both of them focused on the auditory system. Several more-recent studies have used a different methodology, functional magnetic resonance imaging (fMRI), to reveal activity patterns in the brains of gay and straight people while they were viewing potentially arousing images. These images have included photographs of male and female faces,[17] video clips of male–male and female–female couples engaged in sexual behavior,[18] and photographs of male and female genitals in a state of arousal.[19]

[†] PET scans produce an estimate of how neuronal activity varies over time in many small regions (called voxels) throughout the brain. In the Swedish study the scans were performed while the subjects were not engaged in any specific mental activity. To the extent that any two regions tend to be active simultaneously in this circumstance, there is likely to be a functional connection between them. The demonstration of a functional connection does not specify exactly how the two regions are connected anatomically.

In men, these fMRI studies have revealed that certain widely distributed brain systems are active during the viewing of erotic images, so long as those images are appropriate to the viewer's sexual orientation. That is, roughly the same brain regions are active when straight men view female images as when gay men view male images, and similarly for lesbian and straight women.[20] Some brain regions thought to be involved in the processing of negative emotions are active when subjects view images that don't correspond to their sexual orientations, for example, when straight men view videos of male–male sex. None of these findings are particularly surprising. Some differences have been reported, however, suggesting that gay and straight people of the same sex don't process erotic stimuli in precisely equivalent ways.[21]

Using methods discussed in Chapter 1, it has been found that women, unlike men, respond with equal genital and subjective arousal to erotic videos showing male–male and female–female couples, regardless of their own sexual orientations.[22] In the brain too, the response patterns of lesbians and straight women are much less orientation-specific than is the case with gay and straight men.[23] But in another study of arousal, in which images of male and female genitals in a state of arousal were used as the stimuli, female subjects responded more as one would expect: Lesbians were aroused by female genitals, and straight women by male genitals.[24] Ponseti's group extended these observations to patterns of brain activity and found that again, activity patterns differed between lesbian and straight women in a way that one would expect based on their sexual orientations.[25] It does therefore seem that, at least in women, there is something special about images of genitals that triggers "automatic" arousal patterns directly connected with individuals' sexual orientations, whereas other sexual images may elicit more-cognitive processing.

The amygdala is of particular interest in the context of sexuality. Neural activity in this brain region is strongly influenced by the emotional salience of a stimulus.§ For example, activity in the amygdala is greater when a person views an image of a face with a happy expression than it is for a face with a neutral expression. This is true even when the image is presented in a fashion that prevents any conscious perception of a face—as, for example, when the image is presented to one eye but is suppressed from consciousness by presentation of a different image to the other eye.[26] This binocular suppression technique is thought to work because two perceptual pathways converge on the amygdala, a conscious pathway that involves the cerebral cortex and an unconscious pathway that involves subcortical structures such as parts of the thalamus and a region called the striatum.[27] In the case where the emotionally laden face is not consciously perceived because of binocular suppression, the pertinent

---

§ The amygdala consists of several distinct regions, some of which are sexually dimorphic. However, functional brain scanning techniques cannot easily resolve these regions.

information reaches the brain by the unconscious, subcortical pathway. You may recall from Chapter 1 that it is possible to ascertain a person's sexual orientation using images of naked men and women that are prevented from reaching consciousness by binocular suppression. Thus it is very plausible that the amygdala is where these orientation-specific images are processed and that the output from this analysis is forwarded to brain regions concerned with physiological sexual arousal, such as the hypothalamus. This idea remains to be tested experimentally, however.

Chemosignals

I have already mentioned the relevance of pheromones to the sex life of the fruit fly, *Drosophila*. Those pheromones are present on the cuticle (hard outer surface) of the fly, and they are detected by other flies through the sense of taste. Mammals too engage in chemical communication. Rodents, for example, produce volatile substances, often derived from steroid sex hormones, that are released from the animals' urine or body secretions into the air. Other rodents of the same species detect these substances via the sense of smell (olfaction) using the *vomeronasal organ,* a small structure within the nose that is specialized for sensing chemical signals. You will often see these substances referred to as "mammalian pheromones," but they differ in significant ways from insect pheromones, and for that reason many researchers now prefer the term chemical signals, or *chemosignals.*[28]

The importance of chemosignals to sexual behavior in rodents has been demonstrated in many studies. For example, Catherine Dulac's group at Harvard University studied mutant mice that were unable to sense any urinary chemosignals.[29] Male mice with this mutation could not tell the difference between males and females; unlike wild-type male mice, which have a strong preference to interact sexually with females, these mutant mice courted and attempted to mount males and females equally. Female mice with the mutation showed the entire sequence of male-typical sexual behaviors, including solicitation, mounting, and pelvic thrusting, and like the mutant males they directed these behaviors indiscriminately toward males and females. Even simply removing the vomeronasal organ in otherwise normal females had the same effect as the mutation.

These findings suggest that chemosignals play an important role in directing the sexual behavior of male and female mice to animals of the opposite sex. They also indicate that the neural circuitry responsible for male-like sexual behavior is present in adult female mice but is normally suppressed by inputs from the vomeronasal organ.

Do chemosignals play a role in the sex lives of humans? There is some evidence against this idea. The olfactory system is much less well developed in

humans than in many other mammals. The vomeronasal organ in particular is
vestigial or absent; it does not contain sensory cells that connect with the brain,
and the genes that code for the vomeronasal receptor molecules in rodents are
nonfunctional, "fossil" genes in humans.[30] What's more, men and women who
have completely lacked the sense of smell since birth—the condition called isolated congenital anosmia—are just as likely to be married, are as satisfied with
their sex lives, and have as many or more children as people who can smell
(although anosmic males do have considerably fewer sexual relationships and
engage in sex less frequently than men with normal olfaction).[31]

On the other hand, there is some evidence that substances suspected of
being human chemosignals may be detected by the main olfactory sense organ
rather than by the vomeronasal organ.[32] And chemosignal enthusiasts point
to a variety of studies in which sniffing body secretions or substances purified
from secretions appears to have some psychological effect, such as improving
the person's mood or affecting his or her judgments of attractiveness.[33]

Human sex chemosignals are thought to be sex steroids that have been
chemically altered by bacteria on the skin. Some researchers hold that to be
considered a chemosignal, a substance must act through unconscious channels, while others refer even to consciously perceived odors as chemosignals
(or pheromones). It's very possible that a substance will have a perceptible odor
at a high concentration but also work as a chemosignal at concentrations too
low to be consciously sensed.

People's sex and sexual orientation affect both their sensitivity to chemosignals and their brain responses to those signals, according to work by Katrin
Lübke and her colleagues at the University of Düsseldorf.[34] Gay men, like
women, are more sensitive than straight men to androstenone, a substance
present in male armpit secretions. One component of the olfactory evoked
potentials—the responses to odors measured in EEGs—occurs faster in gay
men than in straight men when smelling armpit odor from gay men, faster in
straight men than in gay men when smelling armpit odor from straight women,
and faster in lesbians than in straight women when smelling armpit odor from
straight women.

Savic and her colleagues at the Karolinska Institute used PET technology to
visualize brain activity in straight and gay men and women who were exposed
to two compounds that the researchers referred to as "putative human pheromones."[35] One substance, called androstadienone (AND), is a steroid derivative
that is present in armpit secretions of both men and women, but at higher levels
in men.[36] The other, called estratetraenol (EST), is an estrogen-like compound
present in the urine of pregnant women. When sniffed, AND and EST have a
variety of effects on mood. Some of these effects differ between the sexes, but
that doesn't seem to be the case with regard to sexual arousal: Both AND and
EST are reported to enhance sexual arousal in both men and women.[37] Smelling

AND, however, causes straight women to increase their ratings of men's attractiveness, even in the presence of a masking odor that prevents them from being conscious of AND's presence.[38]

Savic's group found that some brain regions were activated by the "putative pheromones" in a similar fashion in all subjects, regardless of their sex or sexual orientation. These regions included cortical areas known to be involved in the processing of odors as well as the amygdala. A more interesting pattern, however, was seen in the hypothalamus—specifically, in a zone at the front of the hypothalamus that included the medial preoptic area (where INAH3 is located) as well as nuclei behind the medial preoptic area that are also thought to be involved in the regulation of sexual behaviors. (The PET technique lacks the resolution to image individual hypothalamic nuclei, unfortunately.) This zone was active in straight men when they smelled EST but not AND, while straight women showed the exact opposite pattern: The zone was active when they smelled AND but not EST. In gay men this area responded to AND but not EST, just as in straight women and in sharp contrast to straight men. In lesbians, as in straight men, this zone did not respond to AND. It did respond to EST, but not as strongly as it did in straight men. Thus the response pattern in lesbians was strikingly different from that in straight women but not precisely the same as that in straight men. The same group reported that hypothalamic responses in male-to-female transexual subjects resembled those of natal women and gay men.[39]

The concentration of the chemosignals in these studies was poorly controlled; it was probably much higher than people would experience in real life. A group at the Vrije Universiteit in Amsterdam re-examined hypothalamic responses to AND at a range of lower concentrations.[40] At one relatively high concentration straight women's responses were higher than straight men's (in accordance with Savic's results), but at another concentration it was the other way round.

Using the concentration at which women responded more strongly, the Dutch group went on to test prepubertal children and adolescents, some of whom were conventionally gendered and others of whom had been diagnosed with gender dysphoria.[41] In both prepubertal and adolescent conventional children the hypothalamic responses were the same as in adults; thus the development of these sex-differentiated responses does not depend on the hormonal changes of puberty. The gender-dysphoric adolescents responded according to their experienced gender, not their birth sex. This was not true for the younger gender-dysphoric subjects, however, so in terms of the hypothalamic responses it seems that gender-dysphoric children deviate from their same-sex peers in late childhood or early adolescence. Of course, it wasn't possible to know which of those prepubertal children would become transexual, gay, or straight adults.

Savic's group also studied chemosignal responses in women with moderate or severe congenital adrenal hyperplasia.[42] The women had masculinized digit ratios and a history of male-typical play behavior in childhood, consistent with other studies (see Chapter 6). No doubt Savic expected the PET scans to show male-typical patterns of activation by AND and EST, but in fact the CAH women's responses were the same as those of unaffected women. It was a small study, and only a few of the women were non-heterosexual. Still, the findings drop a fly into the ointment of neurohormonal theory.

Regarding all these chemosignal studies, it is not known whether the reported differences between gay and straight people arise during early development—and thus possibly help determine a person's sexual orientation—or whether they result from people's experience of sexual contacts with one sex or the other.

Stress Responses

The stress hormone cortisol is secreted by the adrenal glands, but the release of this hormone is under the control of cell groups in the hypothalamus. (The pituitary gland is an intermediary in this control pathway.) When subjected to standardized social stresses in a laboratory setting, men typically secrete more cortisol than women. In a study led by Robert-Paul Juster of the Fernand-Seguin Research Centre in Montreal, gay and bisexual men had weaker cortisol responses than straight men, and lesbian and bisexual women had stronger responses than straight women.[43] In other words, the cortisol responses of both non-heterosexual men and non-heterosexual women were shifted toward those typical of the other sex (see Figure 8.3). This was true even though all four groups reported the same subjective levels of stress.

The authors of the study interpret these differences between gay and straight individuals in terms of the different life experiences of gay and straight people. Still, it is difficult to understand how these experiences would affect lesbians and gay men in opposite ways, particularly when there were no group differences in the subjective levels of stress. It is perhaps more plausible to believe that that the brain circuitry responsible for the cortisol response develops in a sex-atypical fashion in gay and bisexual men and women. As with the chemosignal studies, however, it would take further studies to tease these possibilities apart.

Brain Lateralization

At first glance the cerebral cortex appears bilaterally symmetrical: The right hemisphere looks like a mirror image of the left. In fact, however, there are

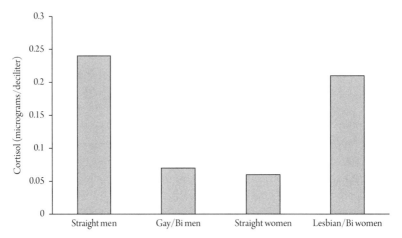

Figure 8.3 Stress responses and sexual orientation. This figure shows the average concentrations of free cortisol in the saliva of straight and gay/bisexual men and women 40 minutes after exposure to a standardized social stress. Based on data from Juster et al. (2015).

differences between the two sides of the brain in gross anatomy and neural connections. Even more striking are the asymmetries in function: A well-known example is the localization of basic language functions to the left hemisphere.

In general these anatomical and functional asymmetries are more marked in men than in women. There are also some reported differences between the brains of gay and straight people of the same sex. In these cases, the brain organization of gay people resembles or is shifted toward that of straight people of the opposite sex. We've already discussed one such difference above: In heterosexual men the right amygdala has more-widespread connections to other brain regions than the left amygdala, whereas in heterosexual women the left amygdala has more-widespread connections. In gay people it's the converse: The left amygdala has more-widespread connections in gay men, and the right amygdala has more-widespread connections in lesbians.[44] Here are some other examples:

- In men the right hemisphere is typically larger than the left, whereas in women the two hemispheres are about the same size. Conversely, in gay men the two hemispheres are about the same size, whereas in lesbians the right hemisphere is larger than the left.[45]
- Heterosexual men rely mainly on the right hemisphere for analyzing the emotions visible in images of female faces, whereas heterosexual women use the two hemispheres about equally. In addition, men who are less psychologically masculine are less right-biased than men who are more masculine.[46]

Gay men are also less right-biased than straight men, according to a study by Qazi Rahman and Sifat Yusuf.[47]

- Heterosexual men are more strongly left-biased for language than heterosexual women. Gay men resemble heterosexual women in this respect.[48]
- Left-handedness and mixed handedness are associated with less-marked cerebral lateralization for some functions.[49] As discussed in Chapter 5, both gay men and women are more likely to be left-handed or mixed-handed than straight men or women, which is consistent with less-marked cerebral lateralization in gay men and women.

Sheep

As discussed in Chapter 3, about 8% of male domestic sheep (rams) prefer to mate with other rams than with ewes. This is the only well-documented example of a nonhuman species in which substantial numbers of individuals could be said to have a durable homosexual orientation. Thus even though sheep are not ideal laboratory animals, several researchers have focused on them with a view to understanding the biological basis of male sexual orientation.

As with other mammals, the sheep's hypothalamus contains a cell group that is typically larger in males than in females; it is named *oSDN* (ovine sexually dimorphic nucleus). This sex difference is present before birth and is brought about by the influence of testosterone on the developing brain.[50]

According to studies by Anne Perkins of Carroll College in Montana, Charles Roselli of Oregon Health and Science University, and their colleagues, the brains of homosexual rams differ in several important respects from those of heterosexual rams:

- As I reported for its human equivalent, the oSDN is smaller in homosexual rams than it is in heterosexual rams (Figure 8.2D).[51]
- The levels of the enzyme aromatase in the oSDN are lower in homosexual rams than in heterosexual rams.[52]
- The levels of receptors for estrogen in the amygdala are lower in homosexual rams than in heterosexual rams.[53]

The sheep, like the rat, is a species in which conversion of testosterone to estrogen (by aromatase) and the binding of estrogen to its receptors are thought to be important for masculinization of the brain during fetal life, at least with regard to some traits.[54] The brain differences between heterosexual and homosexual rams therefore suggest that homosexual rams may have experienced

lower levels of testosterone, and of estrogen formed from it, during the prenatal sexual differentiation of the brain, and that their brains may therefore
have been masculinized to a lesser degree than is typically the case. There cannot have been a global absence of masculinization, however, because except for
their choice of partners, most of the sexual behaviors of the homosexual rams
are typically male.

Roselli's group examined the effect of treating pregnant ewes with an
aromatase-blocking drug.[55] The idea was that the drug would block conversion of testosterone to estrogen in the brains of male fetuses, possibly
leading to homosexual partner choice in adulthood. The results were quite
mild, however: The treated rams showed less mounting behavior but did
not choose male sex partners. The authors conjectured that the dosage of
the aromatase blocker might not have been sufficient to cause homosexual
behavior. Another possibility is that testosterone by itself plays an important role in the development of sexual orientation in sheep, even without
conversion to estrogen.

Be that as it may, the existence of an animal model for male sexual orientation that quite closely parallels what is seen in humans offers a variety of
possibilities for exploring the underlying mechanisms in ways that would be
difficult with human subjects. For example, it should be possible to compare
gene activity, neurotransmitter distribution, neural connections, and synaptic architecture in homosexual and heterosexual sheep and, based on the
findings, to form hypotheses about how the gross brain differences already reported translate into circuitry that mediates sexual behavior with male or female partners.

Inhibition and Sexual Orientation

Some observations suggest that male heterosexuality might involve not just
the existence of sexual attraction to the opposite sex but also the active suppression of sexual attraction to the same sex. Most of the evidence comes
from animal studies. Damage to the medial preoptic area in male rats or ferrets changes their preference from female sex partners to male partners, suggesting that SDN-POA might normally both activate attraction to females and
suppress attraction to males.[56] Conversely, as mentioned earlier, removing
the vomeronasal organ in female mice causes them to court both males and
females, as if the input from this organ usually suppresses courtship toward
females.[57]

There is some evidence in humans too—at least in men—that the brain
circuitry serving same-sex attraction is actively suppressed in heterosexual
individuals. Homosexual attraction and behavior can appear in previously

heterosexual men afflicted by Klüver-Bucy syndrome, which is caused by damage to structures in the temporal lobe including the amygdala, a major source of input to the medial preoptic area.[58] Homosexual attraction can also appear in heterosexual men who undergo surgical or chemical castration for prostate cancer[59] or who take female hormones as a prelude to sex reassignment surgery.[60] It is certainly only a minority of men in these categories who experience novel homosexual attraction, but the fact that this change occurs at all suggests that the brain circuitry serving attraction to males does exist in at least some heterosexual men, albeit in a functionally suppressed form.

The predominant neurotransmitter used by the neurons of the rat's SDN-POA appears to be gamma-aminobutyric acid (GABA), which generally has an inhibitory action on other neurons.[61] Thus it is conceivable that the neurons of SDN-POA (or INAH3 in humans) directly inhibit cell groups elsewhere in the hypothalamus that promote attraction to males; the resulting suppression of attraction to males may be lifted when the medial preoptic area is damaged or deprived of its neural or hormonal inputs. This idea is highly speculative and could be entirely wrong—I mention it simply to point out that there are possible biological mechanisms for setting up sexual attraction to one sex that depend primarily on *preventing* attraction to the other sex.

Overview

There is growing evidence for structural and functional differences between the brains of gay and straight people. These involve brain systems that could well be involved in the regulation of sexual attraction to one sex or the other, such as the hypothalamus and amygdala, as well as systems that are unlikely to have any close involvement with sexuality.

With regard to the former, the findings are supportive of the idea already put forward several times in this book, that prenatal sex hormones control the sexual differentiation of brain centers or networks involved in sexual behaviors, and that this process goes forward differently in individuals who become gay and in those who become straight. The brains of pre-gay male fetuses may undergo less masculinization, more feminization, or both than those of pre-straight male fetuses, and vice versa for pre-lesbian female fetuses.

The parallels with the results of animal experiments described in earlier chapters are a large part of the reason for leaning toward this conclusion. Still, some caution is in order. One possible interpretation of Byne's findings on INAH3 is that sexual orientation relates only to the packing density of neurons in the nucleus, not their total number.[62] If this is true, the key difference between gay and straight men with respect to INAH3 might not arise during the early developmental period when, if animal studies are relevant, testosterone promotes the survival of neurons in INAH3. Instead, it might develop during some poorly defined later period when the neurons are elaborating their synaptic connections.

I did not measure neuronal packing density in my own subjects, so I cannot strongly confirm or refute such an interpretation. Still, I am skeptical that changes in packing density alone could explain my results, because for that to be the case, the density would have to be very much increased in the subjects with small INAH3s—and that is something I would have noticed. In fact, several of my gay subjects had virtually *no* detectable INAH3, which is incompatible with possessing a full complement of neurons. Thus I tend to believe that in at least some of the gay subjects, the small size of INAH3 reflected a smaller number of neurons—either because fewer neurons were originally generated or because more neurons underwent programmed cell death.

The differences found between gay and straight people in brain regions that are not obviously concerned with sexuality, such as parts of the cerebral cortex, could be connected with the cognitive differences between these groups discussed in Chapters 4 and 5. Because the brain differences, like the cognitive differences, generally represent shifts toward the other sex, they could be taken as further evidence for sex-atypical brain development in gay people.

In Chapter 4 I mentioned studies by Simon Baron-Cohen and colleagues showing correlations between testosterone levels in fetal amniotic fluid and gendered characteristics in childhood. In a small group of boys they also looked for a correlation between fetal testosterone levels and brain anatomy when the boys were 8–11 years old.[63] They found such correlations in the cerebral cortex, where areas that are typically larger in males than females were larger in the boys who had high fetal testosterone levels than in those with lower fetal testosterone. This finding supports the general idea that fetal testosterone levels drive the sexual differentiation of the brain and contribute to anatomical variations within one sex. Baron-Cohen's group did not find such a correlation in the hypothalamus, however. This could be for a number of reasons: because small cell groups such as INAH3 cannot be visualized on MRI scans, because none of the boys had fetal testosterone levels low enough to affect INAH3 size, or because the mature hypothalamic anatomy is not established until puberty. It is also possible that the variability in hypothalamic anatomy among these boys was caused by variations in the sensitivity of the hypothalamus to fetal testosterone, rather than by variations in testosterone levels themselves.

9

The Body

Are there are any differences between the bodies of gay and straight people, and if so how do they come about? In Chapter 6 I already discussed evidence for one such difference—in finger length ratios. I now look at a broader range of studies. Some focus on easily measured anatomical features, such as height and weight, and others look at more-subtle characteristics, such as facial structure. For some reason, there are many inconsistencies among the studies in this field. Still, it is worth reviewing them, because they may shed additional light on what developmental mechanisms are at work in gay and straight people.

Body Size and Shape

Ray Blanchard of Toronto's Centre for Addiction and Mental Health and his colleague Anthony Bogaert, now at Brock University in Ontario, conducted several studies of the relationship between body size and sexual orientation. They reported that gay men are slightly shorter and lighter than straight men, on average, and in some of these studies lesbians were taller and heavier than straight women.[1]

The differences in height and weight between gay and straight men are already apparent at birth, according to a study conducted in Denmark, where detailed birth records are available for the entire population.[2] In that study gay men—identified by the fact that they entered a same-sex marriage—were significantly shorter and lighter at birth than the general male population. This finding indicates that some factor operating before birth causes (or contributes to) the relationship between men's body size and sexual orientation.

With regard to females, the Danish study did not find any overall relationship between birth length or weight, considered separately, and the likelihood that a woman would enter a same-sex marriage. However, babies who were both heavy and short (a combination that is predictive of being overweight or obese in adulthood) did have an increased likelihood of entering a same-sex marriage. This finding suggests a prenatal biological influence on female sexual orientation, though perhaps only for a subset of females.

Trunk and Limb Length

Men have longer limbs, longer trunks, and wider shoulders than women, but these sex differences are not all in proportion. In men, the limbs are longer in relationship to the dimensions of the trunk than they are in women: Leg length forms a higher fraction of total height, and arm length a higher fraction of total arm span, in males.

Both limb and trunk length are strongly influenced by sex hormone levels during development. This influence involves a direct action of testosterone and estrogen on the skeleton, as well as an indirect action whereby sex hormones influence the secretion of growth hormone from the pituitary gland. The extra growth of the male limb bones occurs primarily before puberty, whereas the extra growth of the male trunk occurs mainly after the onset of puberty.[3] In both males and females, estrogen is responsible for the closure of the growth zones in the limb bones at puberty and thus limits the final length of the limbs.

James Martin and Duc Huu Nguyen of the Western University of Health Sciences in Pomona, California, performed a detailed and fairly large study of gay and straight men and women, taking anatomical measurements of about 100 subjects in each group.[4] They found no differences in the dimensions of the trunk between the straight and gay men or between the straight and lesbian women. In other words, the sex dimorphism in trunk dimensions was just as marked for gay people as for straight people. Martin and Nguyen did, however, find very marked differences in limb length: The limbs of the gay men were significantly shorter, in proportion to their trunk dimensions, than those of the straight men, whereas the limbs of the lesbians were significantly longer than those of the straight women. In other words, both gay men and lesbians were shifted toward the opposite sex in these measures. The differences were more marked for the arms than the legs (Figure 9.1). There were also differences in the length and shape of the hands, again with the values for gay individuals shifted toward those typical for the opposite sex.

Martin and Nguyen interpret their findings to mean that gay men had less exposure to sex steroids during development than did straight men, and that lesbians had greater exposure than did straight women. This conclusion is supported by animal studies. For example, administration of testosterone to newborn female rats (which shifts their sexual partner preference toward

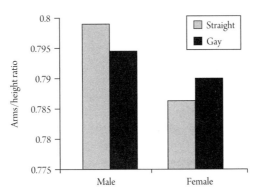

Figure 9.1 Body proportions and sexual orientation. Bars show the ratio of the length of the arms (left and right arms combined) to height. Men generally have a higher ratio than women, but both gay men and lesbians have ratios that are shifted about a third of the way toward the values for the opposite sex. Data from Martin and Nguyen (2004).

females) also increases the lengths of their limb bones compared with un-treated females.[5]

The differential limb growth between gay and straight individuals probably occurs during childhood, because that is when the basic male/female difference arises. The timing of the postulated differences in hormone exposure is less clear. They could take place during childhood, or they could occur during fetal life. In the latter case they would exert a kind of priming effect, probably by influencing the sensitivity of the bones to sex hormones.

Penis Size

Bogaert and Scott Hershberger analyzed unpublished data from the Kinsey studies, in which subjects were asked to measure their own penises at home and mail in the results.[6] According to this analysis, the average length of the straight men's erect penises (measured along the top surface) was 5.99 inches (15.21 cm), whereas the average length of the gay men's penises was 6.32 inches (16.05 cm), or one-third of an inch (0.84 cm) longer. Comparable differences were found in erect circumference and in flaccid length and circumference, al-ways favoring gay men.

Although all these differences were highly significant in statistical terms, there was plenty of room for systematic error. In a recent meta-analysis of studies in which men's penises were measured by health professionals, the average erect length was only 5.17 inches (13.12 cm).[7] This suggests that the average straight man in the Kinsey survey overstated the length of his penis by the best part of an inch. Perhaps the gay men were even more prone to exaggeration: Anyone who has read gay sex ads will acknowledge the legitimacy of this concern.* What's more, in a study that asked gay men to measure their partners' penises on two separate occasions, the reproducibility of the measurements from one test to the other was poor, illustrating the problem with entrusting the task to "amateurs."[8]

Although I'm doubtful about the findings of Bogaert and Hershberger's study, I'm obliged to mention it because it runs counter to expectations based on the simplest interpretation of the prenatal hormone theory: Low prenatal testosterone levels, one might think, would lead to small rather than large penises. Bogaert and Hershberger do subscribe to the hormonal theory, however, and they therefore suggested a couple of workarounds. One was that the usual prenatal peak in testosterone levels occurs earlier than usual in pre-gay fetuses, thus making levels higher during the early period most crucial for genital development but lower during the later period for brain development. The other suggestion was that testosterone levels are indeed low in pre-gay fetuses but that these low levels cause the developing penis to have increased sensitivity to the hormone, so that it grows more than usual when testosterone levels rise at birth or at puberty.

Bogaert and Hershberger's findings, if correct, suggest a biological difference between gay and straight men, most likely involving testosterone levels during development. However, the study needs to be replicated in a modern sample with objective measurement techniques before it can be given much credence.

Structure of the Face

Two studies have used quantitative morphometric techniques to compare facial structure in gay and straight people. One of these, by a group at Brock University that included Bogaert, looked at both sexes, while the other, by a group at Charles University in Prague, compared only gay and straight men.[9]

With regard to men, both studies identified several features that varied with sexual orientation. Both found that gay men have shorter noses than straight men, for example. Some features were sex-atypical in gay people: In the Canadian study, for example, the overall face shape and the position of the nose in lesbians were shifted toward masculine values. Some other features differed between gay and straight people but not in a sex-atypical fashion.

---

* In a recent issue of *Frontiers in LA*, a gay newsmagazine, the mean penis length of 20 advertisers was an implausible 8.37 inches (21.3 cm).

The differences in facial structure between gay and straight people were quite subtle and showed considerable variation among individuals. Bogaert's group titled their study "Facial Structure Predicts Sexual Orientation in Both Men and Women," but this was true only in a limited, statistical sense. Their methodology would do a poor job of picking out the gay individuals from a high school yearbook, a collection of police mug shots, or the obituary pages of the *New York Times*.

Hair Whorl Direction

Most people's scalp hair features a whorl-like arrangement visible on the top of the head. Viewed from above the head, the majority of hair whorls are clockwise, but a minority of people—about 1 in 10—have a counterclockwise whorl. In 2003 a National Cancer Institute geneticist, Amar Klar, claimed that gay men have a greatly elevated rate of counterclockwise whorls. Based on surreptitious observations of men on a gay beach, he reported that 30% of gay men have such a whorl—far higher than the rate among men he observed on a nongay beach. Klar tied this finding in to a hypothesis linking left-handedness, counterclockwise hair whorls, and male homosexuality to a single gene that supposedly controls all these traits.[10]

Given the enormous difference between Klar's data for gay and straight men—statistically speaking, it had less than a 1 in 10,000 likelihood of having arisen by chance—his study attracted considerable attention from the media and from psychologists. Yet two subsequent studies, carried out with much greater scientific rigor, failed to observe any significant difference in hair whorl directions between gay and straight men.[11] Several studies found no correlation between hair whorl direction and handedness either. Klar's data may have been distorted by subjective bias, that is, by the fact that he knew which groups his subjects belonged to when he was assessing the direction of their hair whorls. Statistical tests can't identify problems of this kind.

Gaydar

Gaydar is a colloquial term for the ability to spot people who are gay without the benefit of any explicit information about their sexual orientation. To the extent that gaydar works, there must be something about the discernible characteristics of gay men that distinguishes them from straight men, and something about lesbians that distinguishes them from straight women.

As many studies have reported, gaydar does work, but it is not infallible.[12] From a scientific point of view, though, the interest is not so much in identifying gay individuals as in learning more about the recognizable characteristics that make gaydar possible. Doing so could throw light on the factors that influence the development of sexual orientation. For present purposes, then, I am interested mainly in what gaydar can tell us about the person observed rather than what it can tell us about the observer, although the latter is an interesting issue in itself.[13]

In Chapter 4 I described a study by Gerulf Rieger and his colleagues at Northwestern University in which observers were shown short excerpts from home movies of gay and straight people made when they were children.[14] The observers, who were not told the subjects' sexual orientations, rated the pre-gay boys as much more feminine than the pre-straight boys, and they rated the pre-lesbian girls as more masculine than the pre-straight girls. Because the videos had not been made with research in mind, their content was poorly controlled. Nevertheless, it appears that the judges depended both on the type of activities that the children were engaged in and on ill-defined aspects of the children's demeanor (their "vibes," as one might say). Whatever the exact cues, the pre-gay children were unconsciously "outing" themselves by virtue of gender-atypical behavioral traits.

In the case of adults, a variety of cues, alone or in combination, can be used to assess a person's sexual orientation. This was shown in further studies by Rieger and colleagues.[15] The group video-recorded interviews with gay and straight men and women (20–25 in each of the four groups). From each interview, the researchers extracted a single 5- to 10-second clip, consisting of the first sentence the interviewee spoke in response to a question about his or her interests. The video was modified to emphasize the interviewee's body outline and de-emphasize facial appearance and other details. Raters (a mix of gay and straight men and women) were presented with the video without the sound, the sound without the video, a written transcript of the spoken sentence, a still photograph of the standing interviewee, or the video combined with the sound. For each of these except the written transcript, the raters discerned the interviewees' sexual orientations at levels far above chance; they did best with the combined video plus sound. This suggests that appearance (as seen in the still photo), body motion, and voice all carry independent information about a person's sexual orientation, and that this information can be picked up on with just a few seconds' observation. In fact, forcing raters to make their judgments almost instantaneously leads to more-accurate results than if they are allowed more time.[16] This suggests that gaydar involves automatic mental processes more than reasoned opinions, just as touch-typing gets worse if you start thinking about where the keys are.

There is even some evidence for discernible differences in body odor between gay and straight people—particularly between gay and straight men.[17] This would offer yet another sensory modality through which gaydar could operate About the only modality that hasn't been investigated is touch—which is somewhat ironic, given that the reputed "softness" of gay men has inspired plenty of slang terms for them across the ages, such as the Greek *malakos*, the Latin *mollis*, and its 18th-century English derivative, "molly."

Let's look in more detail at one of these sensory channels—voice quality. Listening to brief passages of neutral speech, most people can distinguish gay from straight men, and lesbians from straight women, with above-chance accuracy.[18] In fact, just a single spoken word (e.g., "food") is sufficient for above-chance discrimination. If the gay and straight speakers are selected because they are more gay- or straight-sounding than most, then just a single, meaningless syllable (e.g., "foo") will do the job, although that's only true for some syllables and not others.[19]

Several groups of researchers have dissected the voices of gay and straight people (most commonly gay and straight men), looking for differences. The fundamental frequency (or pitch) of the voice is no different between gay and straight people of the same sex. There are differences in some *formants*, however. Formants are the frequency bands in which the power of the sound is concentrated; they are modulated by active phenomena such as the position of the tongue.

Formants are primarily characteristic of vowels rather than consonants, and most recognizable gay/straight differences involve vowels. Vowel formants may consist of higher frequencies in gay men than in straight men. Gay men also tend to produce vowels of longer duration, and their vowels are more distinct from one another (they show greater "vowel space dispersion") than those of straight men.[20] These characteristics also differentiate women from men.

Still, some consonants do play a role. Gay men, like straight women, tend to use higher frequencies than straight men when they pronounce the fricative consonant *s*.[21] This also contributes to clearer speech, because using higher frequencies better distinguishes *s* from the lower-frequency fricative *f*. Curiously, this is the opposite of a lisp—a low-frequency misarticulation that centuries of stereotyping have attributed to gay men.

People make mistakes, of course, in judging sexual orientation by vocal characteristics. In general, they don't often guess that the voices of straight people belong to gay people, but they do fairly commonly guess the reverse. This suggests that gay people's voices range across a spectrum from easily recognizable as gay-sounding to not recognizable at all. In fact, one recent Italian–German study found that only a minority of gay people's voices are recognizable by gaydar; these few individuals are so reliably recognized, however, that they confer statistical significance on studies in which the majority of the gay subjects are wrongly judged to be straight.[22]

The voices of gay people—or at least of those gay people who are recognized as such—are shifted in several respects toward the voices of the other sex, but this shift is certainly not global.[23] Gay men's voices, for example, resemble those of straight men in some respects and those of straight women in other respects, and there are other differences between gay and straight male voices that don't represent gender shifts.

Another informative study of gaydar was carried out by psychologist Kerri Johnson (now at UCLA) and her colleagues.[24] This work focused on walking style (gait). The researchers found, first, that raters judged people's *sex* primarily from body shape. "Hourglass-shaped" figures—those with a low *waist/hip ratio*—were judged to female, whereas "tubular" figures—those with roughly similar shoulder, waist, and hip dimensions—were judged to be male. Raters judged the masculinity–femininity of walking figures primarily from the relative motion of the shoulders and hips: The more marked the figures' shoulder motion ("swagger"), the more masculine the figures were judged to be; the more marked their hip motion ("sway"), the more feminine they were judged to be. Computer-generated walking figures that had a male shape and moved with a swagger were judged to be straight men, while those that had a male shape but moved with a sway were judged to be gay men. Conversely, figures that had a female shape and moved with a sway were judged to be straight women, while those that had a female shape but moved with a swagger were judged to be lesbians.

When presented with video clips of real gay and straight men and women walking on a treadmill—clips that had been simplified so as to contain information about body shape and motion and little else—raters identified the figures' sexual orientation at levels well above chance, though certainly not with complete accuracy. Thus it appears that the average person walks with enough of a sex-typical or sex-atypical gait to offer a usable clue to his or her sexual orientation.

Rieger's study of videotaped subjects, mentioned earlier, also pointed to the conclusion that gendered traits are used to judge sexual orientation. In that study, raters were asked how masculine or feminine the persons in the videotapes seemed. There was a strong correlation between judgments of sexual orientation and judgments of masculinity–femininity, even though the judgments were made by separate groups of raters. The more feminine a male subject was judged to be, the more likely he was to be judged as gay, and the more masculine a woman was judged to be, the more likely she was to be judged as lesbian. In fact, the male subjects who were most consistently judged to be gay also judged *themselves* to be the most feminine, and similarly for female subjects and judgments about being masculine. Another study, led by psychologist Minna Lyons of Liverpool Hope University, found evidence that gender atypicality is an important cue when raters judge sexual orientation from photographed faces.[25] All in all, it's pretty clear that gaydar works, at least in large part, by the recognition of gender atypicality—whether in appearance or behavior—in gay people.

Not all studies of gaydar have yielded positive results. One negative study was published in 2015 by psychologist Janet Hyde of the University of Wisconsin–Madison, along with William Cox and two other colleagues.[26] They reported that their subjects were unable to distinguish between the faces of gay and straight men so long as the images were matched for photographic quality.[†] On this basis they concluded that the entire phenomenon of gaydar is a myth grounded in stereotypes. Hyde has built a career around skewering gender-based "myths," so this conclusion is hardly a surprise. It's possible that she and her colleagues are right, but it's also possible that they made what's called a type 2 statistical error—a failure to verify a real effect—particularly as their results did show a trend in the same direction as the studies supporting gaydar.

It's important to make a couple of cautionary points. The first is that seemingly fixed, innate attributes such as facial appearance are not always what they seem. While some researchers have taken pains to standardize photographic procedures, ensure neutral expressions, eliminate makeup and hairstyles, and so on, others (such as Lyons) have used photographs obtained from the Internet that vary widely in pose and expression and that do include the subjects' hair. The subjects in such photographs may communicate their sexual orientations by means other than the actual structure of their faces.

Another point concerns the base rates of homosexuality and heterosexuality in the population. Straight people may be as much as 50 times more common than gay people (see Chapter 1). Thus, as shown formally by Martin Plöderl of the Christian-Doppler Klinik in Salzburg, Austria,[27] if even a very small minority of straight people appear gay, the accuracy of gaydar as a real-life tool will be greatly diminished. When researchers find that gaydar is accurate— which they usually do—they have nearly always sidestepped the base-rate problem by including roughly equal numbers of gay and straight subjects. The base-rate problem limits the usefulness of gaydar in daily life, but it doesn't undermine gaydar's usefulness in a scientific sense—that is, the opportunity it offers to study what differences there may be, on average, between gay and straight people.

Although we can conclude that gaydar works to a considerable extent by the detection of sex-atypical traits, that leaves unresolved the question of how these traits develop. With regard to behavioral traits, conscious or unconscious imitation of the other sex or of other gay people could play an important role. Imitation of the other sex could occur during childhood or adulthood, while

---

[†] Photographic quality was determined by viewers' ratings, but these ratings might have been distorted by irrelevant variables such as the attractiveness or gender atypicality of the subjects.

imitation of other gay people would more likely happen after a person joins a gay community.

Linguists Ron Smyth and Henry Rogers of the University of Toronto, who are the authors of some of the studies just discussed, believe that gay male speech develops by imitation of female speech during childhood.[28] They believe this because first, speech in general is acquired by imitation, and second, "gay" vocal qualities involve phonetic characteristics that are not constrained by anatomy or physiology. (They don't, for example, involve differences in fundamental frequency, which is tied to the mass and dimensions of the vocal cords.)

Without denying the likelihood that imitation plays some role in gay people's adoption of sex-atypical behaviors, this may not be the whole story. Although, for example, both men and women are physiologically capable of adjusting the duration of their vowel sounds, which would allow social learning to influence this variable, the sex difference in vowel duration has been observed in native speakers of German, Swedish, and English.[29] This suggests that the gender difference in this trait may be driven by something that transcends the acquisition of a specific language.

Genes could play an important role in the development of unconscious behaviors such as those that are detected by gaydar. Even trivial behavioral characteristics, such as how children hold their hands, are remarkably similar between monozygotic twins and remarkably different between dizygotic twins. Is this because monozygotic twins imitate each other and dizygotic twins don't? No, because when twins are separated very early in life and brought together in adulthood, the monozygotic pairs show the same uncanny similarity in hand posture, while the dizygotic twins are as different from each other as ever.[30] If genes play such an important role in the development of such unconscious behaviors, it means that these behaviors emerge from specific developmental programs in the brain—programs that could easily differ between men and women and between gay and straight people.

Although I have focused on what gaydar tells us about the people observed rather than what it tells us about the observers, there is one point about the observers that is worth mentioning. We might intuitively suppose that gay people would have more accurate gaydar than straight people. After all, gay people have strong motivation and frequent opportunity to hone this skill. For straight people, on the other hand, the skill is largely irrelevant to their lives. Yet most studies have found little or no difference in the accuracy of gay and straight people's gaydar.[31] And people, gay or straight, demonstrate their good gaydar skills with exposure to just brief and highly reduced specimens of speech or movement.

If gaydar were based on the recognition of characteristics that are unique to gay people, this uniformly high performance level would defy explanation. But it isn't. Rather, gaydar appears to involve, by and large, the detection of ordinary gendered traits—traits that distinguish men and women and that are important to anyone's life as a social animal. What turns "gendar" into gaydar, for the most part, is simply the mismatch between some of these discernible gendered traits and a person's physical sex.

Overview

In this chapter I've reviewed studies that focus on the bodies of gay and straight people. These studies looked for differences in stature and body proportions, penis size, and hair whorl direction. I also surveyed studies on the basis of gaydar—what clues to their sexual orientation gay (and straight) people give off in appearance and in ordinary, unconscious behaviors. The results of many of these studies suggest that gay people are gender-atypical in subtle aspects of their anatomy and behavior.

Because of the lack of consistency among studies, some caution is obviously called for interpreting these reports. Even so, they do bolster the conclusions reached in earlier chapters, providing more indications that early development follows somewhat different pathways in gay and straight people, probably because of differences in levels of sex hormones or in the response of the brain or body to those hormones. The reported anatomical differences in height, limb/trunk proportions, facial structure, finger length ratios (described in Chapter 6), and size of the cerebral hemispheres (chapter 8), as well as the behavioral differences in voice quality and gait that are detected by gaydar, all tend to support this model.

I will postpone a more detailed review of these issues until the final chapter of this book. Before that, however, I need to describe a set of studies that point to a different factor that seems to influence sexual orientation, in men at least: birth order.

The Older-Brother Effect

According to Ray Blanchard of Toronto's Centre for Addiction and Mental Health and his colleagues, gay men have more older brothers, on average, than do straight men. This apparent influence of older brothers on the sexual orientation of later-born boys is biological rather than social in nature, the Toronto researchers believe. They hypothesize that the influence of one boy on another is not a direct one but rather is mediated by their mother—more specifically, by their mother's immune system.

The idea that being a later-born member of a family predisposes men to homosexuality was put forward by psychiatrists at London's Maudsley Hospital—Eliot Slater and (separately) Edward Hare* and Pat Moran—in the 1960s and 1970s.[1] But the real heavy lifting in this area has been done by Blanchard, Kenneth Zucker, Anthony Bogaert, and various colleagues. Since the early 1990s they have published at least 25 papers on the topic, many of them being replications of the basic finding in a wide variety of subject groups.

One way to represent a person's birth order position is by use of an index devised by Slater. The *Slater's Index* is the number of the person's older siblings divided by the person's total siblings. Thus a firstborn child has a Slater's Index of 0 and a last-born child has an index of 1. Because a Slater's Index cannot be calculated for only children, other methods of calculating birth order have been proposed, but those methods have problems of their own.[2]

My own Slater's Index, as the second of five children, is 1 divided by 4, or 0.25. The Toronto group has found in study after study that the average Slater's Index is slightly higher for samples of gay men than it is for straight men. Figure 10.1 shows the data for seven such studies.[3]

---

* Edward Hare was stepfather to my four brothers and myself. From oldest to youngest our sexual orientations are gay, gay, straight, straight, and straight—a sequence that's at odds with his theory.

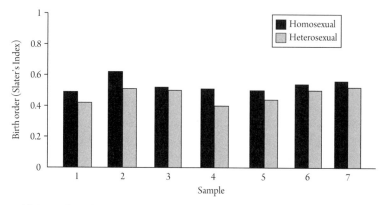

Figure 10.1 Birth order and sexual orientation. The bars show the average Slater's Indexes for gay and straight men in seven samples studied by Blanchard and colleagues. An index of 0 would represent a firstborn child; an index of 1 would represent a last-born child. Single children are excluded, because they cannot be represented by this index. In all samples, gay men are on average later-born than straight men.

If gay men have a higher (later-born) Slater's Index than straight men, this could be for any of four reasons: They could have more older brothers, more older sisters, fewer younger brothers, or fewer younger sisters. As shown in Figure 10.2, an analysis of Blanchard's data showed that all four of these possibilities were true. Gay men had significantly more older brothers and sisters and significantly fewer younger brothers and sisters than did straight men.

This doesn't mean that all four of these factors play a causal role in male homosexuality. If, for example, only older brothers play a causal role, gay men will of course have more older brothers than straight men, but they will also tend to have more older sisters. The reason is that it takes time to produce older brothers, and girls may also be born during that time. The older sisters will "come along for the ride," so to speak. Similarly, gay men will tend to have fewer younger brothers and sisters simply because being later-born means that there will be less time for their mothers to have other children.

The Toronto group used a statistical technique called logistic regression to sort out which of these four factors was playing a causal role and which were "coming along for the ride." The results indicated that only the number of older brothers influenced the men's sexual orientation. The differences in the numbers of older sisters, younger brothers, and younger sisters were all secondary consequences of the increased number of older brothers. Blanchard calls this influence the "fraternal birth order effect," but it is often simply called the *older-brother effect*.

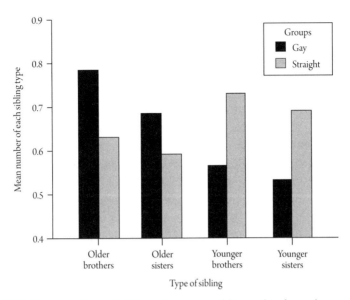

Figure 10.2 Mean numbers of older and younger siblings of each sex for homosexual and heterosexual men. These data represent the unweighted averages of 14 samples, taken from studies by Ray Blanchard's group, that collectively included about 3000 gay men and 7000 straight men. ("Unweighted" means that each sample was treated equally regardless of the number of men in each sample, which varied greatly.) Redrawn from Blanchard (2004).

How Well Established Is the Older-Brother Effect?

Blanchard, Bogaert, and their colleagues have reported observing the older-brother effect in 12 studies by my count, some of which dealt with more than one group of subjects. Four of the studies[4] were based on data collected long ago by Alfred Kinsey, psychoanalyst Irving Bieber, sexologist Alan Bell, and psychologist Marvin Siegelman. Six of the studies were based on groups of North American volunteers recruited by the investigators.[5] One was based on a multinational sample recruited through the Internet.[6] One study was based on two national random-sample surveys—potentially the most accurate kind of study—using British and American subjects.[7] In another national random-sample survey, which involved British subjects, Bogaert failed to observe an older-brother effect.[8] He attributed this failure to insufficiently precise information about the subjects' birth order and siblings.

In addition to gay men, the Toronto researchers have reported an older-brother effect for other, potentially related groups. These included gay male adolescents and feminine (probably pre-gay) boys,[9] androphilic ("homosexual") male-to-female transexuals,[10] and male sex offenders whose victims were adult, pubescent, or prepubescent males.[11] In each case these males had more older brothers than comparable gynephilic males (e.g., male sex offenders whose victims were female).

Two Italian studies, led by Andrea Camperio-Ciani of the University of Padua, obtained results similar to the Toronto group's: Gay men were later-born than straight men, and this was due entirely to an excess of older brothers.[12]

The results of studies by some other researchers, however, have not been in complete accord with the Toronto findings. In a Northwestern University study led by Gene Schwartz, which recruited about 1700 gay and straight male subjects, there was a significant older-brother effect. In addition to having an excess of older brothers, the gay men also had an excess of older and younger sisters.[13] According to a logistic regression analysis the number of younger sisters, and possibly of older sisters as well, had an influence that was independent of the number of older brothers. A British study led by Michael King obtained similar results to the Northwestern study, except that it was the older sisters rather than the younger sisters who influenced the men's sexual orientation independently of the older brothers.[14] Doug VanderLaan and Paul Vasey reported that Samoan fa'afafine (homosexual men—see Chapter 7) have excess older brothers compared with other male Samoans, but they have excess younger brothers and older sisters too, and the older sisters had an influence that was independent of the older-brother effect.[15]

Particularly surprising are the negative results from two very large, apparently well-designed studies. Danish researchers started with all two million Danes who were born in a three-decade time span.[16] They compared the family data of 3500 persons who entered into homosexual marriages with those of nearly half a million persons who entered into heterosexual marriages—gay and straight people respectively, one would assume. The men who entered into same-sex marriages were no more likely to have older brothers than the men who entered opposite-sex marriages.

The other study, by economist Andrew Francis of Emory University, used data from the National Longitudinal Study of Adolescent Health,[17] which has followed about 10,000 American teenagers through to their early 20s. Francis found that men with a single older brother were no more likely to be gay than men with no older brothers. Men with multiple older brothers were slightly more likely to be gay, but the effect didn't reach statistical significance.

Two research groups recently reported a complete failure to detect any older-brother effect among gay men. One study, led by Joseph Currin of Oklahoma State University, was based on a sample of 500 straight and 122 gay men recruited via the Internet.[18] The other, by Mariana Kishida and Qazi Rahman, was based on a sample of 1011 straight and 921 gay British men.[19]

Richard Green studied a large group of male-to-female transexuals.[20] He confirmed the Toronto group's finding that androphilic transexuals have more older brothers than gynephilic transexuals, but as we'll see later, he maintained that his data undercut the theoretical explanation that Blanchard has put forward to explain the older-brother effect. Older-brother effects have also been noted among male-to-female transsexuals in Turkey and Spain.[21]

All in all, the older-brother effect is less robustly established than one would like, especially with respect to studies conducted by researchers other than Blanchard, Bogaert, and their colleagues. Blanchard has spelled out what he considers the weaknesses of some of the negative studies.[22]

How Strong Is the Older-Brother Effect?

The Toronto researchers have put a great deal of effort into quantifying the older-brother effect. They have assessed the strength of the effect in two complementary ways. First, they have asked how much having an older brother increases the likelihood that a man will be gay. Second, they have calculated the percentage of all gay men who owe their sexual orientation to the older-brother effect—a measure that provides an estimate of the importance of the older-brother effect in relation to all the other potential factors that may predispose men to homosexuality.

According to Blanchard and Bogaert, the effect of older brothers on the sexual orientation of their younger brothers is linear: Compared with having no older brothers, each older brother increases the likelihood that a man will be gay by the same fixed percentage of the previous value (i.e., the value for one less brother); they have estimated this percentage as 33%.[23] The results of some large-scale studies, however, suggest that the effect may be nonlinear. One such study, by Schwartz and his colleagues, found that the first and second older brothers have only small effects but that the effect grows rapidly stronger with three or more older brothers.[24] Francis's study, which found no effect of one older brother but a marginally significant trend toward an effect with multiple older brothers, also raises the possibility of a nonlinear effect.[25]

Let's stay with Blanchard's linear model and the 33% estimate, however. This is a sizable influence of an older brother. It is much larger, for example, than the effect of older brothers on gendered traits in childhood, as discussed in Chapter 4.

Looked at another way, however, it's quite a modest effect. According to estimates from Blanchard's group, the rate of homosexuality among men with no older brothers is 2%.[26] Thus having one older brother will raise the likelihood of being gay to less than 3%, and having two brothers will raise it to less than 4%. It would take more than 10 older brothers to give a man a better-than-even chance of being gay by the older-brother effect, but families with 11 or more boys almost never crop up. It's still very possible that some men with just one or two older brothers are gay on account of the older-brother effect, but some other factor would have to be acting in concert with that effect: either another cause of homosexuality, or just a hefty dose of good luck.

Blanchard and Bogaert, along with James Cantor and Andrew Paterson, borrowed statistical techniques from medical epidemiology to estimate the percentage of all gay men who owe their sexual orientation to the older-brother effect.[27] The figure they came up with was 15%, or about one in seven gay men. In a later study, using different samples and methods, Blanchard and Bogaert increased this figure to 29%, meaning that between a quarter and a third of all gay men owe their sexual orientation to their older brothers.[28]

This claim seems to imply that every gay man has one, and only one, cause for his homosexuality. But there is no reason to accept that idea rather than the alternative idea: that fraternal birth order and other factors such as genes can add together or interact in a man's psychosexual development. Thus I interpret Blanchard and Bogaert's statement that 29% of gay men owe their homosexuality to their older brothers simply as a figure of speech intended to convey some idea of the magnitude of the older-brother effect in relation to all factors that influence men's sexual orientation.

There's another problematic aspect of these figures, which has to do with historical trends in family size. Since the early 19th century, the average number of children born to American women has dropped from seven (for White women) or eight (for Black women) to barely more than two today.[29] This drop is part of a global phenomenon known as the *demographic transition*. Thus most American men used to have older brothers, and many had several.[†] Today, on the other hand, few young men have even one. If, even in today's brother-poor society, the older-brother effect is responsible for producing 29% of the gay men in the United States, then the overall rate of male homosexuality should have been much higher two centuries ago than it is now. The same should be true for contemporary societies that have not yet undergone the demographic transition to small family size.

Bogaert has discussed this issue.[30] He believes that the rate of male homosexuality in the United States has indeed declined—he compares a 10% estimate made by UCLA psychiatrist Judd Marmor in 1980[31] with the 2–3% figure from a national random-sample survey carried out in the early 1990s.[32] Yet this supposed decline in little more than a decade is far too precipitous either to be credible in itself or to mesh with the slow decline in family size over the last two centuries. We don't know the rate of male homosexuality early in the 19th century, but it seems unlikely that it was far higher than it is today. Fred Whitam's studies, mentioned in Chapter 1, suggest that the rate of (urban)

[†] Many of these older brothers died early in life, but this fact is irrelevant to Blanchard's theory of the older-brother effect, as we'll see.

homosexuality is similar in the Philippines and Guatemala to what it is in the United States, even though average family size is smaller in the United States.[33]

Thus the older-brother effect, if it is as strong as Blanchard and his colleagues maintain, implies that the rate of homosexuality, and particularly the numbers of men who are gay on account of their older brothers, should have changed significantly across time or should differ between cultures. So far no such differences have been well documented.

The Older-Brother Effect and Handedness

In three studies, Blanchard's group reported a rather surprising finding: The older-brother effect, they said, applies only to right-handed gay men; gay men who are mixed- or left-handed do not have any excess of older brothers.[34] In a very large Internet-based study, Blanchard and Richard Lippa made a similar finding, although it took a fair amount of massaging of the data to see it.[35]

The reason this finding is surprising is that, as described in Chapter 5, gay men in general are slightly left-shifted in handedness compared with straight men. Thus both being non-right-handed and having older brothers are factors that, considered individually, increase the likelihood that a man will be gay. Putting these two factors together in the same man might be expected to increase the likelihood of his being gay even further. Instead, the two factors seem to cancel each other out: Non-right-handed men with older brothers are no more likely to be gay than are men who lack either of these predisposing factors. I'll consider why this might be at the end of the chapter.

Further complicating the issue is a study by Bogaert in which he reported that there are not one but two groups of gay men defined by handedness who don't show the older-brother effect.[36] One group consists of left- and mixed-handed men, as already discussed; the other consists of "extremely right-handed men"—that is, men who use their right hands for just about every task. It's only the men in the middle—the "moderately right-handed" gay men—who show the older-brother effect, according to Bogaert. This finding, if correct, would suggest that there are several developmental mechanisms that lead to male homosexuality.

What Causes the Older-Brother Effect?

One possible explanation of the older-brother effect is that having an older brother doesn't increase a man's chances of experiencing same-sex attraction at all, but merely increases the chances that he will admit to such attraction when asked in a survey or that he will express that attraction in same-sex behavior. Such behaviors might be accounted for by certain personality traits that are thought to distinguish later-born from firstborn sons, such as a greater rebelliousness, openness to experience, and liberality.[37] These personality differences may result from a tendency of parents to impose their expectations on first- or early-born sons but to allow later-born sons more freedom of self-expression.

Some findings support this interpretation. In particular, many (but not all) of the Toronto researchers' studies have been based on archival data that was gathered many years or decades ago, when homosexuality was less familiar and more stigmatized than it is today. In those days a firstborn son's conformist tendencies might have made him especially reluctant to admit to homosexual feelings. Many of the studies that failed to find an older-brother effect were carried out much more recently, and some of them were conducted in places (the United Kingdom and Denmark) whose populations are more accepting of homosexuality than the US population is. At those times and locations early-born sons may not have been subject to the same parental pressure toward heterosexual behavior and identity, so they may have answered sex surveys with the same honesty as later-born sons; thus the older-brother effect disappeared.

If this is the correct explanation for an apparent older-brother effect, one can make a testable prediction regarding the strength of the effect in different American states. The states vary greatly in how forthcoming gay people are about their sexuality, according to the analysis by Christian Rudder that I discussed in Chapter 1. In states where gay people are reluctant to admit that they are gay (such as Mississippi) an older-brother effect should be more apparent than in states where gay people are open about their sexuality (such as Hawaii). I'm not aware of any data bearing on this question, however.

Speaking against this and all other social explanations for the older-brother effect are the findings of a 2006 study by Bogaert.[38] He recruited about 950 gay and straight men (index subjects), many of whom had been brought up in nonstandard families—that is, who had adopted brothers or stepbrothers or were adopted themselves. It turned out that only older brothers who had the same biological mother as the index subjects increased the likelihood that the index subjects would be gay. Adoptive brothers, stepbrothers, and half-brothers who had only the father in common with the index subjects had no such effect. What's more, biological older brothers had an influence even if those brothers never lived with the index subjects (e.g., because the index subjects were adopted out of the birth family).

Given the crucial importance of this study to the interpretation of the older-brother effect, it needs to be replicated by other investigators. As it stands, however, it points strongly away from social explanations for the effect and toward biological ones operating before birth—specifically, to an influence exerted on male fetuses by mothers who previously had at least one male child. For the remainder of this chapter I will assume that this explanation is the correct one.

Blanchard, Bogaert, and their colleagues have proposed that it is the mother's immune system that "remembers" the earlier pregnancy and exerts an influence on subsequent male fetuses.[39] In their maternal-immunity model, women who are pregnant with males may be exposed to certain *antigens* (molecules capable of stimulating an immune response) that are possessed by male but not by female fetuses. The exposure might happen during the pregnancy or because of leakage of fetal cells into the mother's circulation at birth.

The mother may then develop *antibodies* against those male-specific antigens. If so, when her immune system encounters those antigens again—during a later pregnancy with another male fetus—the antibodies will bind to the antigens and block their function. If the usual action of those antigens is to guide brain development in a male-typical direction, the fetus might therefore end up developing in a less stereotypically masculine manner than other boys, which might include a tendency toward homosexuality. Each successive pregnancy with a male fetus will increase the likelihood and strength of such an immunological reaction, heightening the likelihood that the fetus will develop into a gay man.

Bogaert and his colleagues have looked for direct evidence that mothers of gay men carry antibodies against male-specific antigens.[40] They have reported that mothers of gay men who have older brothers carry higher levels of antibodies against an antigen known as NLGN4Y (or NLGN5) than do mothers of heterosexual men. Mothers of gay men who do not have older brothers carry intermediate levels of these antibodies.

NLGN4Y is a neuroligin—a molecule that is located on the receptive side of synaptic connections and that plays a role in the formation of synapses. It is coded for by a gene on the Y chromosome and thus is expressed only in males. (A gene on the X chromosome codes for a very similar neuroligin, but it is different enough that antibodies may exist that bind only to the Y-linked molecule.) Whether the inactivation of NLGN4Y (or any other male-specific antigen) predisposes a boy to grow up gay is not known. It is not a straightforward matter to answer this question, because laboratory animals such as mice do not possess this particular neuroligin.

Regardless of whether NLGN4Y is a key player in the development of male homosexuality or not, the maternal-immunity hypothesis neatly explains why (in most of the Toronto researchers' data, at least) only males exert the effect and why only males are sensitive to it. It also explains why the older-brother effect becomes stronger with increasing numbers of older brothers and why (according to Bogaert's study) older brothers exert an effect even if they've never lived with their younger brothers.

Another relevant finding has to do with birthweight. Several studies have reported that children with older brothers have lower birthweights than children with older sisters. According to Blanchard's group, it is only later-born boys, not girls, who show this effect.[41] What's more, they reported that gay men with older brothers had even lower birthweights than straight men with older brothers. Blanchard and colleagues interpret these findings in the following way. Usually, the anti-male antibodies generated during the first pregnancy have only weak effects: They reduce the birthweight of later-born boys somewhat but don't affect their sexuality. Occasionally the anti-male antibodies have stronger effects, in which case they reduce the weight of later-born boys more and also predispose them to homosexuality.

Somewhat undermining this interpretation are the findings of a more recent and far larger Danish study, which found that older brothers reduce the birthweight of later-born girls as well as boys, although not to the same extent.[42] The Danish researchers do believe in the anti-male antibody mechanism, however: They suppose that the effect on girls results from a kind of innocent-bystander effect that is technically called "determinant spreading."

The Danes made another intriguing observation: If a woman's two sons were fathered by different men, the second son did not show the expected reduction in birthweight. This, the researchers surmise, was because the second son's paternal antigens were different from the first son's and therefore were not recognized by the mother's antibodies. With a large enough sample, it might be possible to assess whether switching fathers also prevents homosexuality in a woman's later-born sons.

Another study of newborns, published in 1979, may be relevant to the older-brother effect. Eleanor Maccoby of Stanford University and colleagues reported that later-born boys have lower testosterone levels at birth than do firstborn sons.[43] The effect was particularly marked for sons born soon after their older siblings. This difference is in the expected direction to increase the likelihood of homosexuality in later-born boys. The researchers did not report that male older siblings had any greater influence on later-born boys' testosterone levels than female older siblings, however, which would have been a key finding supportive of the maternal-immunity hypothesis.

Green pointed out another potential problem with the maternal-immunity hypothesis.[44] As mentioned earlier, he confirmed the older-brother effect in his study of transexuals: Androphilic male-to-female transexuals had more older brothers than did gynephilic transexuals. But the androphilic transexuals with older brothers were not necessarily the last-born males in their families: What about those males who were born even later? Green identified 22 such men, and found that 21 of them were heterosexual and 1 was bisexual. None was homosexual. If the maternal-immunity theory was right, Green reasoned, at least some of these males should have become gay men or androphilic transsexuals, but they didn't.

Green's observation is actually not fatal to the maternal-immunity hypothesis, but it does constrain the hypothesis somewhat. We can think about it this way: We know that most boys with older brothers don't become gay. This could be either because most mothers don't generate anti-male antibodies or because most boys are unaffected by those antibodies. If the former case were true, Green's observation would be a real problem, because the few mothers who generate the antibodies should exercise the same influence on the sexual orientation of all her later-born sons, and they evidently don't. If, on the other hand, most mothers generate antibodies to male fetuses but most fetuses are unaffected by them, there would be no particular reason to expect large numbers of later-born sons to follow their gay brothers toward homosexuality. In that case, Green's observation would not be a showstopper. Thus if Green's observation is found to be generally true, it would suggest that some characteristic of the fetus itself is crucial to whether maternal anti-male antibodies will predispose it to homosexuality or not.

In summary, the maternal-immunity hypothesis offers a credible biological explanation for the older-brother effect. Nevertheless, it is not yet known whether a mother's immune system, once primed by exposure to a male fetus, actually has the capacity to propel a subsequent male fetus toward homosexuality.

Of course, there are plenty of gay men who don't have older brothers: men who are the oldest male sibling or who are only children. With regard to the only children at least, Blanchard and colleagues have suggested than a maternal immune effect is at work here too.[45] They find that gay males who were only children had even lower birthweights than gay men with older brothers (who themselves, as mentioned above, have relatively low birthweights). In addition, mothers whose first pregnancy gave rise to a gay male and who had no live-born children thereafter reported more spontaneous abortions (miscarriages or stillbirths) after their first pregnancy than did any other mothers, including mothers whose only children became straight men. These two findings suggest that a maternal immune response could be involved in the development of gay male only children. It's not clear whether such a mechanism would be the same as that proposed to be operating in gay men with older brothers or whether it would involve some entirely different immunological pathway.

As a general comment on the birth order studies by Blanchard, Bogaert, and their colleagues, it's worth pointing out that they have divided gay men into a remarkable number of subcategories: those who do or do not have older

brothers; those who are firstborn or later-born sons; those who are only children or have siblings; those who are non-right-handed, moderately right-
handed, or extremely right-handed; and various permutations of the above.
Only further research will determine which of these are meaningful divisions
that help us understand the development of sexual orientation.

11

Beyond Gay and Straight

The title of this book suggests a division of humanity into two natural kinds: those who are gay and those who are straight. But it's not that simple, of course. First, there are women and men who are, to a greater or lesser degree, attracted to both sexes, as well as those who are attracted to neither. Second, there is significant sexual diversity among gay and bisexual people, and perhaps among straight people as well—diversity that may be captured by slang terms such as "top/bottom/versatile," or "butch/femme." Finally, there are dimensions of sexual attraction that relate to attributes of a person's preferred partners other than their sex, such as their age.

In this chapter I briefly review these various forms of sexual diversity. My aim is not so much to give a complete accounting of this diversity as to consider what it may tell us about the issues discussed in earlier chapters of this book, especially regarding the "reason why" of sexual orientation.

Bisexuality in Men

If one assesses sexual orientation by asking people about their sexual attraction to males and females, then the distribution of sexual orientations is continuous across the seven-point Kinsey scale or the simplified five-point scale, and this is true both for men and for women. As shown in Figure 1.2, however, there is a striking difference between the sexes. Among men there are more exclusively gay individuals than there are individuals who say that they are equally attracted to both sexes, so the overall distribution is bimodal, with one large peak representing straight men, a much smaller peak representing gay men, and a trough between them representing men who are about equally attracted to both sexes. Among women, on the other hand, there are more individuals who say they are equally attracted to both sexes than there are individuals who say they are attracted only to women, and as a result there is only one peak, representing straight women, with the rest of the distribution simply tailing off in the non-heterosexual direction.

This sex difference, which has been confirmed in large international studies,[1] suggests that there might be something different about bisexuality in men and in women. The taxometric analysis described in Chapter 1 points to the same conclusion: Nearly all the bisexual men fell into the gay male taxon, whereas many of the bisexual women did not fall into the gay female taxon. For that reason I will discuss bisexuality separately for the two sexes, starting with men.

One possible explanation for the male pattern is that men who call themselves bisexual are not in fact sexually attracted to both men and women. The mantra "Gay, straight, or lying," sometimes heard in the gay male community, takes this possibility as fact, although there could be much more to the phenomenon than conscious falsehood.

It is in fact likely that some men who call themselves bisexual are really attracted to only one sex—usually to men. For one thing, calling oneself bisexual is often a transient phase on the path to an openly gay male identity. In a survey conducted in the mid-1990s by sociologist Janet Lever (now at California State University, Los Angeles), about 40% of gay-identified men said that they had called themselves bisexual earlier in their lives, usually between the ages of 16 and 25.[2] For these men it's reasonable to suspect that "bisexual" was simply an expression of uncertainty or a convenient way of avoiding the stigma of the label "gay." Quite a few young male celebrities, such as the British Olympic diver Tom Daley, came out as bisexual but later changed that self-identification to gay.[3]

Another piece of evidence that supports this idea comes from a more recent study by researchers at the online dating site OkCupid.[4] Among the 18-to 22-year-olds on the site who called themselves bisexual, only about 20% sent messages to both men and women; the great majority of the remainder sent all their messages to men. Again, one may guess that most such men were in fact gay and would eventually acknowledge the fact.

It's also possible that some men call themselves bisexual out of a general reluctance to be categorized or to place themselves at an extreme of any spectrum. One finding that could be interpreted in this fashion come from a very large Internet-based study that asked respondents about both their sexual orientation and their handedness.[5] There was a marked association in this study between identifying as bisexual and identifying as ambidextrous. The association could be real, but it could also be a form of response bias reflecting a general "don't pigeonhole me" mentality. This possibility deserves further study.

What happens when the physiological responses of "bisexual" men are tested in the laboratory? In a 2005 study, Gerulf Rieger, Meredith Chivers, and Michael Bailey measured men's genital arousal (i.e., degree of penile erection) while they were viewing erotic videos of males or females.[6] Heterosexual and homosexual men showed genital responses that accorded with their self-declared attractions. Men who identified as bisexual and who reported roughly equal attraction to both sexes, however, did not show equivalent responses to erotic images of men and women. Rather, they responded much more strongly to one sex—usually to men—than to the other. Yet curiously, these men did report roughly equal subjective arousal to the male and female videos during the testing. The researchers speculated that these "bisexual" men might actually only experience attraction and arousal to one sex but were reporting attraction and arousal to both for some nonsexual reason.

That 2005 study provoked considerable pushback from the LGBT community.[7] Perhaps in response to the criticism, Bailey's group carried out a second study, in which they recruited a group of men who met much more stringent criteria for bisexuality:[8] Besides identifying as bisexual, they had to have had at least two sexual relationships with men and two with women, as well as romantic relationships lasting at least three months each with both a man and a woman. Unlike in the previous study, the genital arousal patterns of these men were significantly less biased toward one sex than were the arousal patterns shown by gay or straight men (Figure 11.1). This study suggested that at least some men who call themselves bisexual can be identified as such on the basis of an objective test of sexual arousal.

Another approach was taken by psychologists Jerome Cerny and Erick Janssen.[9] They monitored genital arousal in men who identified as straight, bisexual, or gay while they viewed erotic videos that featured men and women in different combinations. The striking finding concerned videos featuring a man having sex with both a man and a woman: In this case the bisexual men, consistent with their stated identity, were significantly more aroused than were either the straight or gay men.

Further objective evidence for the existence of true male bisexuality comes from viewing-time experiments.[10] In these studies subjects browsed through a series of photographs of attractive near-nude males and females displayed on a computer while the computer unobtrusively recorded the length of time they spend viewing each photo. Straight men spent most of the time looking at female models, whereas gay men spent most of the time looking at male models. Bisexual men, on the other hand, spent more nearly equal time viewing photos of the two sexes.

In Chapter 1 I mentioned that pupil dilation can also be used to assess sexual orientation: People's pupils dilate when they view erotic images featuring persons of their preferred sex. According to studies by Rieger and colleagues, bisexual men differ from both gay and straight men in this kind of test, in that they show more-equal pupil dilation when viewing images of the two sexes.[11]

All in all, it's clear that men who are significantly attracted to and aroused by both men and women do exist, but it may take careful screening to distinguish

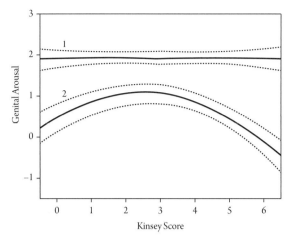

Figure 11.1 Sexual orientation and genital arousal. This figure shows the genital arousal patterns of 100 men of various sexual orientations, from exclusively straight (0 on the Kinsey scale) to exclusively gay (6 on the Kinsey scale), in response to erotic videos of either men or women. Curve 1 plots the men's average genital arousal to videos featuring whichever sex aroused them most; the flatness of this curve shows that straight, bisexual, and gay men all responded to their most arousing sex with about the same degree of arousal. Curve 2 plots the same men's average arousal to their less arousing sex. As one would expect, straight and gay men showed little or no arousal to this sex. Bisexual men, on the other hand, showed significant arousal to their less preferred sex and thus a smaller difference between their arousal to the two sexes. This response provided objective support for their bisexual identity. The dotted lines indicate 95% confidence intervals. From Rosenthal et al. (2011).

them from men who say they are bisexual but are not—at least not in any straightforward meaning of the term.

To complicate matters further, there are also men who are sexually attracted to and have sex with both men and women, but who do not identify as bisexual or do so only because others label them as such. "For society's sake, I'm bisexual . . . but in my brain, I'm just a person who likes people," commented one man in a study of behaviorally bisexual men.[12] "Dictionary-wise I'm bi," said another man, "because I had sex with men and women, but me I just look at what I like, and if I'm attracted to you and it works out then it works out." Such men—and women—may use terms like "pansexual" or "omnisexual" as a way of emphasizing the irrelevance to them of a potential partner's sex or gender identity.

I'm not aware of studies that have explored the sexual responses of such individuals in a laboratory setting. If they are truly unconcerned with their partners' sex one might expect them to be sexually aroused by persons who merge elements of both sexes, such as women with beards or men with breasts. These persons might not be arousing to those of us who use different criteria to judge the attractiveness of men and women.

How does the existence of male bisexuality mesh with the ideas about causation that have been discussed in earlier chapters? One possibility is that bisexual men have the same biological predisposition to either heterosexuality or homosexuality as "monosexual" (straight or gay) men, but also have another personality trait that broadens the scope of their sexual attraction. This "broadening factor" could be a relatively high sex drive, whose effect is to expose a sexual attraction that most men are unaware of or don't consider worth mentioning. Or it could be a nonsexual trait—such as sensation-seeking, novelty-seeking, or curiosity—whose effect in the sexual domain is to widen the horizons of a man's desire.

According to a study by Richard Lippa,[13] a high sex drive in men is not associated with an increased attraction to the non-preferred sex, so it does not appear to be a candidate for a broadening factor. There is some evidence that a nonsexual trait could play that role, however. In one study, men's sexual curiosity was assessed by their agreement or disagreement with statements such as "The idea of partner-swapping is exciting to me."[14] The men's genital arousal was also measured while they viewed erotic videos featuring men or women. Bisexual-identified men who scored high on sexual curiosity showed bisexual genital responses—that is, there was relatively little difference between their responses to men and women. Bisexual-identified men who scored *low* on sexual curiosity, on the other hand, responded genitally in a similar manner to gay men—that is, they were much more aroused by men than by women. Whether greater sexual curiosity was one aspect of a heightened general curiosity was not clear from the results, as the men's curiosity on nonsexual topics was not assessed.

What seems to emerge from these and related studies[15] is that at least two groups of men call themselves bisexual. One group consists of men who are bisexual by objective tests of sexual arousal; it seems likely that personality factors such as heightened sex drive, sexual curiosity, or sensation-seeking contribute to their bisexuality. The other group consists of men who by tests of genital arousal are homosexual; the reason why they say they are attracted to and aroused by both sexes remains unclear and may vary from person to person.

Ritch Savin-Williams and his former graduate student Zhana Vrangalova have studied "mostly straight" men, that is, heterosexual men with a minor but non-negligible interest in male partners.[16] Such men may correspond to group 1 in Kinsey's 0–7 scale of sexual orientation. These men are much less common than "mostly straight" women (4% versus 13% of the respective populations, according to a recent study from the US Centers for Disease Control[17]), but they outnumber men who are equally attracted to both sexes (1.9% in that study) or who are exclusively attracted to men (1.5%). Their numbers are also consistent from culture to culture. Their sexual orientation is fairly consistent over time; when they do change their stated sexual orientation, it is usually to an exclusively straight identity rather than to a bisexual or gay identity. In this sense a mostly straight identity is different from a transitional bisexual identity, which as mentioned above is a common steppingstone to coming out as gay. Older adult men are much less likely than younger men to describe themselves as mostly straight, either because they belong to a more conservative cohort or because their sex drive has weakened to the point that they are no longer aware of this minor component of their sexuality.

Besides *sexual* attraction—the desire to have sexual contact with someone—there is also *romantic* attraction, which is the desire for emotional intimacy. For most men these two kinds of attraction are aligned: They are sexually and romantically attracted to persons of one and the same sex, either women or men. Some men, however, may experience sexual attraction only to one sex and romantic attraction only to the other. This discordance, which has been described as a kind of bisexuality,[18] might account for why some men call themselves bisexual while showing genital arousal only to one sex. It's not clear to me why romantic attraction in the complete absence of sexual attraction should be considered sexual at all, or why it should be taken into account when assessing a person's sexual orientation. Sexual/romantic discordance is an interesting phenomenon that deserves further study, but it's not evidence of bisexuality—at least not in my use of the term.

Where do bisexual men stand with respect to the differences between straight and gay men that have been discussed in previous chapters? Unfortunately, many of those studies have omitted bisexual men, have included too few of them for meaningful analysis, or have lumped them together with gay men as "non-heterosexual." Also, few studies have probed deeper into the men's sexual orientation than simply asking what they call themselves or to whom they are attracted.

With those provisos, there is evidence that bisexual men score somewhere between straight and gay men in tests of some gendered traits. When tested on the male-favoring cognitive skill of mental rotation, for example, bisexual men scored significantly worse than straight men but significantly better than gay men[19] (Figure 5.1). Another example comes from Lippa's work on occupational preferences: The average preferences of bisexual men were more feminine than those of straight men but not as feminine as those of gay men[20] (Figure 5.4). Lippa found the same thing for the personality trait of agreeableness.

On some other measures, bisexual men have scored about the same as gay men. With regard to jealousy, for example, both bisexual and gay men are much less concerned with their partners' sexual infidelity than are straight men.[21]

And with regard to self-assessed masculinity–femininity, Lippa reported that bisexual men are about as feminine as gay men (actually, slightly *more* feminine).[22]

With traits that are gendered but in which gay men score the same as straight men, such as otoacoustic emissions,[23] bisexual men also score like straight men. What I haven't come across—though there may well be examples somewhere in the literature—is a gendered trait that differentiates straight and gay men for which bisexual men score like straight men.

In other words, when gay men are gender-shifted with respect to straight men, bisexual men are shifted in the same direction, but not always to the same extent. Of course this statement refers to averages: It's likely that some bisexual men (or some *kinds* of bisexual men) are gender-shifted to the same degree as gay men whereas others are not gender-shifted at all.

One final study on male bisexuality deserves mention. In a study of genital arousal conducted by researchers at the University of Georgia in the 1970s,[24] men defined as bisexual had to fulfill quite rigorous criteria: They had to call themselves bisexual, say that they were equally sexually aroused by men and women, and say that they had had roughly equal numbers of male and female sex partners. The study also included gay and straight men. The basic results were similar to those of Rieger's 2005 study: When viewing erotic videos, the bisexual men said they were about equally aroused by male and female images, but they showed genital arousal only to the male images; in fact, there was no difference between the genital responses of the bisexual men and the gay men.

In addition, however, the men were asked to estimate how erect their penises were during the videos. (They could not actually see their penises during the measurements.) Here the results differed markedly between the bisexual and gay men: The gay men stated (correctly) that their penises were erect during the male videos but not during the female videos, whereas the bisexual men stated (incorrectly) that their penises were erect during both the male and the female videos.

If the bisexual men's statements reflected their honest beliefs, it seems strange that they would believe their penises to be erect when they were not. One possibility is that they simply couldn't accept the reality of their "gay" genital arousal pattern, conflicting as it did with their stated bisexual orientation; this would be an example of the phenomenon that psychologists call cognitive dissonance. A more interesting possibility, however, is that their genital arousal was regulated by a neural mechanism to which they had no conscious access. Might then the key difference between gay men and "bisexual" men with gay genital arousal patterns be a lack of feedback, in the "bisexual" men, from the neural circuits mediating genital arousal to cortical circuits involved in the conscious evaluation of arousal? That is one of many ideas about male bisexuality that remain to be tested.

Bisexuality in Women

The findings concerning bisexuality in women are almost the reverse of those just described for men: According to some laboratory studies, *more* women are bisexual than identify as such.

Meredith Chivers has been an important contributor in this area—first as a graduate student in Bailey's lab and more recently in her own lab at Queen's University in Ontario.[25] I have already described Chivers's findings briefly in Chapter 8. According to Chivers's group, when sexual arousal is assessed by measuring vasocongestion in the walls of the vagina, both self-identified heterosexual and bisexual women are aroused about equally by erotic videos featuring men and by those featuring women. Lesbians, on the other hand, are more aroused by videos featuring women than by those featuring men. In other words, the genital responses of straight women are much broader than would be expected based on their stated sexual attraction. Their response levels are influenced more by the nature of the sexual behaviors that are being shown than by who is doing the behavior; in fact, they even show genital responses to videos of copulation by bonobos—videos that are not at all arousing to men.[26]

Some other studies support the idea that sexual arousal is nonspecific or "bisexual" in straight women. In viewing-time studies, for example, Lippa and Travis Patterson found that straight women, unlike straight men, spent about equal time looking at male and female swimsuit models[27]; the straight women also said that they were about equally attracted to the male and female models. Lesbians, however, spend more time viewing same-sex than opposite-sex models.[28]

The findings just mentioned could be taken as supporting Lisa Diamond's concept of fluidity in women's sexual orientation, at least with regard to straight and bisexual women (see Chapter 1). That concept has been the subject of considerable popular interest over the last few years. Yet according to more-recent studies, aspects of genital responsiveness in straight women are indeed gender-specific. Chivers's group, led by her students Jessica Spape and Amanda Timmers, had straight women and straight men view images of male and female genitals that were in an aroused state (i.e., erect penises and vasocongested vulvas) or in a non-aroused state (flaccid penises and female pubic triangles without vasocongestion).[29] When the subjects viewed non-aroused genitals the findings matched those of earlier studies: The women's own genitals responded to images of both male and female genitals about equally, whereas the men's genitals responded maximally to the female genitals. When viewing *aroused* genitals, however, straight women showed genital responses that were as sex-specific as those of straight men: They were evoked by male genitals far more than by female genitals. The women's subjective arousal showed the same pattern. Thus these very explicitly erotic visual stimuli seem to tap into a woman's sexual orientation more directly than do other visual stimuli.

Most studies of women's genital arousal, including the ones just mentioned, have assessed arousal by measuring vasocongestion in the walls of the vagina. A group led by Martin Lalumière has measured another aspect of genital arousal—lubrication at the vaginal opening.[30] Lubrication responses, according to this group, are not closely correlated with vaginal vasocongestion and are more congruent with a woman's stated sexual orientation. In particular, heterosexual women lubricate more to videos showing male–female sex than to any other sexual stimuli.[31]

The fact that some aspects of genital arousal in straight women are congruent with their sexual orientation means that their heterosexuality is not simply a matter of subjective interpretation or social labeling. Nevertheless, straight women differ from straight men in that some aspects of their genital responses—vasocongestion in particular—are not restricted to occasions in which they experience sexual attraction or psychological arousal. Thus it may be that the measurement of genital responses is not a very effective means to understand women's sexual orientation.

It could be relevant that women are more likely than men to engage in sexual intercourse when they unmotivated (or even averse) to doing so, and such circumstances may have been more common during human history and prehistory, when male sexual expression was less subject to social controls. Thus some researchers have suggested that women's genital arousal is, in part, a nonspecific protective response to signs that sex is in the offing—a mechanism, in other words, to reduce the likelihood of genital injury regardless of a woman's psychological arousal or the lack of it. Still, not all observations are consistent with this idea.[32]

Bisexual women score like lesbians or somewhere between lesbians and straight women on the various gendered traits that have been discussed in earlier chapters. So, for example, bisexual women have intermediate scores on tests of mental rotation and occupational preference, and similar scores to lesbians on tests of technological interests and systemizing.

Although Lippa found that a high sex drive does not broaden sexual attraction in men, he did find it to do so in women.[33] Thus a high sex drive may be at least part of the reason why some women are attracted to both sexes.

In spite of the studies just described, the nature and origins of bisexuality in men and women are still poorly understood. What is clear is that sexual orientation is a continuum across the Kinsey scale in both women and men, and that any theory of sexual orientation must take account of that fact. Still, the Kinsey distribution in men is much closer to dichotomous (i.e., either straight or gay) than it is in women. And even in women, taxometric analysis suggests that there are two underlying categories.

The existence of bisexuality is often taken—by nonscientists especially—as evidence against the idea that genes account for people's sexual orientation. Genes *aren't* the whole story, as I've made clear in Chapter 7. Still, the existence of bisexuality is irrelevant to whether genes are the whole story or not. There are not only black cats and white cats but also gray cats, and gray fur color is just as genetically determined as any other. Genes, in other words, can produce a spectrum of phenotypes, just as nongenetic factors can. The only thing that bisexuality proves about genes is that sexual orientation cannot be fully determined by a single either–or genetic switch—but that much is evident from the genetic studies themselves.

Asexuality

The Kinsey scale suggests that all people experience sexual attraction to the same degree, differing from each other only in how they apportion that attraction between the sexes. As was pointed out by pioneering sex researcher Magnus Hirschfeld, however, sexual orientation is really a two-dimensional construct: The strengths of same-sex and opposite-sex attraction can vary independently. Thus individuals can be attracted very strongly to both sexes, can be attracted strongly to one sex but weakly or not at all to the other, or can experience little or no sexual attraction to either sex.[34] Those men and women who never experience sexual attraction to anyone (or anything) are called *asexual*.

Asexuality has drawn increasing attention in recent years, in part on account of activism by asexual individuals and by the organization Asexuality Visibility and Education Network. Here's a brief summary of what's known about asexuality, based on the work of Lori Brotto of the University of British Columbia and others[35]:

- About 1% of the population—women more commonly than men—is asexual.
- Asexuality is not a "cover" for closeted gay people.
- Asexuality is lifelong.
- Some asexual people do experience romantic (but not sexual) attraction.
- About half of asexual people masturbate.
- Asexual men exhibit low genital arousal to sexual stimuli.
- Asexual people are not distressed by being asexual.
- There is little evidence that asexuality is a mental disorder, but there may be a link between asexuality and Asperger syndrome or autism spectrum disorders.

There is some evidence for biological markers associated with asexuality.[36] These include an increased rate of left-handedness or mixed-handedness in asexual women. There are also birth order effects: Asexual men are more likely to have older brothers than straight men, but (as has been reported for gay men) this is true only for those asexual men who are right-handed. Asexual women have fewer older brothers and older sisters than straight women. So far, there appear not to be differences in digit ratios between asexual and sexual people, but this negative finding could be a result of limited sample sizes.

These findings suggest that biological factors might underlie asexuality. If so, those same factors might help regulate the strength of sexual attraction experienced by the general population. The birth order findings hint at some commonality between the development of asexuality and homosexuality, in men at least. Much more work needs to be done to explore the basis of asexuality.

Age Preference and Pedophilia

Yet another dimension of sexual attraction has to do with the age of one's preferred sex partners. As with sexual orientation, there is a continuous spectrum ranging from pedophilia (primary attraction to prepubescent children) to gerontophilia (primary attraction to the elderly). Unlike with sexual orientation, however, most people cluster somewhere near the middle—that is, they find young adults most sexually attractive.

As with sexual orientation, women are more fluid in their age preferences than men. The average straight man finds women in their early 20s to be the most physically desirable, and this preference doesn't change over a man's life span. The average straight woman, on the other hand, is attracted to progressively older men as she herself ages—at least until she reaches the age of about 40.[37] Another striking sex difference between the sexes is that nearly all pedophiles are men.

There is some evidence that pedophilia is influenced by biological factors, just as homosexuality is. Much of this research has been conducted by James Cantor of Toronto's Centre for Addiction and Mental Health and his colleagues.[38] Pedophiles are much more likely to be left-handed and are shorter, on average, than non-pedophiles. They are more likely to report having suffered head injuries during childhood, and are about 10 IQ points less intelligent, on average. Three research groups have reported on differences in brain structure between pedophiles and non-pedophiles, but the three studies were not in agreement. Cantor's group found reductions in white matter in the temporal and parietal lobes. Two other groups found differences in gray matter in various structures, but the structures were not the same in those two studies.[39]

It should be borne in mind that most studies of pedophiles (including Cantor's) have involved individuals accused or convicted of molesting children. Many pedophiles have not molested children or have done so without being caught. In fact, a recent German study reported that only those pedophiles who have molested children differ in brain anatomy from non-pedophiles.[40] Thus the brain markers that have been linked to pedophilia might actually reflect personality traits that make it more likely that pedophiles will molest children, such as impulsiveness or low intelligence.

Butch–Femme and Top–Bottom

In the lesbian community, "butch" and "femme" are colloquial expressions referring to different kinds of women. Butch lesbians are thought of as relatively masculine in their gender identity and in the way they present themselves to the world (their gender role), whereas femme lesbians are thought of as more typically feminine. The butch/femme distinction doesn't necessarily define sexual behavior, but butch lesbians are often thought to take a leading or active role in sexual interactions, especially if their partners are femme.

During some historical periods the butch/femme distinction was the organizing principle of lesbian society, and all lesbian relationships were expected to consist of butch–femme pairs. At other times the distinction has been downplayed, ignored, or treated playfully. Not all contemporary lesbians identify as butch or femme, but many do: In one study of 207 lesbians surveyed at an LGBT street fair by Marc Breedlove's group, 43% identified as butch, 42% identified as femme, and 15% did not identify as either.[41]

The butch/femme distinction is widely assumed to be the province of queer theory rather than science, and only a few of the research studies discussed earlier in this book have tackled the issue. In Chapter 6 I did mention a couple of studies that found higher testosterone levels in butch than in femme lesbians, but testosterone levels in adults are too variable to say much about development. It has also been reported that butch lesbians have a higher waist/hip ratio (i.e., they are wider around the waist in comparison with the hips) than do femme lesbians.[42] Here again, though, the waist/hip ratio varies over the life span under the influence of various social factors and is therefore not likely to be a useful developmental marker.

One interesting study was done by Breedlove's group, however. In Chapter 6 I mentioned their finding that digit ratios in lesbians are shifted, on average, in a male-typical direction. They conducted a follow-up (the street-fair study just mentioned) in which they asked subjects not only about their sexual orientation but also, in the case of lesbians, about their identification as butch or femme. It turned out that the 2D:4D ratios of the butch-identified lesbians were shifted in a male-typical direction, but those of femme-identified lesbians did not differ significantly from those of straight women. Another study, published only in abstract form, made the same observation.[43] These reports could be taken to bolster the idea that butch lesbians are a biologically different entity from femme lesbians—specifically, that butch lesbians were exposed to unusually high androgen levels prenatally, whereas femme lesbians were not. More studies, however, are needed to verify the butch/femme difference in finger length ratios.

In gay male culture, "tops" and "bottoms" are somewhat analogous to butch and femme lesbians. The top/bottom distinction is concerned more directly with sexual behavior, however: Tops are defined by a preference to take the insertive role in anal intercourse, whereas bottoms prefer to take the receptive role. "Versatile" gay men don't have a preference, and some gay men have no desire to engage in any kind of anal intercourse. Among men who do engage in anal intercourse, about one-quarter are tops, one-quarter are bottoms, and one-half are versatile.[44]

The characteristics of tops and bottoms have been investigated by David Moskowitz of New York Medical College and others.[45] According to their studies, tops have larger penises, prefer the insertive role in other sexual behaviors (e.g., fellatio), and have more masculine and dominant personalities in general as compared with bottoms. They also recall having been more masculine during childhood. In another study, gay men who reported a history of childhood femininity scored better on tests of olfactory ability than gay men who reported a more conventionally gendered childhood.[46] This is another hint that there are objectively different subtypes of gay men. Yet another relevant observation, mentioned in Chapter 7, is that pairs of monozygotic male twins who are both gay also resemble each other in their masculinity or femininity, as if genes predispose not just to homosexuality but also to certain *kinds* of homosexuality.[47]

It is tempting to think of gay male bottoms (or very feminine gay men) and butch lesbians as the "biologically fated" gay people, and gay male tops (or more masculine gay men) and femme lesbians as having a more fluid orientation. Consistent with this idea, in Independent Samoa the very feminine *fa'afafine* are sexually attracted only to conventionally masculine men, but those masculine men who partner with *fa'afafine* are also sexually attracted to women.[48] The same was probably true for feminine homosexual men and their partners in Native American cultures.[49] However, a recent study found that lesbians were more aroused by female than male erotic images, no matter where they stood on a scale of masculinity–femininity.[50]

In contemporary Western culture there certainly are men who seem conventionally masculine and identify as tops yet are exclusively attracted to men. Still, it's difficult to know how many of these men are truly masculine by the kind of criteria discussed in this book, and how many are *acting* masculine for the purpose of erotic self-gratification, overcoming shame, or attracting partners. The scientific studies on different kinds of gay people are so few in number that it's not yet possible to have any well-grounded opinion on the topic, beyond the obvious fact that it needs further study.

Transgender/Transexuality

As laid out in earlier chapters, not only is homosexuality a gender-atypical trait in itself; it also is often accompanied by a variety of other gender-atypical traits that may not themselves be sexual in nature. So it's worth asking whether people who are commonly more gender-atypical than gays or lesbians, namely, those who are transgender or transexual, show some of the same traits and markers as gay people—perhaps even to an exaggerated degree.

There are not a large number of studies comparing trans and non-trans people from a biological perspective. Also, this area of research is complicated by the fact that there are two very different kinds of male-to-female transexuals.* One kind corresponds to the traditional idea of a "man trapped in a woman's body" who is very feminine in many respects. Transexuals of the other kind are not especially feminine but seek to transition because they are sexually aroused by the idea of themselves in a woman's body; such individuals have been called autogynephilic transexuals.[51]

Family and twin studies support the existence of genetic factors predisposing to male-to-female transexuality.[52] In monozygotic twin pairs in which one twin is transexual, the likelihood that the other twin will also be transexual is about 20–30% (but higher for biologically male than for biologically female pairs). One monozygotic twin pair has been reported in which the two boys were reared apart from birth, not knowing of each other's existence, yet both became male-to-female transexuals.[53] In dizygotic twin pairs in which one twin is transexual, on the other hand, the likelihood that the other twin will also be transexual is very low. These data are consistent with a substantial genetic influence on gender identity, roughly similar in magnitude to the genetic influence on sexual orientation (see Chapter 7).

There is evidence for the involvement of one specific gene—the gene that codes for the androgen receptor—in gender identity. Male-to-female transexuals tend to carry versions of this gene that are less efficient at signaling the presence of testosterone than are the versions found in conventionally gendered men, according to a UCLA research group.[54] (A Spanish research group

---

* I use the phrase "male-to-female transexual" for clarity and because it corresponds to the terminology used in the scientific literature. A more contemporary term is "transwoman."

failed to confirm this finding, perhaps because the two studies recruited different kinds of transexuals.[55]). A less efficient androgen receptor might cause the brains of male-to-female transexuals to end up less masculinized than those of non-transexual men. There is also some evidence for the involvement of one of the estrogen-receptor genes in male-to-female transexuality[56] and for the involvement of a gene that influences sex steroid levels in female-to-male transexuality.[57]

Regarding brain organization, the most interesting finding is that the size of INAH3 (the sexually dimorphic cell group in the hypothalamus) in male-to-female transexuals is about half what it is in straight men and not significantly different from its size in straight women. This finding, made by a Dutch group,[58] is the same as the one I made when comparing gay and straight men (see Chapter 8). It therefore suggests that gay men and male-to-female transexuals have a shared history of sex-atypical brain development, at least with respect to the hypothalamus. Differences between transexual and non-transexual subjects have also been reported in other brain regions.[59]

Regarding finger length ratios, there are reports that the 2D:4D ratios of transexuals are gender-atypical—that is, shifted from the ratios typical for their birth sex toward those typical for their experienced gender.[60] Some studies have failed to find differences of this kind, however.

The similarity between the biological findings in gay and transexual people reinforces the notion that homosexuality is a form of gender-atypical development likely mediated by genetic and neurohormonal mechanisms.

12

Conclusions

Sexual orientation is an aspect of gender that emerges from the prenatal sexual differentiation of the brain. Whether a person ends up gay, straight, or bisexual depends in large part on how this process of biological differentiation goes forward, the lead actors being genes, sex hormones, and the brain systems that they influence.

No single piece of evidence is the clincher or proof that the foregoing statements are correct. In fact, the concept of "proof" is not in most scientists' vocabulary. Rather, the previous paragraph represents a unified set of ideas (a theory) that has spurred numerous predictions (hypotheses), many of which have been confirmed by observation and experiment. It is far from a complete understanding of how sexual orientation develops, but it provides a solid basis for future research on the topic.

I should emphasize that this is not *my* theory of sexual orientation. It was proposed in rough outline by Magnus Hirschfeld a century ago, and it has been developed by many others over the intervening decades. Currently, in some form or another, it represents a near-consensus view among scientists who study sexual orientation.

The biological perspective on sexual orientation stands in marked contrast to traditional beliefs, which have remained largely silent on the origin of heterosexuality while ascribing homosexuality to family dynamics, learning, early sexual experiences, or free choice. As I discussed in Chapter 2, there is no actual evidence to support any of those ideas, although we cannot completely rule out that they play some role.

Differences of opinion on this score often result from differences in what we understand by the term "sexual orientation." Biological factors give us a sexual orientation in the sense of a disposition or capacity to experience sexual attraction to one sex or the other, or to both. Other factors influence what we do with those feelings.

Two theories that invoke environmental factors in the development of sexual orientation merit special consideration because they intersect with the biology in interesting ways. Günter Dörner's prenatal stress theory (Chapter 6) emerged from research in rats. Such stress has been reported to alter the timing of the prenatal testosterone surge in male rat fetuses, leading to "demasculinization" of the brain and to atypical sexual behavior in adulthood. These animal studies offer a rational background for investigating the effect of prenatal stress in humans. Yet carefully controlled studies have not been able to document any analogous effect in men. Apparently, human mothers and human fetuses are resistant to this kind of stress effect.

The other interesting idea is Daryl Bem's proposal that genes predispose to childhood gender nonconformity and that interactions with peers propel the gender-nonconformist child toward homosexuality in adulthood (Chapter 4). There is no evidence, however, that modifying peer interactions affects the likelihood that a gender-nonconformist child will grow up gay. Again, then, Bem's "exotic becomes erotic" theory lacks empirical support.

Sexual Orientation Is Linked to Other Gendered Traits

If there is one idea that does have empirical support, it is that homosexuality is part of a package of gender-atypical traits. Some characteristics of the bodies and minds of gay men are shifted in a female direction as compared with straight men, and some characteristics of the bodies and minds of lesbians and bisexual women are shifted in a male direction as compared with straight women.

It's important to stress that these shifts are, for the most part, only shifts and not complete gender reversals, and they don't affect *every* gendered trait. Gay men don't have women's bodies, otherwise they would *be* women. Nor do they have women's minds; otherwise they would be transwomen. Similarly, lesbians don't have the bodies or minds of men. What is impressive is not so much the size of these gender shifts but their number and variety. Here is a quick synopsis of some of the reported findings that I have described earlier in this book:

- *The body.* The ratio of limb length to trunk length—a sexually differentiated trait—is shifted in a sex-atypical direction in both gay men and lesbians. Finger length ratios are gender-shifted in lesbian and bisexual women, and possibly in gay men too. Facial structure is partially gender-shifted in both gay men and lesbians. Both gay men and lesbians are gender-shifted in aspects of body function, including gait and voice quality, that are recognized by "gaydar."
- *The brain.* Gay men are gender-shifted in the size of INAH3, the sexually dimorphic cell group in a region of the hypothalamus concerned with male-typical sexual behavior. They are also gender-shifted in the relative sizes

of the left and right cerebral hemispheres. Both gay men and lesbians are gender-shifted in their brain responses to compounds thought to be sex-specific chemosignals, as well as in the functional connectivity of their amygdalas. Lesbians and bisexual women are gender-shifted in their auditory physiology. Both lesbians and gay men are gender-shifted in their hormonal responses to stress.

• *Childhood characteristics*. Pre-gay children are gender-nonconformist in a variety of traits, including physical aggressiveness, engagement in rough-and-tumble play and sports, preference for the company of same- or opposite-sex peers, interests, and unconscious behaviors that allow raters to judge them as gender-nonconformist from home videos.

• *Cognitive traits*. Gay men and lesbians are gender-shifted in a variety of male-favoring visuospatial traits, such as mental rotation, targeting, and navigation, as well as female-favoring tasks such as verbal fluency. Gay men are gender-shifted in the female-favoring trait of object-location memory.

• *Personality*. Gay men consider themselves less masculine and lesbians consider themselves less feminine than do straight men and women, respectively. Both gay men and lesbians have gender-shifted occupational preferences. Gender shifts have also been reported in physical aggressiveness, instrumentality, empathy, expressiveness, and aesthetic and technological interests.

Gay people remain gender-*typical* in a variety of traits, especially those related to sexuality, such as gay men's high interest and lesbians' low interest in casual sex.

A very few shifts have been reported among gay men that seem to be in the opposite, "hypermasculine" direction. These traits are penis size (gay men's penises were reported in a single study to be larger than straight men's), auditory evoked potentials (some aspects of gay men's evoked potentials have been reported to be shifted in a direction away from the female-typical pattern), and handedness (gay men have been reported to show more left-handedness than straight men).

There is reason for concern about the validity or interpretation of all three of these findings, however. As discussed in Chapter 9, men overstate the size of their penises, and gay men may well do so more than straight men. Regarding auditory evoked potentials, as discussed in Chapter 6, Dennis McFadden's group recently failed to verify the basic sex difference in these potentials that they had previously reported. Similarly, as discussed in Chapter 4, Richard Lippa has reported that there is no basic difference in handedness between heterosexual men and women. Thus auditory potentials and handedness may not be shifted in a hypermasculine direction. All in all, the evidence for hypermasculine traits in gay men is weak.

A Common Origin for Gender-Shifted Traits?

To understand why gay people are gender-shifted in so many and such diverse traits besides their sexual orientations, it makes sense to look to the processes that are responsible for differences between men and women in general. Chief among these is the hormonally mediated sexual differentiation of the body and brain.

In humans, testosterone is the major hormone responsible for sexual differentiation during early development. Before focusing on this hormone, it's worth recalling that other factors play contributory roles, as discussed in Chapter 3. Anti-müllerian hormone (AMH), secreted by the testes, prevents development of the female reproductive tract in males, and (in rodents at least) it contributes to the sexual differentiation of the hypothalamus. It is also responsible for at least one sex difference in behavior—the greater degree of exploratory behavior shown by male rodents. Another factor is the internal chromosomal sex (XX or XY) of brain cells, which contributes to the sex difference in aggressive behavior (in mice, again). It is quite possible that future research will uncover more ways in which these and other "minor" factors influence the sexual differentiation of the brain, perhaps including brain systems responsible for sexual feelings and behaviors.

The central role of testosterone, however, has been amply demonstrated in nonhuman animals by experiments in which this hormone has been administered or had its action blocked in fetal or newborn animals. When present at high levels (during early and mid-pregnancy in humans), it drives development in a male direction; when present at low levels during that same time span, it permits development to proceed in a female direction. Although testosterone can be converted into estrogen within the human brain by the enzyme aromatase, suggesting some role for estrogen in male brain development that remains to be identified, observations on males who are insensitive to estrogen or who lack aromatase have not pinpointed any effects on psychosexual development or gender identity.

To judge from the animal experiments described in Chapter 3, testosterone exerts organizing effects on brain systems that contribute to a wide variety of gendered traits, including sexual behaviors and sexual partner preference. The same seems to be true in humans, according to observations on persons with congenital adrenal hyperplasia and other conditions that affect fetal androgen levels or sensitivity to androgens (Chapter 6).

Thus the most parsimonious biological explanation for the development of sexual orientation is this: If testosterone levels during a critical prenatal period are high, the brain is organized in such a way that the person is predisposed to become typically masculine in a variety of gendered traits, including sexual attraction to females. If testosterone levels are low during that same period, the brain is organized in such a way that the person is predisposed to become typically feminine in gendered traits, including sexual attraction to males. Bisexuality might result from intermediate levels of testosterone, although there is little direct evidence bearing on this.

A closely related alternative hypothesis is that there is no difference between pre-gay and pre-straight fetuses in the actual circulating levels of testosterone, but that their brains respond to testosterone in different ways because of differences in hormone receptors or other molecules that are involved in translating the hormonal signal into neuronal architecture. In this case the same level of testosterone might drive brain development strongly in a male direction in a pre-straight male fetus but less so in a pre-gay male fetus, and similarly for female fetuses.

We don't have definitive information that would allow us to choose between these two models. Because they are so closely related I lump them together into a "prenatal hormonal" model for the development of sexual orientation. However, some of the gendered traits associated with sexual orientation (such as limb/trunk ratios and finger length ratios) involve the body rather than the brain. Thus if we wish to identify a single "decision point" in the development of sexual orientation, we should look to elements that are common to the development of the body and the brain, not to a specifically brain-related element. Actual testosterone levels or receptor mechanisms that respond to testosterone seem better candidates in that regard than brain-specific growth factors, neurotransmitter mechanisms, or the like.

Probably most sex researchers believe at this point that a prenatal hormonal mechanism of this kind is operative in the development of sexual orientation. Otherwise it is too difficult to explain the association of sexual orientation with all the other gendered traits that I've listed. However, there remains considerable uncertainty about the strength of the effect—in other words, about whether these prenatal hormonal factors decide if a person will experience sexual attraction to males or females or whether they rather provide a predisposition that other factors, such as parenting and life experiences, can modify. Because the evidence for these other factors seems so weak, I am inclined to place most of the developmental control in the hands of prenatal hormones. But I do acknowledge that certain observations— such as the fact that CAH women are shifted only partially in the direction of homosexuality—could be interpreted to mean that other factors play important roles.

As mentioned in Chapter 3, there is increasing evidence that the brain undergoes organizational changes not only before birth but also at puberty. What the latter changes might mean for the development of sexual orientation is not clear. Given that pre-gay and pre-straight children differ from each other well before puberty, it is not likely that sexual orientation is determined by events occurring at puberty. Still, it may be that puberty has some role to play beyond the simple "turning on" of a predetermined sexuality.

The Role of Genes

The prenatal hormonal theory is not an ultimate explanation of how people become straight or gay, because it leaves unexplained how hormone levels might come to differ between fetuses of the same sex. There are many ways in which this could happen, but one likely possibility is that genes help set these levels.

The family and twin studies discussed in Chapter 7 provide evidence that genetic differences between individuals account for a substantial fraction of the differences in sexual orientation that are observed in the population. Estimates of the heritability of homosexuality have been quite variable but range around 30–50% for both sexes, which is similar to heritability estimates for many other psychological traits.[1] (Some studies suggest a lower heritability in women.)

Twin studies, especially the Finnish study discussed in Chapter 7, suggest that a common set of genes predisposes both to gender-nonconformist characteristics in childhood and to homosexuality in adulthood.[2] If so, it is likely that these genes work through the hormonal pathway, because childhood gendered characteristics seem to be strongly influenced by prenatal hormones (Chapters 4 and 6).

Working on this assumption, Dean Hamer and others looked for differences in the genes that code for two key hormone-related molecules, the androgen receptor and aromatase, but drew a blank (see Chapter 7). However, a very large number of genes are involved one way or another in the pathway by which sex hormones influence their target tissues. These include genes for enzymes involved in the synthesis and metabolism of the hormones; genes for several kinds of receptors, coactivators, and corepressors; and the many genes whose activity is regulated by sex hormones. The evidence for the involvement of the neurotransmitter GABA in the sexual differentiation of the hypothalamus[3] introduces another collection of genes—those involved in GABA transmission—as possible contributors to the heritability of sexual orientation. Thus there is every reason to test for the involvement of other candidate genes.

In general, few major genes have been identified in the field of behavioral genetics; most heritable psychological traits seem to be influenced by multiple genes, each of modest effect. This could well be true for sexual orientation too. If so, different individuals might carry different complements of "gay genes" and thus exhibit different kinds of homosexuality. For example, one gay person might carry genes that influence limb/trunk ratio in addition to sexual orientation, another person might have psychological gender-shifted traits but not bodily ones, and yet another person might be gay but lack other gender-shifted traits altogether. And single genes might be decisive in some families (as suggested by the family tree in Figure 7.1) but play no role in others.

The biological factors that predispose to homosexuality in men and women do not have to be the same. Marc Breedlove has argued that genes are the key players in men whereas prenatal sex hormones have that role in women.[4] Some of the evidence indeed supports a difference of that kind. For example, most studies point to a stronger genetic influence on sexual orientation in men than in women. Conversely, finger length ratios—a likely indicator of prenatal testosterone levels—are clearly sex-atypical in lesbians but only slightly so, or possibly not at all, in gay men.

Still, the difference is probably not as clear-cut as Breedlove suggests. Genes do influence sexual orientation in women, even if not as strongly as in men. And prenatal hormone levels may themselves be controlled by genes. That is obviously true in congenital adrenal hyperplasia, for example: The high prenatal androgen levels in CAH-affected fetuses result from a genetic mutation.

Does the Older-Brother Effect Work Through Prenatal Hormones?

In Chapter 10 I discussed the work of Ray Blanchard, Anthony Bogaert, and their colleagues indicating that having older brothers increases the chances that a man will be gay. Those authors have presented evidence that this older-brother effect is biological rather than social. They propose that a woman may generate an immune response to male-specific antigens during her first pregnancy with a male fetus and that this response has an effect on the development of later male fetuses.

One question this proposal raises is whether this immunological process works by lowering testosterone levels in the later male fetuses. Blanchard and his colleagues suggest that it does.[5] I would be happy to believe that, except for the observation by Qazi Rahman that older brothers have no effect on childhood gender characteristics or mental rotation.[6] The topic merits further research, but at this point it seems that the older-brother effect does not involve the broad gender shift that would be expected if was mediated by lowered fetal testosterone levels. It may therefore work through some other mechanism, involving a more specific effect on the brain circuitry responsible for sexual orientation. Blanchard and colleagues' recent findings on the possible involvement of a brain-specific neuroligin (Chapter 10) also point in that direction.

Is There a Random Biological Influence?

In Chapter 3 I mentioned the idea that random biological processes can influence psychosexual development. The example I cited was the uterine proximity effect in rodents: Female fetuses that by chance are located next to males pick up testosterone from those males and are partially masculinized in their sexual behavior. Actually, many developmental processes are probabilistic or stochastic, meaning that the results are not rigidly determined but are subject to random variability or "noise."

Perhaps the strongest clue that probabilistic processes influence sexual orientation comes from monozygotic twins. If one such twin is gay, there are roughly even odds that the co-twin will be gay or straight. How can this be the case if the twins possess the same genome, developed in the same uterus at the same time, and experienced very similar rearing conditions? If early sexual experiences determine sexual orientation, those experiences might differ between twins of different sexual orientation: One twin might have been sexually molested and the other not, for example. However, the evidence speaks against an influence of molestation or sexual experiences in general on sexual orientation, as discussed in Chapter 2.

Lynn Hall of New York University School of Medicine and Craig Love of Brown University performed a study that may throw light on how monozygotic twins can wind up with differing sexual orientations.[7] They examined the finger length ratios of seven pairs of monozygotic female twins who were discordant for sexual orientation: One sister in each pair was lesbian, and the other was straight. Hall and Love found that in each pair, the 2D:4D ratio of the lesbian twin was lower (i.e., male-shifted) in comparison with the straight twin. In another study, Hall identified another consistent anatomical difference between discordant monozygotic female twin pairs—a lower total number of ridges in the fingerprints of the lesbian twin.[8] In both studies, pairs of *concordant* monozygotic twins showed no differences of this kind.

Given the small numbers of subjects, these studies need to be replicated. Nevertheless, they suggest that when monozygotic female twins are discordant for sexual orientation, the lesbian twin experienced higher levels of testosterone prenatally than her heterosexual sister did, or her tissues were more sensitive to testosterone than her sister's. In other words, the same biological factor—prenatal testosterone levels or the response to them—appears to guide the development of sexual orientation in discordant monozygotic twins as in gay and straight people generally; but in the case of these twins there is no apparent prior cause for the different hormone levels.

If the recent work on discordant male twins by Tuck Ngun and colleagues is correct (Chapter 7), different patterns of epigenetic labeling may be a prior cause for discordance in sexual orientation in monozygotic twins. But what causes those different patterns in the first place? Probing further and further back along the pathway of deterministic causation, we may end up in a fog of random events.

How Does Sexual Orientation Become Categorical?

Most gendered traits are dimensional: An individual's verbal-fluency score, for example, can lie anywhere along a broad spectrum, although women tend to outscore men. Sexual orientation, on the other hand, is categorical. Using taxometric analysis to distinguish categorical from dimensional variables, a Washington State University group found that there is a homosexual taxon (category) in men, to which gay men and most bisexual men belong (see Chapter 1). They found evidence for a similar taxon in women, which included lesbians but only a minority of bisexual women.

One could imagine that the categorical nature of sexual orientation results from an entirely deterministic process of development. For example, there might be a "gay gene" and a "straight gene," and possession of one or the other drives an individual to a sexual orientation at one or the other end of the Kinsey scale. That would be a delightfully simple model, but it doesn't seem very likely to be correct, at least for the population as a whole. For one thing, intermediate factors such as prenatal testosterone levels probably vary continuously: There's no evidence, for example, that there are two sets of male fetuses with clearly distinct, non-overlapping testosterone levels. Also, if male sexual orientation were rigidly determined in this way, we would expect much tighter associations with other gendered traits than are actually observed.

It is more likely that some developmental process takes a broad spread of individual trajectories and forces them into just two channels, one leading to heterosexuality and one leading to homosexuality. For example, it might be that male fetuses whose prenatal testosterone levels are above some threshold value or tipping point are steered down the "straight" channel, while those whose testosterone levels are below that threshold are steered down the "gay" channel. Thus two fetuses whose testosterone levels are quite similar but on different sides of the threshold would end up with radically different sexual orientations.

This two-channel model implies that something must be keeping the channels separate—a developmental wall or ridge, if you like. What could that correspond to in biological terms? One possibility is that it involves mutual (reciprocal) inhibition between neural centers or circuits responsible for sexual attraction to males and to females. Even when the input signals are continuous variables, mutual inhibition produces a "winner take all" situation in which there can be only one of two outcomes. If a mutual inhibitory mechanism is at work, the greater prevalence of bisexuality in women suggests that it is less strongly active in females than in males. Some observations in rats suggest that there might indeed be a sex difference of this kind: Inhibitory processes in several sex-related regions of the hypothalamus are stronger in males than in females.[9]

Mutual inhibition might operate only during development, and in such a way as to set up a single dominant channel in any particular individual while the other channel simply withers away and ceases to exist. That could be part of the reason why organizational effects of hormones are limited to a certain period of development.

Alternatively, the mutual inhibition might continue to operate—perhaps in an attenuated fashion—throughout life. This latter idea is more compatible with the observation that under certain circumstances sexual partner preference can change. In Chapter 8 I mentioned two examples from animal studies: In adult female mice, destruction of the vomeronasal organ uncovers an entire suite of male-typical sexual behaviors, including mounting of females, that the animals did not previously show,[10] and in adult male ferrets and rats, destruction of the medial preoptic area (including SDN-POA) changes their partner preference from female to male.[11]

Although sexual orientation usually remains stable in humans, I have mentioned that homosexual feelings can sometimes emerge spontaneously in previously heterosexual women, as well as in previously heterosexual men who undergo hormone treatments or castration or who experience brain damage. Thus there are suggestions that brain circuitry capable of mediating sexual attraction to the non-preferred sex does exist in adult animals and humans but is functionally disabled by inhibition from brain centers concerned with attraction to the preferred sex.

If such mutually inhibitory circuitry does operate, its neuronal basis remains to be identified. Even so, it is tempting to speculate that INAH3 (in humans) and SDN-POA (in rats and ferrets) represent one element of the circuitry—namely, the source of inhibition exerted by the male-typical channel on the female-typical channel. SDN-POA is rich in cells that are sensitive to testosterone and that use the inhibitory transmitter GABA.[12] The observation that damage to this region in male rats and ferrets changes the animals' partner preference, as mentioned above, is also consistent with this idea. Where the other elements of this hypothetical control system might be located is unknown, but several other regions of the hypothalamus are actively involved in the regulation of male and female sexuality, including regions in the medial preoptic area near INAH3 as well as a region further back in the hypothalamus known as the ventromedial nucleus.

Rather than relying on mutual inhibition, another model invokes feedback. In this model, testosterone levels exceeding a certain threshold trigger positive feedback (in the form of an autocatalytic loop) in the target cells that drives them toward complete male-typical development; if testosterone levels do not reach that threshold, no such triggering occurs, and brain development is allowed to follow a female-typical pathway. Such a model has been proposed to account for all-or-nothing sexual differentiation at the neuronal level in *Drosophila*.[13]

Unconscious Processes in Sexual Attraction and Arousal

It doesn't take much of a brain to be gay or straight, if some of the findings mentioned in earlier chapters are correct. One example concerns chemosignals and the olfactory system. According to a study mentioned in Chapter 8, straight women who were exposed to the chemosignal androstadienone (AND) rated men as more attractive, even though the women were not aware of this substance's presence in the air they were breathing.[14] This finding is not surprising, perhaps: Olfactory signals can reach sites such as the amygdala and the hypothalamus without being relayed through the region of the cerebral cortex that's responsible for the conscious perception of odors (the orbitofrontal cortex). Yet according to Ivanka Savic's studies (also discussed in Chapter 8), hypothalamic responses to AND are orientation-specific: Exposure to this substance evokes activity in the anterior hypothalamus in straight women and gay men, but not in straight men or lesbians.

More surprising are studies showing that visual information relevant to sexual orientation can also bypass consciousness. As I mentioned in Chapter 1, two studies have reported that subjects pay more attention to photos of naked individuals of their preferred sex than to individuals of the other sex—even when they are prevented from consciously seeing any photos by means of a binocular suppression paradigm.[15] The amygdala can show distinct reactions to some emotionally laden images even when conscious awareness of those images is suppressed.[16] There have been suggestions that visual information sufficient to generate emotional responses can reach the amygdala via a "low road" within the brain that bypasses the cerebral cortex altogether.[17]

In experimental animals, removal of the cerebral cortex does not prevent organized sexual activity. Decorticate male rats, for example, will investigate other rats, and if those rats smell and act like females the males will mount them, copulate, and sire pups.[18] Nothing like this could happen in humans. Still, we do possess sex-specific subcortical pathways relating to sexuality, and it seems that the activity mediated by these pathways is sex-atypical in gay people.

Given what we know, it might be possible to trigger orientation-specific genital arousal through unconscious channels—through a combination of masked chemosignals and suppressed erotic images, for example. Such a highly simpli-fied "functional backbone" of sexual orientation, stripped of its many cogni-tive complications, could offer unique opportunities to understand the brain mechanisms of sexual orientation. It's not that conscious thoughts and feel-ings are irrelevant to sexual attraction—in the usual circumstances they are at the center of the action. But when those aspects of the mind are sidestepped, something important and illuminating may remain.

Changes in the Prevalence and Nature of Homosexuality

People often assume that if the prevalence or nature of a trait like homosex-uality varies across cultures, or across history in the same culture, then that trait must be a cultural phenomenon. Biological factors are assumed to be a fixed attribute of human populations that could not contribute to such diver-sity in space or time. In reality, however, biological factors may be closely in-volved in these differences.

I have already discussed one such example in Chapter 10 with respect to the older-brother effect. The demographic transition has led to a dramatic re-duction in family size over the last two centuries, such that men with older brothers—the majority of all men in the early 19th century—are an endan-gered species today. Thus the number of gay men who owe their homosexuality to the older-brother effect should have declined markedly.

Another possible effect of the demographic transition on homosexuality relates to the fertile female hypothesis, discussed in Chapter 7. According to this idea, genes predisposing to male homosexuality increase the fecundity (number of children) of gay men's female relatives, and this increased female fecundity is what keeps gay genes in the population. Yet before the demographic transition, women were pregnant so often that they didn't have a great deal of spare reproductive capacity. This fact would have limited the positive effect of gay genes on fecundity. The situation is quite different now: Most women could have half a dozen more children than they actually give birth to, and those extra children would almost certainly survive, so there is a great deal of room for genes to increase reproductive success. Thus to the extent that the fertile fe-male hypothesis is correct, genes for male homosexuality should have become more prevalent in the population over the last two centuries.

If the older-brother effect and the "fertile female" genes predispose to dif-ferent *kinds* of male homosexuality (accompanied by different levels of gender nonconformity, for example), then the overall quality of male homosexuality might have changed perceptibly over the past two centuries—all thanks to an interaction between a cultural process, the demographic transition, with human biology.

Social and biological changes over an even longer term may have influenced the prevalence of homosexuality. Economic historians such as Oded Galor of Brown University and Gregory Clark of the University of California, Davis, have argued that human nature changed over the long "Malthusian era" between the Agrarian Revolution and the Industrial Revolution, as social factors promoted the reproductive success of men who were less violence-prone and more disposed to care for their children.[19] The spread of "feminizing" genes could well be an element of this change. If Edward Miller's theory of gay genes, discussed in Chapter 7, is correct, the increasing prevalence of these feminizing genes would in turn have increased the prevalence of male homosexuality. Such ideas turn the existence of gay men into a kind of byproduct or accident—a felicitous accident, to be sure, but not one that needs to be adaptive in an evolutionary sense.

Very little attention has been paid to comparable issues regarding sexual orientation in women. The blurred lines between heterosexuality, bisexuality, and homosexuality in many women; the evidence for women's sexual fluidity; the partial separation between a woman's genital arousal and her conscious desires and identity; and the close connection in women between sexual attraction and a broader desire for intimacy—all these complexities make female sexual orientation a more daunting topic than male sexual orientation to investigate from a biological or evolutionary perspective.

One clue to a possible origin for female non-heterosexuality is offered by an apparent similarity between women's sexuality and that of one of our close primate relatives, the bonobos (Chapter 3). Among female bonobos homosexual behavior is not indicative of a homosexual orientation; rather, it acts as a kind of social glue, facilitating the formation of female–female alliances, which in turn raise the status of females and help them establish dominance over males. It has been suggested that women's capacity for same-sex attraction and behavior has played a similar adaptive role.[20] Few if any human societies have been dominated by women, but some societies may have been more gender-egalitarian than they would have been in the absence of female–female sexual contacts. In modern times, sexual bonds between women played a significant role in second-wave feminism; what role they may have played in earlier history and prehistory is largely unknown.

Still, there are plenty of women who are truly lesbian and have no interest in sex with men, and the existence of such women does not fit the bonobo-inspired model. It may, however, be explicable in terms of Miller's "byproduct" ideas. In such a model, a variety of masculine traits might have helped women secure male partners—as the work of Brendan Zietsch has suggested[21]—but when enough "masculinizing" genes coincided in one woman, she would be likely to become a lesbian. As with male homosexuality, this model represents lesbianism as a happy accident rather than an adaptation.

Have women become more masculine over the centuries and millennia—
and men more feminine—not just as a result of social pressures but also as part
of an evolutionary process? If so, has this process increased the prevalence of
homosexuality in both sexes? And what will happen in the distant future: Will
the adaptive value of male femininity and female masculinity continue to increase, leading to a new equilibrium in which the gender lines are increasingly
blurred and the prevalence of homosexuality is even greater than it is today?
None of us will be around to learn the answer. The only prediction one can
make with some confidence is that homosexuality is not going to go away.

What Is Sexual Orientation?

At the beginning of this book I defined sexual orientation in terms of the balance of same-sex and opposite-sex attraction. Many variables other than the
sex of potential sex partners can affect sexual attraction, of course: their age,
their race, and so on. Aren't these other variables also dimensions of sexual
orientation, or sexual orientations in themselves?

Plenty of members of sexual minorities, such as pedophiles, asexual men
and women, and practitioners of various "kinks," would like their forms of
sexuality (or the lack of one) to be considered sexual orientations. That would
conform to their sense that their sexuality is a central, inborn aspect of their
personhood, one that neither changes over their life span nor feels like a disorder. They may also feel that calling their forms of desire "orientations" legiti-
mizes them, putting them on the same level as the now more or less accepted
categories of lesbians and gay men.

Some of these dimensions of attraction—age preference in particular—
do seem quite like sexual orientation in the conventional sense. The main
reason not to consider them aspects of sexual orientation is that the phrase
"sexual orientation" already has a universally understood meaning both in
general discourse and in the scientific literature. To change that meaning
would cause endless confusion. Still, the terms "sexual age orientation" and
"asexual orientation" are clear and have already seen limited use in the literature.[22] Perhaps this kind of phraseology could be expanded to other forms
of sexual expression without incorporating assumptions about causation,
pathology, or legitimacy.

Sexual Orientation and Gender: The Social Fallout

I have discussed the social implications of a biological perspective on sexual
orientation in an earlier book,[23] and I will not attempt another review of the

topic here. One facet of the science deserves comment from a social perspective, however. That is the idea that sexual orientation is linked with a broader collection of gendered traits. Does this concept stigmatize gay people by reinforcing stereotypes of mannish lesbians and "queeny" gay men?

Children who are gender-nonconformist do tend to suffer for it, not merely during childhood itself[24] but also years later. According to Katarina Alanko and her colleagues, when such children reach adulthood they are at increased risk of psychiatric problems such as anxiety and depression, and this is true for both boys and girls and regardless of whether they end up gay or straight.[25] Gender nonconformity in adulthood can also lead to stigmatization and resulting psychological distress, but gay men suffer more distress than do lesbians, according to a study by Michael Bailey's group[26]—perhaps because any masculine traits that lesbian or bisexual women may exhibit are more socially acceptable or advantageous than are feminine traits in gay men.

Whether gender-nonconformist children experience psychological problems is strongly affected by how they are treated. When parents have cold or controlling attitudes toward these children the chances of psychological distress in adulthood are greatly increased, but a warm parent–child relationship reduces the likelihood of such distress.[27] No doubt the same is true for relationships with siblings, peers, teachers, and society in general.

Some critics, such as social psychologist Peter Hegarty of the University of Surrey in England, have taken the position that research into the relationship between gender nonconformity (especially during childhood) and homosexuality tends to "medicalize" gay people as well as gender-nonconformist children and thus perhaps increases their risk of suffering psychological problems.[28] The fact that "gender identity disorder of childhood" is a diagnosable medical condition may worsen the situation for these children.

Still, there may be practical advantages to keeping the diagnosis. This is how Richard Pillard made the case to me some years ago: "If these same kids grew up in a culture that had a place for them, they would not be in conflict or distress, and no diagnosis would be relevant. That said, these children are still suffering and can benefit from sensitive treatment. And having a diagnosis allows the psychiatrist to get paid."

There have always been gay men who resent any attempt to identify a connection between male homosexuality and gender-nonconformist traits. Benedict Friedländer, cofounder of a German gay-rights organization in the early years of the 20th century, asserted that Magnus Hirschfeld's biological approach reduced homosexuality to a mental disorder. He wrote:

> As long as the love for a male being is presented as a specific and exclusively feminine characteristic . . . there remains an unavoidable image

of a partial hermaphrodite, that is, a kind of psychic malformation. Here too one cannot claim respect, but only at most beg for pity and at best tolerance.[29]

Here's a more recent example. In 2009 Sergio Garcia, an 18-year-old gay senior at Fairfax High School in Los Angeles, ran successfully for prom queen against several female candidates.[30] His action elicited this comment from gay playwright Vincent James Arcuri:

> [B]ecause Garcia is gay, that places him in the feminine role? Are we expected to accept and align "gay" with "girl"? . . . [C]rowning this young man as the prom "queen" only conveys the wrong message, one that accepts and perpetuates an archaic stereotype of homosexuality and reinforces an inaccurate portrayal of gay men as feminine, girlie caricatures.[31]

Gay men may adopt this point of view because they themselves are not particularly feminine or because they are all *too* feminine, having struggled all their lives to present a more masculine image to the world. Arcuri, for example, underwent speech therapy to modify his voice, which he says transitioned at puberty from that of a "girl" to that of a "raging homosexual."[32] "Femiphobia"—the dislike or fear of femininity in a man—is rampant in our society, and when internalized by gay men it may be more destructive even than homophobia.[33]

In my opinion, the finding that gay and straight people tend to differ in a wide variety of sex-differentiated traits offers a valuable insight into the origins of sexual orientation and thus helps us understand this important facet of human diversity. No approach that ignores this reality is going to advance our understanding.

What's more, the kaleidoscopic blend of gender-variant and gender-typical traits that characterizes gay people is exactly what enables us to make our own unique contributions to society. It's the reason that we should be valued, celebrated, and welcomed into society rather than merely being tolerated.

NOTES

Chapter 1

1. van Anders, 2015.
2. Lippa et al., 2010; Lippa, 2016.
3. Jiang et al., 2006; Légère et al., 2016.
4. Rieger & Savin-Williams, 2012.
5. Mock & Eibach, 2012.
6. Dickson et al., 2003.
7. Diamond, 2003, 2008.
8. Diamond, 2016.
9. Marcus, 1992.
10. Neglia, 2009.
11. Haldeman, 1994.
12. American Psychiatric Association, 2007.
13. Kinsey et al., 1948.
14. Laumann et al., 1994; Wellings et al., 1994; Smith et al., 2003; Statistics Canada, 2004; Chandra et al., 2011; Hayes et al., 2012.
15. Chandra et al., 2011.
16. Coffman et al., 2013.
17. Rudder, 2014.
18. Stephens-Davidowitz, 2013.
19. YouGov, 2015; YouGov UK, 2015.
20. Haslam, 1997; Gangestad et al., 2000; Norris et al., 2015.
21. Barthes et al., 2015.
22. Whitam, 1983.
23. Norton, 1999.
24. Dover, 1978.
25. Reynolds, 2002.
26. W. L. Williams, 1986; Nanda, 1998; Vasey & Bartlett, 2007.
27. Lame Deer & Erdoes, 1972.
28. W. L. Williams, 1986.
29. Murray, 2000.
30. Kennedy & Davis, 1983; Faderman, 1991.

Chapter 2

1. Freud, 1905/1975.
2. Bell et al., 1981.
3. Isay, 1989.

    4. Green, 1987.
    5. J. Taylor, 1992.
    6. Socarides, 1978.
    7. Nicolosi & Nicolosi, 2002.
    8. Freud, 1920/1955.
    9. Eysenck, 1985.
   10. Churchill, 1967.
   11. Cameron & Cameron, 1995.
   12. McGuire et al., 1965.
   13. Tomeo et al., 2001.
   14. Herdt, 1981.
   15. Wellings et al., 1994.
   16. Corliss et al., 2002; A. L. Roberts et al., 2010; Andersen & Blosnich, 2013.
   17. A. L. Roberts et al., 2012.
   18. A. L. Roberts et al., 2013.
   19. D. H. Bailey & Bailey, 2013; Rind, 2013; D. H. Bailey et al., 2014; A. L. Roberts et al., 2014.
   20. Andersen & Blosnich, 2013.
   21. Xu & Zheng, 2015a.
   22. Tooby & Cosmides, 1992.
   23. Eckes & Trautner, 2000.
   24. Money et al., 1957; Money & Ehrhardt, 1971.
   25. M. Diamond & Sigmundson, 1997.
   26. Colapinto, 2000.
   27. Bradley et al., 1998.
   28. Reiner & Gearhart, 2004.
   29. Anderssen et al., 2002.
   30. Brakefield et al., 2014.
   31. Mehren, 2004.
   32. Conservapedia, 2015.
   33. Lever, 1994, 1995.
   34. Shidlo & Schroeder, 2002; Spitzer, 2012.

Chapter 3

    1. Gazzaniga, 2008.
    2. Gorski et al., 1978; Gorski, 1985.
    3. Commins & Yahr, 1984; Tobet et al., 1986; Byne, 1998; Roselli et al., 2004a; Vasey & Pfaus, 2005.
    4. Allen et al., 1989; LeVay, 1991; Byne et al., 2001; Garcia-Falgueras & Swaab, 2008.
    5. Goldstein et al., 2001; Cahill, 2005.
    6. Joel et al., 2015
    7. Chekroud et al., 2016
    8. Raznahan et al., 2014; Ruigrok et al., 2014.
    9. Ingalhalikar et al., 2014.
   10. Cosgrove et al., 2007.
   11. Schneider et al., 2011.
   12. Hines et al., 1992; Cooke et al., 1999; Mori et al., 2008.
   13. Luine & Dohanich, 2007.
   14. Eggers & Sinclair, 2012.
   15. Wilhelm et al., 2007.
   16. Asby et al., 2009.
   17. Rodeck et al., 1985.
   18. Gorski, 1985; Goto et al., 2005; Sakuma, 2009.
   19. Scott et al., 2015.

20. E. C. Davis et al., 1996b; Forger, 2009.
21. Rhees et al., 1990a, 1990b; E. C. Davis et al., 1995.
22. Dugger et al., 2008.
23. Habert & Picon, 1984.
24. E. C. Davis et al., 1996a; Yang et al., 2004.
25. R. R. Buss et al., 2006.
26. Arai et al., 1996.
27. Forger et al., 2004; Forger, 2009.
28. McEwen, 1998.
29. Cooke & Woolley, 2005a.
30. Arnold & Breedlove, 1985; McCarthy & Konkle, 2005.
31. Romeo, 2003; Koshibu et al., 2004; Ahmed et al., 2008; De Lorme et al., 2013; Juraska et al., 2013; Mohr & Sisk, 2013; Sisk & Berenbaum, 2013.
32. Cooke et al., 1999.
33. Morris et al., 2008a, 2008b.
34. Phoenix et al., 1959.
35. Goy et al., 1988.
36. de Jonge et al., 1988.
37. Vega Matuszczyk et al., 1988.
38. Adkins-Regan, 2002.
39. Signoret, 1970; Ford, 1983.
40. Mansukhani et al., 1996; Adkins-Regan, 2005.
41. Becker et al., 2002.
42. Bodo & Rissman, 2007; Zuloaga et al., 2008.
43. Bakker et al., 1993; Zuloaga et al., 2008.
44. Olvera-Hernandez et al., 2015.
45. Grumbach & Auchus, 1999.
46. P. Y. Wang et al., 2009; Wittmann & McLennan, 2013.
47. Bramble et al., 2016.
48. Arnold et al., 2004; Gatewood et al., 2006; Majdic & Tobet, 2011.
49. Compaan et al., 1994.
50. Lephart et al., 2001.
51. Kudwa & Rissman, 2003.
52. vom Saal & Bronson, 1980; Pei et al., 2006.
53. Clemens et al., 1978; Pei et al., 2006.
54. Medland et al., 2008.
55. Kerchner & Ward, 1992.
56. Ward, 1972; Anderson et al., 1985; Kerchner & Ward, 1992; Meek et al., 2006.
57. Goldfoot et al., 1984.
58. Cooke et al., 2000.
59. LeVay, 1996.
60. Dörner, 1969; Dorner et al., 1991.
61. MacCulloch & Waddington, 1981; Ellis & Ames, 1987.
62. Dörner, 1969.
63. Dörner, 1989/2001.
64. Bagemihl, 1999.
65. Sommer & Vasey, 2006.
66. Kotrschal et al., 2006.
67. Hunt & Warner Hunt, 1977; Hunt et al., 1980; Hunt et al., 1984.
68. Fry, 1993.
69. de Waal, 1995; Fruth & Hohmann, 2006.
70. Vasey, 2006; Leca et al., 2015.
71. Roselli et al., 2011.
72. Geist, 1971.
73. Roselli et al., 2004a.

Chapter 4

1. Simmons, 1965; Levitt & Klassen, 1974; A. Taylor, 1983; Kite & Deaux, 1987; Madon, 1997.
2. Hines, 2010.
3. Eaton & Enns, 1986; Maccoby, 1998.
4. Berenbaum & Snyder, 1995; Serbin et al., 2001.
5. Berman et al., 1977.
6. D. Kimura, 1999.
7. Beer & Fleming, 1989; Kerns & Berenbaum, 1991; D. Kimura, 1999.
8. Halpern, 2011.
9. Goodenough, 1957.
10. Maccoby, 1998.
11. Sachs et al., 1973.
12. Fagot et al., 1992.
13. Rust et al., 2000.
14. Braggio et al., 1978; Ward & Stehm, 1991; Wallen, 1996.
15. Simpson et al., 2016.
16. Alexander & Hines, 2002; Hassett et al., 2008.
17. Lovejoy & Wallen, 1988.
18. Connellan et al., 2001.
19. Spelke, 2005.
20. Moore & Johnson, 2008; Quinn & Liben, 2008.
21. Alexander et al., 2009.
22. Wallen, 1996.
23. E. K. Roberts et al., 2009.
24. Dreger et al., 2012.
25. Money & Ehrhardt, 1971; Berenbaum & Snyder, 1995; Berenbaum et al., 2000; Hines et al., 2003b, 2004; Meyer-Bahlburg et al., 2004, 2006; Pasterski et al., 2007, 2011, 2015b.
26. Jordan-Young, 2012.
27. Wong et al., 2013.
28. Hines et al., 2002.
29. Auyeung et al., 2009.
30. Chapman et al., 2006.
31. Hines et al., 2003b.
32. Grimshaw et al., 1995.
33. White, 1994.
34. Pallone & Steinberg, 1990.
35. Isay, 1999.
36. Alanko et al., 2009.
37. Blanchard et al., 1983.
38. Grellert et al., 1982.
39. J. M. Bailey & Zucker, 1995.
40. Lippa, 2003b; Loehlin & McFadden, 2003; Cardoso, 2008; Lippa, 2008a; Plöderl & Fartacek, 2008; Alanko et al., 2009; Rahman et al., 2012.
41. Cardoso, 2008.
42. Alanko et al., 2009.
43. W. L. Williams, 1986; Nanda, 1998; Vasey & Bartlett, 2007.
44. W. L. Williams, 1986.
45. Rieger et al., 2008.
46. Green, 1987.
47. Bakwin, 1968; Money & Russo, 1979; Zuger, 1984.
48. Drummond et al., 2008.
49. Ristori & Steensma, 2016.
50. Steensma et al., 2013.
51. Bem, 1996, 2000.

52. Green, 1987.
53. Bergen et al., 2007.

Chapter 5

1. Halpern, 2011.
2. Brand & Millot, 2001.
3. Papadatou-Pastou et al., 2008; I. E. Sommer et al., 2008.
4. Del Giudice, 2015.
5. Nettle, 2007.
6. Costa et al., 2001; Lippa, 2005.
7. Wheelwright & Baron-Cohen, 2011.
8. Schmitt et al., 2012.
9. Sagarin et al., 2012; Frederick & Fales, 2014.
10. Laws & O'Donohue, 2008.
11. Greenfeld, 1997.
12. J. M. Bailey et al., 1994; Toro-Morn & Sprecher, 2003.
13. J. M. Bailey et al., 1994; Murnen & Stockton, 1997; Janssen et al., 2003.
14. Gerressu et al., 2008.
15. Buss, 1989, 2000; Schmitt, 2003; Herlitz & Kabir, 2006; Schmitt et al., 2008; Lippa, 2009; Lohman & Lakin, 2009.
16. Costa et al., 2001.
17. C. L. Williams & Meck, 1991.
18. Jozet-Alves et al., 2008.
19. Darmaillacq et al., 2005.
20. Lippa & Hershberger, 1999; Loehlin et al., 2005.
21. Zucker et al., 1996; Berenbaum, 1999; Berenbaum & Bailey, 2003; Hines et al., 2003b; Wisniewski et al., 2004; Cohen-Bendahan et al., 2005; Meyer-Bahlburg et al., 2006; Hampson & Rovet, 2015; Wisniewski, 2015.
22. Berenbaum et al., 2012.
23. D. Kimura, 1994; D. Kimura & Carson, 1995; Loehlin & McFadden, 2003; Kraemer et al., 2006; Lippa, 2006a; Hampson et al., 2008; Wallien et al., 2008; Kraemer et al., 2009.
24. Penton-Voak & Perrett, 2000; Johnston et al., 2001.
25. Gouchie & Kimura, 1991; Yonker et al., 2006.
26. McCormick & Witelson, 1991; Wegesin, 1998a; Loehlin & McFadden, 2003; Rahman & Wilson, 2003a; Peters et al., 2007.
27. Gladue & Bailey, 1995b.
28. Rahman & Wilson, 2003a; van Anders & Hampson, 2005; Peters et al., 2007.
29. Gladue & Bailey, 1995b.
30. J. A. Y. Hall & Kimura, 1995; Rahman & Wilson, 2003a; Rahman et al., 2005; van Anders & Hampson, 2005; Collaer et al., 2007; Canovas & Cimadevilla, 2011.
31. Rahman et al., 2003a.
32. G. Sanders & Wright, 1997.
33. McCormick & Witelson, 1991.
34. Wegesin, 1998a.
35. Neave et al., 1999.
36. Rahman et al., 2003c; Hassan & Rahman, 2007.
37. Weinrich, 1978.
38. Kanazawa, 2012.
39. Papadatou-Pastou et al., 2008.
40. Lalumière et al., 2000.
41. Loehlin & McFadden, 2003.
42. Mustanski et al., 2002; Lippa, 2003b.
43. Lippa, 2003b.

44. McCormick & Witelson, 1991.
45. Bogaert et al., 2007.
46. Novakova et al., 2013.
47. Brand & Millot, 2001.
48. Lippa, 2008b.
49. Lippa, 2005.
50. Schiller & Rosenberg, 1986.
51. Rostker et al., 2011.
52. J. M. Bailey & Oberschneider, 1997.
53. Lippa, 2008b.
54. J. M. Bailey et al., 1997.
55. Faderman, 1991; Chauncey, 1994.
56. Frederick & Fales, 2014.
57. J. M. Bailey et al., 1994.
58. Bell & Weinberg, 1978; Laumann et al., 1994.
59. J. M. Bailey et al., 1994; Lawson et al., 2014.
60. Spengler, 1977; Alison et al., 2001.
61. Tomassilli et al., 2009.
62. Salais & Fischer, 1995; Sergeant et al., 2006; Perry et al., 2013.
63. Nettle, 2007.
64. Nettle, 2007.
65. Nettle, 2007.
66. Ellis et al., 1990; Gladue & Bailey, 1995a; Sergeant et al., 2006.
67. Ellis et al., 1990.
68. VanderLaan & Vasey, 2009.
69. Lippa, 2005, 2008b.
70. J. A. Y. Hall & Kimura, 1995.

Chapter 6

1. LeVay, 1996.
2. Meyer-Bahlburg, 1984.
3. Pearcey et al., 1996; Singh et al., 1999.
4. van Anders & Watson, 2006, 2007; van Anders et al., 2007.
5. Sperling, 2008.
6. Clarkson & Herbison, 2016.
7. Quigley, 2002.
8. Lamminmaki et al., 2012; Pasterski et al., 2015a.
9. Garagorri et al., 2008.
10. Organisation Internationale des Intersexués, 2009.
11. Klein et al., 1994.
12. Meyer-Bahlburg et al., 2008.
13. Hines et al., 2004.
14. Imperato-McGinley et al., 1991; Hines et al., 2003a.
15. Manning et al., 1998.
16. Lippa, 2003a; Manning et al., 2007; Loehlin et al., 2009; Manning et al., 2014.
17. Galis et al., 2010.
18. Stenstrom et al., 2011.
19. Peters et al., 2007.
20. Lutchmaya et al., 2004.
21. Brown et al., 2002b; Ökten et al., 2002; Ciumas et al., 2009; Rivas et al., 2014.
22. Buck et al., 2003.
23. Cattrall et al., 2005.
24. van Anders et al., 2006; Voracek & Dressler, 2007.

25. Talarovicova et al., 2009.
26. T. J. Williams et al., 2000; McFadden & Shubel, 2002; Rahman & Wilson, 2003b; Puts et al., 2004; Rahman, 2005; Kraemer et al., 2006.
27. Manning et al., 2007.
28. Lippa, 2003b; Hall & Schaeff, 2008.
29. Kangassalo et al., 2011.
30. Grimbos et al., 2010.
31. McFadden & Shubel, 2002; Lippa, 2003a; Manning et al., 2007; Hall & Schaeff, 2008; Kangassalo et al., 2011; Xu & Zheng, 2015b.
32. Robinson & Manning, 2000; Rahman & Wilson, 2003b; Puts et al., 2004; Rahman, 2005.
33. T. J. Williams et al., 2000; Voracek et al., 2005; Kraemer et al., 2006.
34. Manning et al., 2007.
35. Grimbos et al., 2010.
36. L. S. Hall & Love, 2003; Hiraishi et al., 2012.
37. A. A. Bailey & Hurd, 2005; Collaer et al., 2007; McIntyre et al., 2007; Manning & Fink, 2008; Loehlin et al., 2009.
38. Puts et al., 2004; Lippa, 2006a.
39. McFadden et al., 2005.
40. McFadden, 1998.
41. Bilger et al., 1990; McFadden, 1998; Snihur & Hampson, 2011.
42. Wisniewski et al., 2014.
43. Berninger, 2007.
44. McFadden et al., 2006, 2009.
45. McFadden et al., 2009.
46. McFadden et al., 1996.
47. Wisniewski et al., 2014.
48. McFadden, 2000; Snihur & Hampson, 2012a, 2012b.
49. McFadden & Pasanen, 1998, 1999.
50. Burke et al., 2014b.
51. McFadden & Champlin, 2000.
52. Wisniewski et al., 2014.
53. Rahman et al., 2003b.
54. Swerdlow et al., 1993.
55. Grumbach & Auchus, 1999.
56. Auger & Jessen, 2009.
57. Jeong et al., 2008.
58. Wright et al., 2008.
59. McCarthy et al., 2015.
60. Galanopoulou, 2008; Cellot & Cherubini, 2013.
61. A. M. Davis et al., 2000.
62. Ward & Weisz, 1984.
63. Morgan & Bale, 2011.
64. Dörner et al., 1980, 1983.
65. Schmidt & Clement, 1990.
66. de Rooij et al., 2009.
67. J. M. Bailey et al., 1991.
68. Ellis et al., 1988.

Chapter 7

1. J. Taylor, 1992.
2. Pillard et al., 1981; LeVay, 1996.
3. Pillard et al., 1982; Pillard & Weinrich, 1986; Pillard, 1990.

4. J. M. Bailey & Bell, 1993; J. M. Bailey & Benishay, 1993; Hamer et al., 1993; J. M. Bailey et al., 1999; Schwartz et al., 2010.
5. J. M. Bailey & Bell, 1993.
6. Pillard et al., 1982; Pillard & Weinrich, 1986.
7. J. M. Bailey & Benishay, 1993; Hamer et al., 1993; Pattatucci & Hamer, 1995; J. M. Bailey et al., 1999; Schwartz et al., 2010.
8. Dawood et al., 2000.
9. Pattatucci & Hamer, 1995.
10. Hamer et al., 1993; J. M. Bailey et al., 1995.
11. J. Bouchard et al., 1999.
12. J. M. Bailey & Pillard, 1991; J. M. Bailey et al., 1993.
13. Whitam et al., 1993.
14. Kirk et al., 2000.
15. Långström et al., 2010.
16. Alanko et al., 2009.
17. Hershberger, 1997.
18. Kendler et al., 2000.
19. J. M. Bailey & Pillard, 1991; J. M. Bailey et al., 2000; Alanko et al., 2009.
20. van Beijsterveldt et al., 2006.
21. Alanko et al., 2009.
22. Eckert et al., 1986.
23. Whitam et al., 1993.
24. Segal, 2000.
25. Hershberger, 1997.
26. Macke et al., 1993.
27. DuPree et al., 2004.
28. Wang et al., 2012.
29. Hamer et al., 1993.
30. Camperio-Ciani et al., 2004; Rahman et al., 2008.
31. Bailey et al., 1999; McKnight & Malcolm, 2000.
32. Schwartz et al., 2010.
33. S. Hu et al., 1995; Rice et al., 1999; Mustanski et al., 2005; Ramagopalan et al., 2010.
34. A. R. Sanders et al., 2015.
35. Mandiyan et al., 2005.
36. Butcher et al., 2008.
37. Drabant et al., 2012.
38. Forger, 2016.
39. Gordon et al., 2012.
40. Whitelaw et al., 2010.
41. Bocklandt et al., 2006.
42. Nugent et al., 2015.
43. Cited by Balter, 2015.
44. Gill, 1963.
45. Ryner et al., 1996.
46. Ito et al., 1996.
47. Demir & Dickson, 2005.
48. Yamamoto, 2007.
49. K. Kimura et al., 2008.
50. Finley et al., 1997; Grosjean et al., 2001; Svetec et al., 2005; Shirangi et al., 2006; Yamamoto, 2007; Grosjean et al., 2008; Liu et al., 2008.
51. Grosjean et al., 2008.
52. Liu et al., 2008.
53. Liu et al., 2009.
54. Ferveur et al., 1997.
55. Gatewood et al., 2006; Arnold, 2009.

56. Bocklandt & Vilain, 2007.
57. National Library of Medicine, 2008.
58. Weinrich, 1987a.
59. Yankelovich Partners, 1994.
60. Iemmola & Camperio-Ciani, 2009.
61. King et al., 2005.
62. Vasey et al., 2014.
63. King et al., 2005.
64. Wilson, 1975.
65. Vasey et al., 2007; Vasey & VanderLaan, 2008, 2009, 2010a, 2010b; VanderLaan & Vasey, 2012.
66. Bobrow & Bailey, 2001; Rahman & Hull, 2005.
67. King et al., 2005.
68. Trivers, 1974; Hamer & Copeland, 1994.
69. Camperio-Ciani et al., 2004; Iemmola & Camperio-Ciani, 2009; Camperio Ciani & Pellizzari, 2012.
70. Camperio Ciani et al., 2008.
71. Eblex Sheep Better Returns Program, 2008.
72. Stellflug & Berardinelli, 2002.
73. Barthes et al., 2013, 2015.
74. Barthes et al., 2014; VanderLaan et al., 2014.
75. Miller, 2000.
76. Zietsch et al., 2008.

Chapter 8

1. Saper & Lowell, 2014.
2. Swanson, 2003.
3. Hooker et al., 2006.
4. Simerly, 2002; Shah et al., 2004; Choi et al., 2005.
5. Cooke & Woolley, 2005b.
6. Byne, 1998.
7. LeVay, 1991.
8. Byne et al., 2000, 2001.
9. Garcia-Falgueras & Swaab, 2008.
10. Swaab & Hofman, 1990.
11. Allen & Gorski, 1992.
12. Lasco et al., 2002.
13. Luders et al., 2014.
14. Witelson et al., 2008.
15. Ponseti et al., 2007.
16. Savic & Lindström, 2008.
17. Kranz & Ishai, 2006.
18. Safron et al., 2007; S. H. Hu et al., 2008.
19. Ponseti et al., 2006, 2009.
20. Stoleru et al., 2012.
21. Safron et al., 2007; S. H. Hu et al., 2008.
22. Chivers et al., 2004; Suschinsky et al., 2009.
23. Sylva et al., 2013.
24. Spape et al., 2014.
25. Ponseti et al., 2006.
26. M. A. Williams et al., 2004.
27. Ponseti et al., 2006.
28. Petrulis, 2013.

29. Stowers et al., 2002; Kimchi et al., 2007.
30. Trotier et al., 2000; Kouros-Mehr et al., 2001; Besli et al., 2004; Mast & Samuelsen, 2009.
31. Croy et al., 2012, 2013.
32. Knecht et al., 2003; Savic et al., 2009.
33. Kohl et al., 2001; Preti et al., 2003.
34. Lübke et al., 2009, 2012; Lübke & Pause, 2015.
35. Savic et al., 2001, 2005; Berglund et al., 2006.
36. Gower et al., 1994; Lübke & Pause, 2015.
37. Bensafi et al., 2004.
38. Saxton et al., 2008.
39. Berglund et al., 2008.
40. Burke et al., 2012.
41. Burke et al., 2014a.
42. Ciumas et al., 2009.
43. Juster et al., 2015.
44. Savic & Lindström, 2008.
45. Savic & Lindström, 2008.
46. Bourne & Maxwell, 2010.
47. Rahman & Yusuf, 2015.
48. Wegesin, 1998b.
49. Vingerhoets et al., 2012.
50. Roselli et al., 2007; Roselli & Stormshak, 2010; Reddy et al., 2015.
51. Roselli et al., 2004a.
52. Roselli et al., 2004b.
53. Perkins et al., 1995.
54. Masek et al., 1999.
55. Roselli et al., 2006.
56. Paredes & Baum, 1995; Kindon et al., 1996; Paredes et al., 1998.
57. Kimchi et al., 2007.
58. Trimble et al., 1997.
59. Wassersug et al., 2014.
60. Daskalos, 1998.
61. Gao & Moore, 1996.
62. Byne et al., 2001.
63. Lombardo et al., 2012.

Chapter 9

1. Blanchard & Bogaert, 1996a; Bogaert & Blanchard, 1996; Bogaert, 1998; Bogaert & Friesen, 2002; Bogaert, 2010; Bogaert & Liu, 2013.
2. Frisch & Zdravkovic, 2010.
3. Maresh, 1955; Marshall & Tanner, 1974.
4. Martin & Nguyen, 2004.
5. Jansson et al., 1985.
6. Bogaert & Hershberger, 1999.
7. D. Veale et al., 2015.
8. Harding & Golombok, 2002.
9. Valentova et al., 2014; Skorska et al., 2015.
10. Klar, 2005.
11. Rahman et al., 2009; Schwartz et al., 2010.
12. Gaudio, 1994; Linville, 1998; Ambady et al., 1999; Smyth et al., 2003; Johnson et al., 2007; Rendall et al., 2008; Smyth & Rogers, 2008; Rieger et al., 2010.
13. Shelp, 2002; Woolery, 2007.
14. Rieger et al., 2008.

15. Rieger et al., 2010, 2011.
16. Rule, 2016.
17. Martins et al., 2005; Lübke & Pause, 2015.
18. Munson, 2007; Valentova & Havlicek, 2013.
19. Tracy et al., 2015.
20. Smyth et al., 2003; Pierrehumbert et al., 2004; Smyth & Rogers, 2008.
21. Munson et al., 2006; Mack & Munson, 2012.
22. Sulpizio et al., 2015.
23. Munson et al., 2006.
24. Johnson & Tassinary, 2005; Johnson et al., 2007.
25. Lyons et al., 2014.
26. Cox et al., 2016.
27. Plöderl, 2014.
28. Smyth & Rogers, 2008.
29. Smyth & Rogers, 2008.
30. Bouchard, 1984.
31. Lyons et al., 2014.

Chapter 10

1. Slater, 1962; E. H. Hare & Moran, 1979.
2. Berglin, 1982; Blanchard, 2014.
3. Blanchard & Zucker, 1994; Zucker & Blanchard, 1994; Blanchard & Bogaert, 1996a, 1996b, 1998; Blanchard et al., 1998; Ellis & Blanchard, 2001.
4. Blanchard & Zucker, 1994; Zucker & Blanchard, 1994; Blanchard & Bogaert, 1996a; Blanchard et al., 1998.
5. Blanchard & Bogaert, 1996b; Purcell et al., 2000; Ellis & Blanchard, 2001; Bogaert, 2003, 2006a; Blanchard & Lippa, 2007.
6. Blanchard & Lippa, 2007.
7. Bogaert, 2003.
8. Bogaert, 2010.
9. Blanchard et al., 1995.
10. Blanchard & Sheridan, 1992; Zucker & Blanchard, 1994.
11. Bogaert et al., 1997; Blanchard & Bogaert, 1998; Blanchard et al., 2000.
12. Camperio-Ciani et al., 2004; Iemmola & Camperio-Ciani, 2009.
13. Schwartz et al., 2010.
14. King et al., 2005.
15. Vasey & VanderLaan, 2007; VanderLaan & Vasey, 2013.
16. Frisch & Hviid, 2006.
17. Francis, 2008.
18. Currin et al., 2015.
19. Kishida & Rahman, 2015.
20. Green, 2000.
21. Gomez-Gil et al., 2011; Bozkurt et al., 2015.
22. Blanchard, 2004, 2007a, 2007b.
23. Blanchard & Bogaert, 1996b.
24. Schwartz et al., 2010.
25. Francis, 2008.
26. Cantor et al., 2002.
27. Cantor et al., 2002.
28. Blanchard & Bogaert, 2004.
29. Haines, 2008.
30. Bogaert, 2004b.
31. Marmor, 1980.

32. Laumann et al., 1994.
33. Whitam, 1983.
34. Blanchard et al., 2006; Bogaert et al., 2007; Blanchard & Lippa, 2008.
35. Blanchard & Lippa, 2007.
36. Bogaert, 2007.
37. Sulloway, 1996; Paulhus et al., 1999.
38. Bogaert, 2006a.
39. Blanchard & Bogaert, 1996b.
40. Bogaert et al., 2015.
41. Blanchard & Ellis, 2001; Cote et al., 2003.
42. Nielsen et al., 2008.
43. Maccoby et al., 1979.
44. Green, 2000.
45. Blanchard et al., 2016.

Chapter 11

1. Peters et al., 2007.
2. Lever, 1994.
3. S. Roberts, 2014.
4. Rudder, 2010.
5. Blanchard & Lippa, 2007.
6. Rieger et al., 2005.
7. *The Advocate*, 2005.
8. Rosenthal et al., 2011.
9. Cerny & Janssen, 2011.
10. Ebsworth & Lalumiere, 2012; Lippa, 2013; Rullo et al., 2014.
11. Rieger & Savin-Williams, 2012; Rieger et al., 2015a.
12. Baldwin et al., 2015.
13. Lippa, 2006b.
14. Rieger et al., 2013.
15. Stief et al., 2014.
16. Vrangalova & Savin-Williams, 2012; Savin-Williams & Vrangalova, 2013.
17. Copen et al., 2016.
18. Weinrich, 1987b.
19. Peters et al., 2007.
20. Lippa, 2008b.
21. Frederick & Fales, 2014.
22. Lippa, 2008b.
23. McFadden & Pasanen, 1999.
24. Tollison et al., 1979.
25. Chivers et al., 2004; Suschinsky et al., 2009; Chivers et al., 2010; Rieger et al., 2015b; Huberman & Chivers, 2016.
26. Chivers et al., 2007.
27. Lippa et al., 2010.
28. Rullo et al., 2010.
29. Spape et al., 2014; Chivers, 2016.
30. Dawson et al., 2015; Lalumière, 2016.
31. Sawatsky et al., 2016.
32. Lalumière, 2016.
33. Lippa, 2006b.
34. Hirschfeld, 1914.
35. Bogaert, 2004a; Prause & Graham, 2007; Brotto et al., 2010; Poston & Baumle, 2010; Yule et al., 2014; Brotto, 2016; Semon et al., 2016; Yule et al., 2016.

36. Yule et al., 2014.
37. Rudder, 2014.
38. Cantor et al., 2004, 2007, 2008, 2015.
39. Schiffer et al., 2007; Schiltz et al., 2007.
40. Kargel et al., 2015.
41. Brown et al., 2002a.
42. Singh et al., 1999.
43. Tortorice, 2001.
44. Wegesin & Meyer-Bahlburg, 2000; Hart et al., 2003.
45. Weinrich et al., 1992; McIntyre, 2003; Moskowitz et al., 2008; Moskowitz & Hart, 2011; Moskowitz, 2015.
46. Novakova et al., 2013.
47. Dawood et al., 2000.
48. Petterson et al., 2015.
49. W. L. Williams, 1986.
50. Rieger et al., 2015b.
51. Blanchard, 1991; Lawrence, 2004.
52. Veale et al., 2010; M. Diamond, 2013.
53. Segal & Diamond, 2014.
54. L. Hare et al., 2009.
55. Fernandez et al., 2014.
56. Henningsson et al., 2005.
57. Bentz et al., 2008.
58. Garcia-Falgueras & Swaab, 2008.
59. Kruijver et al., 2000; Rametti et al., 2011a, 2011b; Kreukels & Guillamon, 2016.
60. Veale et al., 2010.

Chapter 12

1. Bouchard, 2004.
2. Alanko et al., 2009.
3. Auger et al., 2001.
4. Breedlove, 2016.
5. Blanchard et al., 2006.
6. Rahman, 2005a.
7. L. S. Hall & Love, 2003.
8. L. S. Hall, 2000.
9. Searles et al., 2000.
10. Kimchi et al., 2007.
11. Paredes & Baum, 1995; Paredes et al., 1998.
12. Searles et al., 2000.
13. Sato & Yamamoto, 2014.
14. Saxton et al., 2008.
15. Jiang et al., 2006; Légère et al., 2016.
16. M. A. Williams et al., 2004.
17. LeDoux, 1996.
18. Whishaw & Kolb, 1985; Merker, 2007.
19. Galor & Moav, 2002; Clark, 2007.
20. Kuhle & Radtke, 2013; Fleischman et al., 2015.
21. Zietsch et al., 2008.
22. Bogaert, 2006b; Seto, 2012.
23. LeVay, 1996.
24. Bailey & Zucker, 1995; van Beijsterveldt et al., 2006.
25. Alanko et al., 2009.

26. Skidmore et al., 2006.
27. Alanko et al., 2009.
28. Hegarty, 2009.
29. Quoted in Oosterhuis & Kennedy, 1991.
30. Bloomekatz, 2009.
31. Arcuri, 2009b.
32. Arcuri, 2009a.
33. Isay, 1989.

GLOSSARY

2D:4D ratio The length of the index finger divided by the length of the ring finger.

activational effect The functional activation during postnatal life of a brain system whose basic organization was established earlier in development.

age-stratified relationship A sexual relationship characterized by a substantial age difference between the partners.

amygdala A group of nuclei in the temporal lobe of the brain involved in the processing of emotion, sexuality, and social functions.

androgen insensitivity syndrome (AIS) A congenital condition in which the androgen receptor is nonfunctional, causing affected XY fetuses to develop with the outward appearance of females.

androgens Sex hormones such as testosterone that tend to drive development in a male direction.

androphilic Sexually attracted to men.

anterior commissure A small band of fibers that interconnects the temporal lobes of the left and right cerebral hemispheres; it crosses the midline of the brain in the region of the anterior hypothalamus.

antibody A molecular component of the immune system that recognizes and binds to a specific antigen.

antigen A substance that is capable of triggering an immune response.

anti-müllerian hormone (AMH) A hormone secreted by the developing testes that suppresses development of the female reproductive tract.

aromatase An enzyme that converts testosterone to estrogen.

asexual Never experiencing sexual attraction

auditory evoked potentials Electrical signals that can be recorded from the scalp that reflect the activity of auditory systems of the brain in response to a sound.

AvPv A nucleus in the preoptic area of the hypothalamus that is larger in females than in females; it helps regulate the reproductive cycle, at least in rodents.

bisexual Sexually attracted to persons of either sex.

bottom In gay slang, a man who prefers to take the receptive role in anal sex.

butch masculine or dominant, usually in reference to a lesbian.

chemosignal A chemical substance that serves as a means of social communication (sometimes called a pheromone).

coactivator An intracellular molecule that enhances the action of a hormone.

cochlea The auditory sense organ in the inner ear.

cognitive Of or related to information-processing aspects of the mind such as perception, as distinct from emotions or personality.

concordance rate The probability that both members of a twin pair will exhibit some trait given that one member does.

congenital adrenal hyperplasia (CAH) A genetic condition in which the adrenal gland secretes excess androgens during prenatal development.

conversion therapy Psychological treatment intended to change a person's sexual orientation.

corepressor An intracellular molecule that inhibits the action of a hormone.

corpus callosum The largest band of white matter that interconnects the left and right cerebral hemispheres.

critical period A period during which the development of a certain brain system is particularly sensitive to the influence of hormones or other factors.

crossing over The exchange of genetic material between chromosomes during development of a sperm or ovum.

demographic transition The marked decrease in the number of offspring born to the average woman that has accompanied industrialization and other social changes in many countries.

dimensional Forming a continuous distribution; opposite of categorical.

discordant Of twins, not sharing a trait, such as homosexuality.

dizygotic Of twins, arising from two different fertilized ova.

dopamine A neurotransmitter with a variety of functions within the brain; it is particularly associated with motivation and reward.

egalitarian relationship A homosexual relationship between two persons who are similar in age and gender characteristics.

emotional jealousy Fear that one's partner is emotionally involved with a third party.

epigenetic effect An effect mediated by chemical changes to DNA (such as the addition of methyl groups), or to proteins associated with DNA, that do not involve changes to the DNA sequence itself.

ethologist A scientist who studies animal behavior in nature.

eye-blink auditory startle response A reflex blinking of the eyes in response to an unexpected sound.

fa'afafine A homosexual male in Samoa, who may or may not be transgender.

feminizing genes Hypothetical genes that promote the development of feminine characteristics in males.

femme feminine, usually in reference to a lesbian.

flehmen response In some mammals, a curling of the upper lip that facilitates detection of chemosignals by the vomeronasal organ.

frequency In audition, the number of sinusoidal pressure oscillations per second, corresponding roughly to perceived pitch.

fruitless (fru) A gene in fruit flies that regulates the development of brain regions responsible for sexual behavior.

fundamental frequency The lowest periodic component in a complex sound such as a voice; it is the main contributor to the perceived pitch of the voice.

gamma-aminobutyric acid (GABA) A neurotransmitter that has an inhibitory action in adults but may be excitatory during development.

gay Homosexual.

gaydar The ability to identify a person as gay on the basis of his or her appearance or unconscious behaviors.

gender dysphoria Severe dissatisfaction with one's biological sex.

gendered Differing between the sexes, usually in reference to mental or behavioral traits.

gender-stratified relationship A homosexual relationship characterized by a marked difference in gender characteristics between the partners.

gene A stretch of DNA that is expressed as a functional unit; a unit of inheritance.

genome An individual's entire genetic endowment.

genome-wide association study A search for a gene influencing a certain trait that involves scanning numerous variable sites across the genome. If the variants at a given site differ consistently between individuals who have and who lack the trait, that site is likely to be near a gene of interest.

glutamate A common excitatory neurotransmitter in the brain.

gray matter Brain tissue containing neurons and synapses, as contrasted with white matter.

growth factor A molecule that signals certain target cells to increase their rate of growth.

gynephilic Sexually attracted to women.

heritability The fraction of the variability in a trait within a population that is attributable to genetic differences between individuals.

heterosexual Sexually attracted to persons of the other sex.

heterozygous advantage The condition in which it is more advantageous to have two different versions of a gene than two identical copies.

heterozygous state The state in which an individual has inherited different versions of a particular gene from his or her parents.

homosexual Sexually attracted to persons of one's own sex; gay.

homozygous state The state in which the same version of a gene was inherited from both parents and therefore is present on two homologous chromosomes.

hormone A substance that is secreted by a gland into the bloodstream and that influences the activity or development of tissues elsewhere in the body.

hwame In Mohave culture, a girl who rejects the female role.

hypothalamus A small region at the base of the brain on either side of the third ventricle; it contains cell groups concerned with sexuality and other basic functions.

INAH3 (third interstitial nucleus of the anterior hypothalamus) A cell group in the hypothalamus that differs in size between men and women and between gay and straight men.

index subject A person initially recruited into a study, as opposed to a person drawn into the study later because of a relationship to an index subject.

instrumentality A collection of traits, including assertiveness, competitiveness, aggressiveness, and independence, that tend to be more developed in men than in women.

Kinsey scale A seven-point scale of sexual orientation devised by Alfred Kinsey; it ranges from 0 (exclusively heterosexual) to 6 (exclusively homosexual).

lesbian Homosexual, gay (of women only); a homosexual woman.

linkage study A method of searching for genes that influence a trait. It involves finding genomic markers that are shared at an above-chance frequency by relatives who share the trait. The method can typically identify only regions of interest, not individual genes.

lordosis reflex A sexual behavior, typically shown by female rodents in response to being mounted, in which the animal raises its rump to allow penetration.

mental rotation The ability to tell whether two 2-dimensional drawings represent the same 3-dimensional object viewed from different angles.

monozygotic Of twins, arising from a single fertilized ovum (and thus genetically identical or near-identical).

NELL2 A growth factor involved in the development of the hypothalamus.

neuron A nerve cell—a cell within the nervous system that participates in the processing of information—along with its extensions (axon and dendrites).

nucleus In neuroanatomy, a consistently recognizable cluster or mass of neurons in the brain.

Oedipal homosexuality In psychoanalytic theory, homosexuality resulting from a failure to emerge from the Oedipal phase of psychosexual development.

Oedipal phase In psychoanalytic theory, a period during infancy when a boy is sexually fixated on his mother.

older-brother effect The increased probability of homosexuality in men who have one or more older brothers.

organizational effect An effect of a hormone on the developing brain that influences behavior in later life.

oSDN The sexually dimorphic nucleus in the medial preoptic area of the hypothalamus in sheep.

otoacoustic emission (OAE) A weak sound produced by the cochlea; it may be spontaneous or it may be evoked by clicks.

paraphilia An unusual sexual interest or behavior that is sufficiently distressing or harmful to be considered a mental disorder.

perirhinal cortex An area of cerebral cortex within the temporal lobe that is involved in the encoding of memory, spatial information, and olfaction.

pre-gay children Children who become gay adults.

pre-Oedipal homosexuality In psychoanalytic theory, homosexuality that results from a failure to enter the Oedipal phase.

prepulse inhibition Reduction in the strength of the eye-blink auditory startle response when the startling sound is preceded by a fainter sound.

programmed cell death The "planned" death of a cell or class of cells as the end product of an organized sequence of gene expression.

receptor A molecule or molecular assembly that responds to the presence of a hormone or neurotransmitter.

recessive gene A version of a gene that has little or no apparent effect when present as a single copy.

reparative therapy See *conversion therapy*.

reproductive success The total number of an individual's offspring that survive to maturity.

sex-biased Differing at least to a small degree between the sexes.

sex hormone A hormone that helps regulate sexual function or development. Several important sex hormones are steroids.

sex pheromone A substance produced or released by one individual that affects the sexual feelings or behavior of another individual of the same species.

sexual jealousy Fear that one's partner is physically involved with a third party.

sexually antagonistic model A model explaining the persistence of a gene in which a negative effect of the gene on the reproductive success of one sex is counterbalanced by a positive effect on the reproductive success of the other sex.

sexually dimorphic Differing in structure between males and females.

sexually dimorphic nucleus of the preoptic area (SDN-POA) A cluster of neurons in the medial preoptic area of the hypothalamus that is typically larger in males than in females.

shared environment Any nongenetic influences that promote a trait in both members of a twin pair.

sickle cell anemia A form of anemia caused by the inheritance of two copies of an abnormal gene for hemoglobin.

single-nucleotide polymorphism (SNP) A site in the genome where the identity of a single nucleotide ("letter" of the genetic code) may vary from individual to individual.

Slater's Index A numerical representation of a person's birth order within a sibship, calculated as the number of the person's older siblings divided by his or her total number of siblings.

SRY A gene on the Y chromosome that confers maleness.

standard social science model The idea, prevalent through much of the 20th century, that the human mind starts out as a "blank slate" that is written on by learning and culture.

steroid A class of fatty molecules derived from cholesterol and including the sex hormones testosterone, estrogen, and progesterone.

straight Heterosexual.

suprachiasmatic nucleus A cell group in the hypothalamus that regulates circadian rhythms.

systemizing In the terminology of Simon Baron-Cohen, a male-typical trait involving interest in rule-governed systems.

taxometric analysis A statistical method to look for hidden categories underlying a data set.

testosterone A sex hormone secreted by the testes and the adrenal gland; it is the principal androgen.

thalamus A large group of forebrain nuclei that receive sensory inputs from the neural periphery and are reciprocally connected with the cerebral cortex.

third ventricle A fluid-filled space that occupies the midline of the brain, separating the left and right hypothalami.

top In gay slang, a man who prefers to take the insertive role in anal sex.

transexual (or transsexual) A transgender person who wishes to transition to the other sex or who has already done so.

transgender Having the subjective identity or the social role of a person of the other sex.

trend In statistics, a difference between samples that fails to satisfy a minimum criterion for significance, perhaps because the samples were too small.

two-spirit person In Native American culture, a person who is transgender or who exhibits a mix of male and female characteristics.

unshared environment Any nongenetic influences that promote a trait in one member of a twin pair but not the other.

vomeronasal organ A sensory structure within the nasal cavity of some animals that is involved in the detection of pheromones.

waist/hip ratio The circumference of the body at the waist divided by the circumference of the body at the hips.

white matter Brain tissue containing connecting fibers (axons) but no neuronal cell bodies or synapses.

winkte A biologically male Lakota Indian who adopts a female or mixed-gender role.

X chromosome A sex chromosome of which females in many species, including humans, possess two, while males possess one.

X-linked Of or related to a gene located on the X chromosome, or caused by such a gene.

Y chromosome The smaller of the two sex chromosomes, of which males in many species, including humans, possess one, while females possess none.

BIBLIOGRAPHY

Adkins-Regan, E. (2002). Development of sexual partner preference in the zebra finch: A socially monogamous, pair-bonding animal. *Archives of Sexual Behavior, 31,* 27–33.

Adkins-Regan, E. (2005). *Hormones and animal social behavior.* Princeton University Press.

The Advocate (2005). Outrage over bisexual study. August 30.

Ahmed, E. I., Zehr, J. L., Schulz, K. M., Lorenz, B. H., DonCarlos, L. L. & Sisk, C. L. (2008). Pubertal hormones modulate the addition of new cells to sexually dimorphic brain regions. *Nature Neuroscience, 11,* 995–997.

Alanko, K., Santtila, P., Witting, K., Varjonen, M., Jern, P., Johansson, A., von der Pahlen, B. & Kenneth Sandnabba, N. (2009). Psychiatric symptoms and same-sex sexual attraction and behavior in light of childhood gender atypical behavior and parental relationships. *Journal of Sex Research, 46,* 494–504.

Alexander, G. M. & Hines, M. (2002). Sex differences in response to children's toys in non-human primates (*Cercopithecus aethiops sabaeus*). *Evolution and Human Behavior, 23,* 467–479.

Alexander, G. M., Wilcox, T. & Woods, R. (2009). Sex differences in infants' visual interest in toys. *Archives of Sexual Behavior, 38,* 427–433.

Alison, L., Santtila, P., Sandnabba, N. K. & Nordling, N. (2001). Sadomasochistically oriented behavior: Diversity in practice and meaning. *Archives of Sexual Behavior, 30,* 1–12.

Allen, L. S. & Gorski, R. A. (1992). Sexual orientation and the size of the anterior commissure in the human brain. *Proceedings of the National Academy of Sciences of the United States of America, 89,* 7199–7202.

Allen, L. S., Hines, M., Shryne, J. E. & Gorski, R. A. (1989). Two sexually dimorphic cell groups in the human brain. *Journal of Neuroscience, 9,* 497–506.

Ambady, N., Hallahan, M. & Conner, B. (1999). Accuracy of judgments of sexual orientation from thin slices of behavior. *Journal of Personality and Social Psychology, 77,* 538–547.

American Psychiatric Association (2007). *Just the facts about sexual orientation and youth.* (http://www.apa.org/pi/lgbt/resources/just-the-facts.aspx)

Andersen, J. P. & Blosnich, J. (2013). Disparities in adverse childhood experiences among sexual minority and heterosexual adults: Results from a multi-state probability-based sample. *PLoS One, 8,* e54691.

Anderson, D. K., Rhees, R. W. & Fleming, D. E. (1985). Effects of prenatal stress on differentiation of the sexually dimorphic nucleus of the preoptic area (SDN-POA) of the rat brain. *Brain Research, 332,* 113–118.

Anderssen, N., Amlie, C. & Ytteroy, E. A. (2002). Outcomes for children with lesbian or gay parents. A review of studies from 1978 to 2000. *Scandinavian Journal of Psychology, 43,* 335–351.

Arai, Y., Sekine, Y. & Murakami, S. (1996). Estrogen and apoptosis in the developing sexually dimorphic preoptic area in female rats. *Neuroscience Research, 25*, 403–407.

Arcuri, V. J. (2009a). Channeling Laverne DeFazio. (https://www.frontiersmedia.com/Other/PDF/BackIssues/2726.pdf)

Arcuri, V. J. (2009b). Don't call me queen! (http://becoming-butch.blogspot.com/2009/10/dont-call-me-queen.html)

Arnold, A. P. (2009). Mouse models for evaluating sex chromosome effects that cause sex differences in non-gonadal tissues. *Journal of Neuroendocrinology, 21*, 377–386.

Arnold, A. P. & Breedlove, S. M. (1985). Organizational and activational effects of sex steroids on brain and behavior: A reanalysis. *Hormones and Behavior, 19*, 469–498.

Arnold, A. P., Xu, J., Grisham, W., Chen, X., Kim, Y. H. & Itoh, Y. (2004). Minireview: Sex chromosomes and brain sexual differentiation. *Endocrinology, 145*, 1057–1062.

Asby, D. J., Arlt, W. & Hanley, N. A. (2009). The adrenal cortex and sexual differentiation during early human development. *Reviews in Endocrine and Metabolic Disorders, 10*, 43–49.

Auger, A. P. & Jessen, H. M. (2009). Corepressors, nuclear receptors, and epigenetic factors on DNA: A tail of repression. *Psychoneuroendocrinology, 34(Suppl 1)*, S39–S47.

Auger, A. P., Perrot-Sinal, T. S. & McCarthy, M. M. (2001). Excitatory versus inhibitory GABA as a divergence point in steroid-mediated sexual differentiation of the brain. *Proceedings of the National Academy of Sciences of the United States of America, 98*, 8059–8064.

Auyeung, B., Baron-Cohen, S., Ashwin, E., Knickmeyer, R., Taylor, K., Hackett, G. & Hines, M. (2009). Fetal testosterone predicts sexually differentiated childhood behavior in girls and in boys. *Psychological Science, 20*, 144–148.

Bagemihl, B. (1999). *Biological exuberance: Animal homosexuality and natural diversity.* St. Martin's Press.

Bailey, A. A. & Hurd, P. L. (2005). Finger length ratio (2D:4D) correlates with physical aggression in men but not in women. *Biological Psychology, 68*, 215–222.

Bailey, D. H. & Bailey, J. M. (2013). Poor instruments lead to poor inferences: Comment on Roberts, Glymour, and Koenen (2013). *Archives of Sexual Behavior, 42*, 1649–1652.

Bailey, D. H., Ellingson, J. M. & Bailey, J. M. (2014). Genetic confounds in the study of sexual orientation: Comment on Roberts, Glymour, and Koenen (2014). *Archives of Sexual Behavior, 43*, 1675–1677.

Bailey, J. M. & Bell, A. P. (1993). Familiality of female and male homosexuality. *Behavior Genetics, 23*, 313–322.

Bailey, J. M. & Benishay, D. S. (1993). Familial aggregation of female sexual orientation. *American Journal of Psychiatry, 150*, 272–277.

Bailey, J. M., Bobrow, D., Wolfe, M. & Mikach, S. (1995). Sexual orientation of adult sons of gay fathers. *Developmental Psychology, 31*, 124–129.

Bailey, J. M., Dunne, M. P. & Martin, N. G. (2000). Genetic and environmental influences on sexual orientation and its correlates in an Australian twin sample. *Journal of Personality and Social Psychology, 78*, 524–536.

Bailey, J. M., Gaulin, S., Agyei, Y. & Gladue, B. A. (1994). Effects of gender and sexual orientation on evolutionarily relevant aspects of human mating psychology. *Journal of Personality and Social Psychology, 66*, 1081–1093.

Bailey, J. M., Kim, P. Y., Hills, A. & Linsenmeier, J. A. (1997). Butch, femme, or straight acting? Partner preferences of gay men and lesbians. *Journal of Personality and Social Psychology, 73*, 960–973.

Bailey, J. M. & Oberschneider, M. (1997). Sexual orientation and professional dance. *Archives of Sexual Behavior, 26*, 433–444.

Bailey, J. M. & Pillard, R. C. (1991). A genetic study of male sexual orientation. *Archives of General Psychiatry, 48*, 1089–1096.

Bailey, J. M., Pillard, R. C., Dawood, K., Miller, M. B., Farrer, L. A., Trivedi, S. & Murphy, R. L. (1999). A family history study of male sexual orientation using three independent samples. *Behavior Genetics, 29*, 79–86.

Bailey, J. M., Pillard, R. C., Neale, M. C. & Agyei, Y. (1993). Heritable factors influence sexual orientation in women. *Archives of General Psychiatry, 50*, 217–223.

Bailey, J. M., Willerman, L. & Parks, C. (1991). A test of the maternal stress theory of human male homosexuality. *Archives of Sexual Behavior, 20*, 277–293.

Bailey, J. M. & Zucker, K. J. (1995). Childhood sex-typed behavior and sexual orientation: A conceptual analysis and quantitative review. *Developmental Psychology, 31*, 43–55.

Bakker, J., Brand, T., van Ophemert, J. & Slob, A. K. (1993). Hormonal regulation of adult partner preference behavior in neonatally ATD-treated male rats. *Behavioral Neuroscience, 107*, 480–487.

Bakwin, H. (1968). Deviant gender-role behavior in children: Relation to homosexuality. *Pediatrics, 41*, 620–629.

Baldwin, A., Dodge, B., Schick, V., Hubach, R. D., Bowling, J., Malebranche, D., Goncalves, G., Schnarrs, P. W., Reece, M. & Fortenberry, J. D. (2015). Sexual self-identification among behaviorally bisexual men in the Midwestern United States. *Archives of Sexual Behavior, 44*, 2015–2026.

Balter, M. (2015). Can epigenetics explain homosexuality puzzle? *Science, 350*, 148.

Barthes, J., Crochet, P. A. & Raymond, M. (2015). Male homosexual preference: Where, when, why? *PLoS One, 10*, e0134817.

Barthes, J., Godelle, B. & Raymond, M. (2013). Human social stratification and hypergyny: Toward an understanding of male homosexual preference. *Evolution and Human Behavior, 34*, 155–163.

Barthes, J., Godelle, B. & Raymond, M. (2014). Response to comment on "Human social stratification and hypergyny: Toward an understanding of male." *Evolution and Human Behavior, 35*, 448–450.

Becker, J. B., Breedlove, S. M., Crews, D. & McCarthy, M. M. (Eds.) (2002). *Behavioral endocrinology (2nd ed.).* MIT Press.

Beer, J. & Fleming, P. (1989). Effects of eye color on the accuracy of ball throwing of elementary school children. *Perceptual and Motor Skills, 68*, 163–166.

Bell, A. P. & Weinberg, M. S. (1978). *Homosexualities: A study of diversity in men and women.* Simon and Schuster.

Bell, A. P., Weinberg, M. S. & Hammersmith, S. K. (1981). *Sexual preference: Its development in men and women.* Indiana University Press.

Bem, D. J. (1996). Exotic becomes erotic: A developmental theory of sexual orientation. *Psychological Review, 103*, 320–335.

Bem, D. J. (2000). Exotic becomes erotic: Interpreting the biological correlates of sexual orientation. *Archives of Sexual Behavior, 29*, 531–548.

Bensafi, M., Brown, W. M., Khan, R., Levenson, B. & Sobel, N. (2004). Sniffing human sex-steroid derived compounds modulates mood, memory and autonomic nervous system function in specific behavioral contexts. *Behavioural Brain Research, 152*, 11–22.

Bentz, E. K., Hefler, L. A., Kaufmann, U., Huber, J. C., Kolbus, A. & Tempfer, C. B. (2008). A polymorphism of the *CYP17* gene related to sex steroid metabolism is associated with female-to-male but not male-to-female transsexualism. *Fertility and Sterility, 90*, 56–59.

Berenbaum, S. A. (1999). Effects of early androgens on sex-typed activities and interests in adolescents with congenital adrenal hyperplasia. *Hormones and Behavior, 35*, 102–110.

Berenbaum, S. A. & Bailey, J. M. (2003). Effects on gender identity of prenatal androgens and genital appearance: Evidence from girls with congenital adrenal hyperplasia. *Journal of Clinical Endocrinology and Metabolism, 88*, 1102–1106.

Berenbaum, S. A., Bryk, K. L. & Beltz, A. M. (2012). Early androgen effects on spatial and mechanical abilities: Evidence from congenital adrenal hyperplasia. *Behavioral Neuroscience, 126*, 86–96.

Berenbaum, S. A., Duck, S. C. & Bryk, K. (2000). Behavioral effects of prenatal versus postnatal androgen excess in children with 21-hydroxylase-deficient congenital adrenal hyperplasia. *Journal of Clinical Endocrinology and Metabolism, 85*, 727–733.

Berenbaum, S. A. & Snyder, E. (1995). Early hormonal influences on childhood sex-typed activity and playmate preferences: Implications for the development of sexual orientation. *Developmental Psychology, 31*, 31–42.

Bergen, S. E., Gardner, C. O. & Kendler, K. S. (2007). Age-related changes in heritability of behavioral phenotypes over adolescence and young adulthood: A meta-analysis. *Twin Research and Human Genetics*, *10*, 423–433.

Berglin, C. G. (1982). Birth order as a quantitative expression of date of birth. *Journal of Epidemiology and Community Health*, *36*, 298–302.

Berglund, H., Lindström, P., Dhejne-Helmy, C. & Savic, I. (2008). Male-to-female transsexuals show sex-atypical hypothalamus activation when smelling odorous steroids. *Cerebral Cortex*, *18*, 1900–1908.

Berglund, H., Lindström, P. & Savic, I. (2006). Brain response to putative pheromones in lesbian women. *Proceedings of the National Academy of Sciences of the United States of America*, *103*, 8269–8274.

Berman, P. W., Monda, L. C. & Myerscough, R. P. (1977). Sex differences in young children's responses to an infant: An observation within a day-care setting. *Child Development*, *48*, 711–715.

Berninger, E. (2007). Characteristics of normal newborn transient-evoked otoacoustic emissions: Ear asymmetries and sex effects. *International Journal of Audiology*, *46*, 661–669.

Besli, R., Saylam, C., Veral, A., Karl, B. & Ozek, C. (2004). The existence of the vomeronasal organ in human beings. *Journal of Craniofacial Surgery*, *15*, 730–735.

Bilger, R. C., Matthies, M. L., Hammel, D. R. & Demorest, M. E. (1990). Genetic implications of gender differences in the prevalence of spontaneous otoacoustic emissions. *Journal of Speech and Hearing Research*, *33*, 418–432.

Blanchard, R. (1991). Clinical observations and systematic studies of autogynephilia. *Journal of Sex and Marital Therapy*, *17*, 235–251.

Blanchard, R. (2004). Quantitative and theoretical analyses of the relation between older brothers and homosexuality in men. *Journal of Theoretical Biology*, *230*, 173–187.

Blanchard, R. (2007a). Older-sibling and younger-sibling sex ratios in Frisch and Hviid's (2006) national cohort study of two million Danes. *Archives of Sexual Behavior*, *36*, 860–863; discussion 864–867.

Blanchard, R. (2007b). Supplementary analyses regarding Langevin, Langevin, and Curnoe's (2007) findings on fraternal birth order in homosexual men. *Archives of Sexual Behavior*, *36*, 610–614; discussion 615–616.

Blanchard, R. (2014). Detecting and correcting for family size differences in the study of sexual orientation and fraternal birth order. *Archives of Sexual Behavior*, *43*, 845–852.

Blanchard, R., Barbaree, H. E., Bogaert, A. F., Dickey, R., Klassen, P., Kuban, M. E. & Zucker, K. J. (2000). Fraternal birth order and sexual orientation in pedophiles. *Archives of Sexual Behavior*, *29*, 463–478.

Blanchard, R. & Bogaert, A. F. (1996a). Biodemographic comparisons of homosexual and heterosexual men in the Kinsey Interview Data. *Archives of Sexual Behavior*, *25*, 551–579.

Blanchard, R. & Bogaert, A. F. (1996b). Homosexuality in men and number of older brothers. *American Journal of Psychiatry*, *153*, 27–31.

Blanchard, R. & Bogaert, A. F. (1998). Birth order in homosexual versus heterosexual sex offenders against children, pubescents, and adults. *Archives of Sexual Behavior*, *27*, 595–603.

Blanchard, R. & Bogaert, A. F. (2004). Proportion of homosexual men who owe their sexual orientation to fraternal birth order: An estimate based on two national probability samples. *American Journal of Human Biology*, *16*, 151–157.

Blanchard, R., Cantor, J. M., Bogaert, A. F., Breedlove, S. M. & Ellis, L. (2006). Interaction of fraternal birth order and handedness in the development of male homosexuality. *Hormones and Behavior*, *49*, 405–414.

Blanchard, R. & Ellis, L. (2001). Birth weight, sexual orientation and the sex of preceding siblings. *Journal of Biosocial Science*, *33*, 451–467.

Blanchard, R. & Lippa, R. A. (2007). Birth order, sibling sex ratio, handedness, and sexual orientation of male and female participants in a BBC Internet research project. *Archives of Sexual Behavior*, *36*, 163–176.

Blanchard, R. & Lippa, R. A. (2008). The sex ratio of older siblings in non-right-handed homosexual men. *Archives of Sexual Behavior, 37*, 970–976.

Blanchard, R., McConkey, J. G., Roper, V. & Steiner, B. W. (1983). Measuring physical aggressiveness in heterosexual, homosexual, and transsexual males. *Archives of Sexual Behavior, 12*, 511–524.

Blanchard, R. & Sheridan, P. M. (1992). Sibship size, sibling sex ratio, birth order, and parental age in homosexual and nonhomosexual gender dysphorics. *Journal of Nervous and Mental Disease, 180*, 40–47.

Blanchard, R., VanderLaan, D. P., Skorska, M., Zucker, K. J. & Bogaert, A. F. (2016). Possible separate etiology of homosexuality in gay male only-children. *Archives of Sexual Behavior (in preparation)*.

Blanchard, R. & Zucker, K. J. (1994). Reanalysis of Bell, Weinberg, and Hammersmith's data on birth order, sibling sex ratio, and parental age in homosexual men. *American Journal of Psychiatry, 151*, 1375–1376.

Blanchard, R., Zucker, K. J., Bradley, S. J. & Hume, C. S. (1995). Birth order and sibling sex ratio in homosexual male adolescents and probably prehomosexual feminine boys. *Developmental Psychology, 31*, 22–30.

Blanchard, R., Zucker, K. J., Siegelman, M., Dickey, R. & Klassen, P. (1998). The relation of birth order to sexual orientation in men and women. *Journal of Biosocial Science, 30*, 511–519.

Bloomekatz, A. B. (2009). Fairfax High's prom queen is a guy. *Los Angeles Times*, May 28.

Bobrow, D. & Bailey, J. M. (2001). Is male homosexuality maintained via kin selection? *Evolution and Human Behavior, 22*, 361–368.

Bocklandt, S., Horvath, S., Vilain, E. & Hamer, D. H. (2006). Extreme skewing of X chromosome inactivation in mothers of homosexual men. *Human Genetics, 118*, 691–694.

Bocklandt, S. & Vilain, E. (2007). Sex differences in brain and behavior: Hormones versus genes. *Advances in Genetics, 59*, 245–266.

Bodo, C. & Rissman, E. F. (2007). Androgen receptor is essential for sexual differentiation of responses to olfactory cues in mice. *European Journal of Neuroscience, 25*, 2182–2190.

Bogaert, A. F. (1998). Physical development and sexual orientation in women: Height, weight, and age of puberty comparisons. *Personality and Individual Differences, 24*, 115–121.

Bogaert, A. F. (2003). Number of older brothers and sexual orientation: New tests and the attraction/behavior distinction in two national probability samples. *Journal of Personality and Social Psychology, 84*, 644–652.

Bogaert, A. F. (2004a). Asexuality: Prevalence and associated factors in a national probability sample. *Journal of Sex Research, 41*, 279–287.

Bogaert, A. F. (2004b). The prevalence of male homosexuality: The effect of fraternal birth order and variations in family size. *Journal of Theoretical Biology, 230*, 33–37.

Bogaert, A. F. (2006a). Biological versus nonbiological older brothers and men's sexual orientation. *Proceedings of the National Academy of Sciences of the United States of America, 103*, 10771–10774.

Bogaert, A. F. (2006b). Toward a conceptual understanding of asexuality. *Review of General Psychology, 10*, 241–250.

Bogaert, A. F. (2007). Extreme right-handedness, older brothers, and sexual orientation in men. *Neuropsychology, 21*, 141–148.

Bogaert, A. F. (2010). Physical development and sexual orientation in men and women: An analysis of NATSAL-2000. *Archives of Sexual Behavior, 39*, 110–116.

Bogaert, A. F., Bezeau, S., Kuban, M. & Blanchard, R. (1997). Pedophilia, sexual orientation, and birth order. *Journal of Abnormal Psychology, 106*, 331–335.

Bogaert, A. F. & Blanchard, R. (1996). Physical development and sexual orientation in men: Height, weight and age of puberty differences. *Personality and Individual Differences, 21*, 77–84.

Bogaert, A. F., Blanchard, R. & Crosthwait, L. E. (2007). Interaction of birth order, handedness, and sexual orientation in the Kinsey interview data. *Behavioral Neuroscience, 121*, 845–853.

Bogaert, A. F. & Friesen, C. (2002). Sexual orientation and height, weight, and age of puberty: New tests from a British national probability sample. *Biological Psychology, 59,* 135–145.

Bogaert, A. F. & Hershberger, S. (1999). The relation between sexual orientation and penile size. *Archives of Sexual Behavior, 28,* 213–221.

Bogaert, A. F. & Liu, J. (2013). Physical size and sexual orientation: Analysis of the Chinese Health and Family Life Survey. *Archives of Sexual Behavior, 42,* 1555–1559.

Bogaert, A. F., Skorska, M., Wang, C., Gabrie, J., Zucker, K., VanderLaan, D. & Blanchard, R. (2015). A test of the maternal immune hypothesis of men's sexual orientation. Abstracts, Puzzle of Sexual Orientation Conference, University of Lethbridge, p. 27.

Bouchard, T. J., Jr. (1984). Twins reared together and apart: What they tell us about human diversity. In: Fox, S. W. (Ed.), *Individuality and determinism.* Plenum Press.

Bouchard, T. J. (2004). Genetic influence on human psychological traits: A survey. *Current Directions in Psychological Science, 13,* 148–151.

Bouchard, J., Foulon, C., Storm, N., Nguyen, G. H. & Smith, C. L. (1999). Analyzing genomic DNA discordance between monozygotic twins. In: Crusio, W. E. & Gerlai, R. T. (Eds.), *Handbook of molecular-genetic techniques for brain and behavior research (Techniques in the behavioral and neural sciences, vol. 13).* Elsevier.

Bourne, V. J. & Maxwell, A. M. (2010). Examining the sex difference in lateralisation for processing facial emotion: Does biological sex or psychological gender identity matter? *Neuropsychologia, 48,* 1289–1294.

Bozkurt, A., Bozkurt, O. H. & Sonmez, I. (2015). Birth order and sibling sex ratio in a population with high fertility: Are Turkish male to female transsexuals different? *Archives of Sexual Behavior, 44,* 1331–1337.

Bradley, S. J., Oliver, G. D., Chernick, A. B. & Zucker, K. J. (1998). Experiment of nurture: Ablatio penis at 2 months, sex reassignment at 7 months, and a psychosexual follow-up in young adulthood. *Pediatrics, 102,* e9.

Braggio, J. T., Nadler, R. D., Lance, J. & Miseyko, D. (1978). Sex differences in apes and children. *Recent Advances in Primatology, 1,* 529–532.

Brakefield, T. A., Mednick, S. C., Wilson, H. W., De Neve, J. E., Christakis, N. A. & Fowler, J. H. (2014). Same-sex sexual attraction does not spread in adolescent social networks. *Archives of Sexual Behavior, 43,* 335–344.

Bramble, M. S., Roach, L., Eskin, A., Lipson, A., Ngun, T., Vashist, N., Klein, S., Gosschalk, J. E., Barseghyan, H., Arboleda, V. A. & Vilain, E. (2016). Sex-specific-effects of testosterone on the sexually dimorphic transcriptome of embryonic neural stem progenitor cells. *(In preparation.)*

Brand, G. & Millot, J. L. (2001). Sex differences in human olfaction: Between evidence and enigma. *Quarterly Journal of Experimental Psychology B: Comparative and Physiological Psychology, 54,* 259–270.

Breedlove, S. M. (2016). The science of sexual orientation: Where are we and where are we going? *Archives of Sexual Behavior (in preparation).*

Brotto, L. A. (2016). Asexuality: Orientation, paraphilia, dysfunction, or none of the above. *Archives of Sexual Behavior (in preparation).*

Brotto, L. A., Knudson, G., Inskip, J., Rhodes, K. & Erskine, Y. (2010). Asexuality: A mixed-methods approach. *Archives of Sexual Behavior, 39,* 599–618.

Brown, W. M., Finn, C. J., Cooke, B. M. & Breedlove, S. M. (2002a). Differences in finger length ratios between self-identified "butch" and "femme" lesbians. *Archives of Sexual Behavior, 31,* 123–127.

Brown, W. M., Hines, M., Fane, B. A. & Breedlove, S. M. (2002b). Masculinized finger length patterns in human males and females with congenital adrenal hyperplasia. *Hormones and Behavior, 42,* 380–386.

Buck, J. J., Williams, R. M., Hughes, I. A. & Acerini, C. L. (2003). In-utero androgen exposure and 2nd to 4th digit length ratio—comparisons between healthy controls and females with classical congenital adrenal hyperplasia. *Human Reproduction, 18,* 976–979.

Burke, S. M., Cohen-Kettenis, P. T., Veltman, D. J., Klink, D. T. & Bakker, J. (2014a). Hypothalamic response to the chemo-signal androstadienone in gender dysphoric children and adolescents. *Frontiers in Endocrinology (Lausanne), 5*, 60.

Burke, S. M., Menks, W. M., Cohen-Kettenis, P. T., Klink, D. T. & Bakker, J. (2014b). Click-evoked otoacoustic emissions in children and adolescents with gender identity disorder. *Archives of Sexual Behavior, 43*, 1515–1523.

Burke, S. M., Veltman, D. J., Gerber, J., Hummel, T. & Bakker, J. (2012). Heterosexual men and women both show a hypothalamic response to the chemo-signal androstadienone. *PLoS One, 7*, e40993.

Buss, D. M. (1989). Sex differences in human mate preference: Evolutionary hypothesis tested in 37 cultures. *Behavioral and Brain Sciences, 12*, 1–149.

Buss, D. M. (2000). *The dangerous passion: Why jealousy is as necessary as love and sex.* Free Press.

Buss, R. R., Sun, W. & Oppenheim, R. W. (2006). Adaptive roles of programmed cell death during nervous system development. *Annual Review of Neuroscience, 29*, 1–35.

Butcher, L. M., Davis, O. S., Craig, I. W. & Plomin, R. (2008). Genome-wide quantitative trait locus association scan of general cognitive ability using pooled DNA and 500K single nucleotide polymorphism microarrays. *Genes, Brain and Behavior, 7*, 435–446.

Byne, W. (1998). The medial preoptic and anterior hypothalamic regions of the rhesus monkey: Cytoarchitectonic comparison with the human and evidence for sexual dimorphism. *Brain Research, 793*, 346–350.

Byne, W., Lasco, M. S., Kemether, E., Shinwari, A., Edgar, M. A., Morgello, S., Jones, L. B. & Tobet, S. (2000). The interstitial nuclei of the human anterior hypothalamus: An investigation of sexual variation in volume and cell size, number and density. *Brain Research, 856*, 254–258.

Byne, W., Tobet, S., Mattiace, L. A., Lasco, M. S., Kemether, E., Edgar, M. A., Morgello, S., Buchsbaum, M. S. & Jones, L. B. (2001). The interstitial nuclei of the human anterior hypothalamus: An investigation of variation with sex, sexual orientation, and HIV status. *Hormones and Behavior, 40*, 86–92.

Cahill, L. (2005). His brain, her brain. *Scientific American, 292*(5), 49–63.

Cameron, P. & Cameron, K. (1995). Does incest cause homosexuality? *Psychological Reports, 76*, 611–621.

Camperio Ciani, A., Cermelli, P. & Zanzotto, G. (2008). Sexually antagonistic selection in human male homosexuality. *PLoS One, 3*, e2282.

Camperio-Ciani, A., Corna, F. & Capiluppi, C. (2004). Evidence for maternally inherited factors favouring male homosexuality and promoting female fecundity. *Proceedings of the Royal Society of London Series B: Biological Sciences, 271*, 2217–2221.

Camperio Ciani, A. & Pellizzari, E. (2012). Fecundity of paternal and maternal non-parental female relatives of homosexual and heterosexual men. *PLoS One, 7*, e51088.

Canovas, R. & Cimadevilla, J. M. (2011). Sexual orientation and spatial memory. *Psicothema, 23*, 752–758.

Cantor, J. M., Blanchard, R., Christensen, B. K., Dickey, R., Klassen, P. E., Beckstead, A. L., Blak, T. & Kuban, M. E. (2004). Intelligence, memory, and handedness in pedophilia. *Neuropsychology, 18*, 3–14.

Cantor, J. M., Blanchard, R., Paterson, A. D. & Bogaert, A. F. (2002). How many gay men owe their sexual orientation to fraternal birth order? *Archives of Sexual Behavior, 31*, 63–71.

Cantor, J. M., Kabani, N., Christensen, B. K., Zipursky, R. B., Barbaree, H. E., Dickey, R., Klassen, P. E., Mikulis, D. J., Kuban, M. E., Blak, T., Richards, B. A., Hanratty, M. K. & Blanchard, R. (2008). Cerebral white matter deficiencies in pedophilic men. *Journal of Psychiatric Research, 42*, 167–183.

Cantor, J. M., Kuban, M. E., Blak, T., Klassen, P. E., Dickey, R. & Blanchard, R. (2007). Physical height in pedophilic and hebephilic sexual offenders. *Sexual Abuse, 19*, 395–407.

Cantor, J. M., Lafaille, S., Soh, D. W., Moayedi, M., Mikulis, D. J. & Girard, T. A. (2015). Diffusion tensor imaging of pedophilia. *Archives of Sexual Behavior, 44*, 2161–2172.

Cardoso, F. L. (2008). Recalled sex-typed behavior in childhood and sports' preferences in adulthood of heterosexual, bisexual, and homosexual men from Brazil, Turkey, and Thailand. *Archives of Sexual Behavior, 38*, 726–736.

Cattrall, F. R., Vollenhoven, B. J. & Weston, G. C. (2005). Anatomical evidence for in utero androgen exposure in women with polycystic ovary syndrome. *Fertility and Sterility, 84*, 1689–1692.

Cellot, G. & Cherubini, E. (2013). Functional role of ambient GABA in refining neuronal circuits early in postnatal development. *Frontiers in Neural Circuits, 7*, 136.

Cerny, J. A. & Janssen, E. (2011). Patterns of sexual arousal in homosexual, bisexual, and heterosexual men. *Archives of Sexual Behavior, 40*, 687–697.

Chandra, A., Mosher, W. D., Copen, C. & Sionean, C. (2011). *Sexual behavior, sexual attraction, and sexual identity in the United States: Data from the 2006–2008 National Survey of Family Growth.* (http://www.cdc.gov/nchs/data/nhsr/nhsr036.pdf)

Chapman, E., Baron-Cohen, S., Auyeung, B., Knickmeyer, R., Taylor, K. & Hackett, G. (2006). Fetal testosterone and empathy: Evidence from the empathy quotient (EQ) and the "reading the mind in the eyes" test. *Social Neuroscience, 1*, 135–148.

Chauncey, G. (1994). *Gay New York: Gender, urban culture and the making of the gay male world.* Basic Books.

Chekroud, A. M., Ward, E. J., Rosenberg, M. D. & Holmes, A. J. (2016). Patterns in the human brain mosaic discriminate males from females. *Proceedings of the National Academy of Sciences of the United States of America, Online ahead of print, March 16.*

Chivers, M. (2016). Sexual psychophysiology and its complicated relationship with women's sexual orientation. *Archives of Sexual Behavior (in preparation).*

Chivers, M. L., Rieger, G., Latty, E. & Bailey, J. M. (2004). A sex difference in the specificity of sexual arousal. *Psychological Science, 15*, 736–744.

Chivers, M. L., Seto, M. C. & Blanchard, R. (2007). Gender and sexual orientation differences in sexual response to sexual activities versus gender of actors in sexual films. *Journal of Personality and Social Psychology, 93*, 1108–1121.

Chivers, M. L., Seto, M. C., Lalumière, M. L., Laan, E. & Grimbos, T. (2010). Agreement of self-reported and genital measures of sexual arousal in men and women: A meta-analysis. *Archives of Sexual Behavior, 39*, 5–56.

Choi, G. B., Dong, H. W., Murphy, A. J., Valenzuela, D. M., Yancopoulos, G. D., Swanson, L. W. & Anderson, D. J. (2005). Lhx6 delineates a pathway mediating innate reproductive behaviors from the amygdala to the hypothalamus. *Neuron, 46*, 647–660.

Churchill, W. (1967). *Homosexual behavior among males: A cross-cultural and cross-species investigation.* Hawthorn Books.

Ciumas, C., Linden Hirschberg, A. & Savic, I. (2009). High fetal testosterone and sexually dimorphic cerebral networks in females. *Cerebral Cortex, 19*, 1167–1174.

Clark, G. (2007). *A farewell to alms: A brief economic history of the world.* Princeton University Press.

Clarkson, J. & Herbison, A. E. (2016). Hypothalamic control of the male neonatal testosterone surge. *Philosophical Transactions of the Royal Society of London Series B: Biological Sciences, 371, Online ahead of print, December 18.*

Clemens, L. G., Gladue, B. A. & Coniglio, L. P. (1978). Prenatal endogenous androgenic influences on masculine sexual behavior and genital morphology in male and female rats. *Hormones and Behavior, 10*, 40–53.

Coffman, K. B., Coffman, L. C. & Marzilli Ericson, K. M., (2013). *The size of the LGBT population and the magnitude of anti-gay sentiment are substantially underestimated.* National Bureau of Economic Research Working Paper no. 19508. (https://www.nber.org/papers/w19508)

Cohen-Bendahan, C. C., van de Beek, C. & Berenbaum, S. A. (2005). Prenatal sex hormone effects on child and adult sex-typed behavior: Methods and findings. *Neuroscience and Biobehavioral Reviews, 29*, 353–384.

Colapinto, J. (2000). *As nature made him: The boy who was raised as a girl.* HarperCollins.

Collaer, M. L., Reimers, S. & Manning, J. T. (2007). Visuospatial performance on an Internet line judgment task and potential hormonal markers: Sex, sexual orientation, and 2D:4D. *Archives of Sexual Behavior, 36*, 177–192.

Commins, D. & Yahr, P. (1984). Adult testosterone levels influence the morphology of a sexually dimorphic area in the Mongolian gerbil brain. *Journal of Comparative Neurology*, *224*, 132–140.

Compaan, J. C., Hutchison, J. B., Wozniak, A., de Ruiter, A. J. & Koolhaas, J. M. (1994). Brain aromatase activity and plasma testosterone levels are elevated in aggressive male mice during early ontogeny. *Brain Research Developmental Brain Research*, *82*, 185–192.

Connellan, J., Baron-Cohen, S., Wheelwright, S., Batki, A. & Ahluwalia, J. (2001). Sex differences in human neonatal social perception. *Infant Behavior and Development*, *23*, 113–118.

Conservapedia (2015). Homosexuality and choice. (http://www.conservapedia.com/ Homosexuality_and_choice)

Cooke, B. M., Chowanadisai, W. & Breedlove, S. M. (2000). Post-weaning social isolation of male rats reduces the volume of the medial amygdala and leads to deficits in adult sexual behavior. *Behavioural Brain Research*, *117*, 107–113.

Cooke, B. M., Tabibnia, G. & Breedlove, S. M. (1999). A brain sexual dimorphism controlled by adult circulating androgens. *Proceedings of the National Academy of Sciences of the United States of America*, *96*, 7538–7540.

Cooke, B. M. & Woolley, C. S. (2005a). Gonadal hormone modulation of dendrites in the mammalian CNS. *Journal of Neurobiology*, *64*, 34–46.

Cooke, B. M. & Woolley, C. S. (2005b). Sexually dimorphic synaptic organization of the medial amygdala. *Journal of Neuroscience*, *25*, 10759–10767.

Corliss, H. L., Cochran, S. D. & Mays, V. M. (2002). Reports of parental maltreatment during childhood in a United States population-based survey of homosexual, bisexual, and heterosexual adults. *Child Abuse and Neglect*, *26*, 1165–1178.

Cosgrove, K. P., Mazure, C. M. & Staley, J. K. (2007). Evolving knowledge of sex differences in brain structure, function, and chemistry. *Biological Psychiatry*, *62*, 847–855.

Costa, P. T., Jr., Terracciano, A. & McCrae, R. R. (2001). Gender differences in personality traits across cultures: Robust and surprising findings. *Journal of Personality and Social Psychology*, *81*, 322–331.

Cote, K., Blanchard, R. & Lalumière, M. L. (2003). The influence of birth order on birth weight: Does the sex of preceding siblings matter? *Journal of Biosocial Science*, *35*, 455–462.

Cox, W. T. L., Devine, P. G., Bischmann, A. A. & Hyde, J. S. (2016). Inferences about sexual orientation: The roles of stereotypes, faces, and the gaydar myth. *Journal of Sex Research*, *53*, 157–171.

Croy, I., Bojanowski, V. & Hummel, T. (2013). Men without a sense of smell exhibit a strongly reduced number of sexual relationships, women exhibit reduced partnership security: A reanalysis of previously published data. *Biological Psychology*, *92*, 292–294.

Croy, I., Negoias, S., Novakova, L., Landis, B. N. & Hummel, T. (2012). Learning about the functions of the olfactory system from people without a sense of smell. *PLoS One*, *7*, e33365.

Currin, J. M., Gibson, L. & Hubach, R. D. (2015). Multidimensional assessment of sexual orientation and the fraternal birth order effect. *Psychology of Sexual Orientation and Gender Diversity*, *2*, 113–122.

Darmaillacq, A.-S., Chichery, R., Shashar, N. & Dickel, L. (2005). Early socialization overrides innate prey preference in newly hatched *Sepia officinalis* cuttlefish. *Animal Behaviour*, *71*, 511–514.

Daskalos, C. T. (1998). Changes in the sexual orientation of six heterosexual male-to-female transsexuals. *Archives of Sexual Behavior*, *27*, 605–614.

Davis, A. M., Grattan, D. R. & McCarthy, M. M. (2000). Decreasing GAD neonatally attenuates steroid-induced sexual differentiation of the rat brain. *Behavioral Neuroscience*, *114*, 923–933.

Davis, E. C., Popper, P. & Gorski, R. A. (1996a). The role of apoptosis in sexual differentiation of the rat sexually dimorphic nucleus of the preoptic area. *Brain Research*, *734*, 10–18.

Davis, E. C., Shryne, J. E. & Gorski, R. A. (1995). A revised critical period for the sexual differentiation of the sexually dimorphic nucleus of the preoptic area in the rat. *Neuroendocrinology*, *62*, 579–585.

Davis, E. C., Shryne, J. E. & Gorski, R. A. (1996b). Structural sexual dimorphisms in the antero-ventral periventricular nucleus of the rat hypothalamus are sensitive to gonadal steroids perinatally, but develop peripubertally. *Neuroendocrinology, 63,* 142–148.

Dawood, K., Pillard, R. C., Horvath, C., Revelle, W. & Bailey, J. M. (2000). Familial aspects of male homosexuality. *Archives of Sexual Behavior, 29,* 155–163.

Dawson, S. J., Sawatsky, M. L. & Lalumière, M. L. (2015). Assessment of introital lubrication. *Archives of Sexual Behavior, 44,* 1527–1535.

de Jonge, F. H., Muntjewerff, J. W., Louwerse, A. L. & van de Poll, N. E. (1988). Sexual behavior and sexual orientation of the female rat after hormonal treatment during various stages of development. *Hormones and Behavior, 22,* 100–115.

De Lorme, K., Bell, M. R. & Sisk, C. L. (2013). The teenage brain: Social reorientation and the adolescent brain—the role of gonadal hormones in the male Syrian hamster. *Current Directions in Psychological Science, 22,* 128–133.

de Rooij, S. R., Painter, R. C., Swaab, D. F. & Roseboom, T. J. (2009). Sexual orientation and gender identity after prenatal exposure to the Dutch famine. *Archives of Sexual Behavior, 38,* 411–416.

de Waal, F. B. M. (1995). Bonobo sex and society. *Scientific American, 272*(3), 82–88.

Del Giudice, M. (2015). Gender differences in personality and social behavior. In: Wright, J. D. (Ed.), *International Encyclopedia of the Social & Behavioral Sciences (2nd ed.), vol. 9.* Elsevier, pp. 750–756.

Demir, E. & Dickson, B. J. (2005). *fruitless* splicing specifies male courtship behavior in *Drosophila. Cell, 121,* 785–794.

Diamond, L. M. (2003). Was it a phase? Young women's relinquishment of lesbian/bisexual identities over a 5-year period. *Journal of Personality and Social Psychology, 84,* 352–364.

Diamond, L. M. (2008). *Sexual fluidity: Understanding women's love and desire.* Harvard University Press.

Diamond, L. M. (2016). Are women more sexually fluid than men? *Archives of Sexual Behavior (in preparation).*

Diamond, M. (2013). Transsexuality among twins: Identity concordance, transition, rearing, and orientation. *International Journal of Transgenderism, 14,* 24–38.

Diamond, M. & Sigmundson, H. K. (1997). Sex reassignment at birth. Long-term review and clinical implications. *Archives of Pediatrics and Adolescent Medicine, 151,* 298–304.

Dickson, N., Paul, C. & Herbison, P. (2003). Same-sex attraction in a birth cohort: Prevalence and persistence in early adulthood. *Social Science and Medicine, 56,* 1607–1615.

Dörner, G. (1969). Zur Frage einer neuroendocrinen Pathogenese, Prophylaxe und Therapie angeborenen Sexualdeviationen. *Deutsche Medizinische Wochenschrift, 94,* 390–396.

Dörner, G. (1989/2001). Proposal for changing the status of homosexuality under the W.H.O.'s classification of diseases. *Neuroendocrinology Letters, 22,* 410.

Dörner, G., Geier, T., Ahrens, L., Krell, L., Munx, G., Sieler, H., Kittner, E. & Muller, H. (1980). Prenatal stress as possible aetiogenetic factor of homosexuality in human males. *Endokrinologie, 75,* 365–368.

Dörner, G., Poppe, I., Stahl, F., Kolzsch, J. & Uebelhack, R. (1991). Gene- and environment-dependent neuroendocrine etiogenesis of homosexuality and transsexualism. *Experimental and Clinical Endocrinology, 98,* 141–150.

Dörner, G., Schenk, B., Schmiedel, B. & Ahrens, L. (1983). Stressful events in prenatal life of bi- and homosexual men. *Experimental and Clinical Endocrinology, 81,* 83–87.

Dover, K. J. (1978). *Greek homosexuality.* Harvard University Press.

Drabant, E. M., Kiefer, A. K., Eriksson, N., Mountain, J. L., Francke, U., Tung, J. Y., Hinds, D. A. & Do, C. B. (2012). *Genome-wide association study of sexual orientation in a large, Web-based cohort.* (http://blog.23andme.com/wp-content/uploads/2012/11/Drabant-Poster-v7.pdf)

Dreger, A., Feder, E. K. & Tamar-Mattis, A. (2012). Prenatal dexamethasone for congenital adrenal hyperplasia: An ethics canary in the modern medical mine. *Journal of Bioethical Inquiry, 9,* 277–294.

Drummond, K. D., Bradley, S. J., Peterson-Badali, M. & Zucker, K. J. (2008). A follow-up study of girls with gender identity disorder. *Developmental Psychology, 44,* 34–45.

Dugger, B. N., Morris, J. A., Jordan, C. L. & Breedlove, S. M. (2008). Gonadal steroids regulate neural plasticity in the sexually dimorphic nucleus of the preoptic area of adult male and female rats. *Neuroendocrinology, 88*, 17–24.

DuPree, M. G., Mustanski, B. S., Bocklandt, S., Nievergelt, C. & Hamer, D. H. (2004). A candidate gene study of *CYP19* (aromatase) and male sexual orientation. *Behavior Genetics, 34*, 243–250.

Eaton, W. O. & Enns, R. (1986). Sex differences in human motor activity level. *Psychological Bulletin, 100*, 19–28.

Eblex Sheep Better Returns Program (2008). Target ewe fertility for better returns. (http://www.eblex.org.uk/wp/wp-content/uploads/2013/05/Manual-11-Target-ewe-fertility-for-better-returns.pdf)

Ebsworth, M. & Lalumière, M. L. (2012). Viewing time as a measure of bisexual sexual interest. *Archives of Sexual Behavior, 41*, 161–172.

Eckert, E. D., Bouchard, T. J., Bohlen, J. & Heston, L. L. (1986). Homosexuality in monozygotic twins reared apart. *British Journal of Psychiatry, 148*, 421–425.

Eckes, T. & Trautner, H. M. (Eds.) (2000). *The developmental social psychology of gender.* Lawrence Erlbaum.

Eggers, S. & Sinclair, A. (2012). Mammalian sex determination—insights from humans and mice. *Chromosome Research, 20*, 215–238.

Ellis, L. & Ames, M. A. (1987). Neurohormonal functioning and sexual orientation: A theory of homosexuality–heterosexuality. *Psychological Bulletin, 101*, 233–258.

Ellis, L., Ames, M. A., Peckham, W. & Ahrens, L. (1988). Sexual orientation of human offspring may be altered by severe maternal stress during pregnancy. *Journal of Sex Research, 25*, 152–157.

Ellis, L. & Blanchard, R. (2001). Birth order, sibling sex ratio, and maternal miscarriages in homosexual and heterosexual men and women. *Personality and Individual Differences, 30*, 543–552.

Ellis, L., Hoffman, H. & Burke, D. M. (1990). Sex, sexual orientation and criminal and violent behavior. *Personality and Individual Differences, 11*, 1207–1211.

Estes, Z. & Felker, S. (2012). Confidence mediates the sex difference in mental rotation performance. *Archives of Sexual Behavior, 41*, 557–570.

Eysenck, H. J. (1985). *Decline and fall of the Freudian empire.* Viking.

Faderman, L. (1991). *Odd girls and twilight lovers: A history of lesbian life in twentieth-century America.* Columbia University Press.

Fagot, B. I., Leinbach, M. D. & O'Boyle, C. (1992). Gender labeling, gender stereotyping, and parenting behaviors. *Developmental Psychology, 28*, 440–443.

Fernandez, R., Esteva, I., Gomez-Gil, E., Rumbo, T., Almaraz, M. C., Roda, E., Haro-Mora, J. J., Guillamon, A. & Pasaro, E. (2014). Association study of *ERbeta, AR*, and *CYP19A1* genes and MtF transsexualism. *Journal of Sexual Medicine, 11*, 2986–2994.

Ferveur, J. F., Savarit, F., O'Kane, C. J., Sureau, G., Greenspan, R. J. & Jallon, J. M. (1997). Genetic feminization of pheromones and its behavioral consequences in *Drosophila* males. *Science, 276*, 1555–1558.

Finley, K. D., Taylor, B. J., Milstein, M. & McKeown, M. (1997). *dissatisfaction*, a gene involved in sex-specific behavior and neural development of *Drosophila melanogaster*. *Proceedings of the National Academy of Sciences of the United States of America, 94*, 913–918.

Fleischman, D. S., Fessler, D. M. & Cholakians, A. E. (2015). Testing the affiliation hypothesis of homoerotic motivation in humans: The effects of progesterone and priming. *Archives of Sexual Behavior, 44*, 1395–1404.

Ford, J. J. (1983). Postnatal differentiation of sexual preference in male pigs. *Hormones and Behavior, 17*, 152–162.

Forger, N. G. (2009). Control of cell number in the sexually dimorphic brain and spinal cord. *Journal of Neuroendocrinology, 21*, 393–399.

Forger, N. G. (2016). Epigenetic mechanisms in sexual differentiation of the brain and behaviour. *Philosophical Transactions of the Royal Society of London Series B: Biological Sciences, 371*, Online ahead of print, February 19.

Forger, N. G., Rosen, G. J., Waters, E. M., Jacob, D., Simerly, R. B. & de Vries, G. J. (2004). Deletion of *Bax* eliminates sex differences in the mouse forebrain. *Proceedings of the National Academy of Sciences of the United States of America, 101,* 13666–13671.

Francis, A. M. (2008). Family and sexual orientation: The family-demographic correlates of homosexuality in men and women. *Journal of Sex Research, 45,* 371–377.

Frederick, D. A. & Fales, M. R. (2014). Upset over sexual versus emotional infidelity among gay, lesbian, bisexual, and heterosexual adults. *Archives of Sexual Behavior, Online ahead of print, December 18.*

Freud, S. (1905/1975). *Three essays on the theory of sexuality.* Basic Books.

Freud, S. (1920/1955). The psychogenesis of a case of homosexuality in a woman. In: Strachey, J. (Ed.), *The standard edition of the complete works of Sigmund Freud, vol. 18.* Hogarth, pp. 147–172.

Frisch, M. & Hviid, A. (2006). Childhood family correlates of heterosexual and homosexual marriages: A national cohort study of two million Danes. *Archives of Sexual Behavior, 35,* 533–547.

Frisch, M. & Zdravkovic, S. (2010). Body size at birth and same-sex marriage in young adulthood. *Archives of Sexual Behavior, 39,* 117–123.

Fruth, B. & Hohmann, G. (2006). Social grease for females? Same-sex genital contacts in wild bonobos. In: Sommer, V. & Vasey, P. L. (Eds.), *Homosexual behavior in animals: An evolutionary perspective.* Cambridge University Press, pp. 294–315.

Fry, M. (1993). The rest of the story. *The Living Bird, 12,* 19.

Galanopoulou, A. S. (2008). Sexually dimorphic expression of KCC2 and GABA function. *Epilepsy Research, 80,* 99–113.

Galis, F., Ten Broek, C. M., Van Dongen, S. & Wijnaendts, L. C. (2010). Sexual dimorphism in the prenatal digit ratio (2D:4D). *Archives of Sexual Behavior, 39,* 57–62.

Galor, O. & Moav, O. (2002). Natural selection and the origin of economic growth. *Quarterly Journal of Economics, 117,* 1133–1191.

Gangestad, S. W., Bailey, J. M. & Martin, N. G. (2000). Taxometric analyses of sexual orientation and gender identity. *Journal of Personality and Social Psychology, 78,* 1109–1121.

Gao, B. & Moore, R. Y. (1996). The sexually dimorphic nucleus of the hypothalamus contains GABA neurons in rat and man. *Brain Research, 742,* 163–171.

Garagorri, J. M., Rodriguez, G., Lario-Elboj, A. J., Olivares, J. L., Lario-Munoz, A. & Orden, I. (2008). Reference levels for 17-hydroxyprogesterone, 11-desoxycortisol, cortisol, testosterone, dehydroepiandrosterone sulfate and androstenedione in infants from birth to six months of age. *European Journal of Pediatrics, 167,* 647–653.

Garcia-Falgueras, A. & Swaab, D. F. (2008). A sex difference in the hypothalamic uncinate nucleus: Relationship to gender identity. *Brain, 131,* 3132–3146.

Gatewood, J. D., Wills, A., Shetty, S., Xu, J., Arnold, A. P., Burgoyne, P. S. & Rissman, E. F. (2006). Sex chromosome complement and gonadal sex influence aggressive and parental behaviors in mice. *Journal of Neuroscience, 26,* 2335–2342.

Gaudio, R. (1994). Sounding gay: Pitch properties in the speech of gay and straight men. *American Speech, 69,* 30–57.

Gaus, S. E., Strecker, R. E., Tate, B. A., Parker, R. A. & Saper, C. B. (2002). Ventrolateral preoptic nucleus contains sleep-active, galaninergic neurons in multiple mammalian species. *Neuroscience, 115,* 285–294.

Gazzaniga, M. S. (2008). *Human: The science behind what makes us unique.* Ecco.

Geist, V. (1971). *Mountain sheep: A study in behavior and evolution.* University of Chicago Press.

Gerressu, M., Mercer, C. H., Graham, C. A., Wellings, K. & Johnson, A. M. (2008). Prevalence of masturbation and associated factors in a British national probability survey. *Archives of Sexual Behavior, 37,* 266–278.

Gill, K. S. (1963). A mutation causing abnormal courtship and mating behavior in males of *Drosophila melanogaster. American Zoologist, 3,* 507.

Gladue, B. A. & Bailey, J. M. (1995a). Aggressiveness, competitiveness, and human sexual orientation. *Psychoneuroendocrinology, 20,* 475–485.

Gladue, B. A. & Bailey, J. M. (1995b). Spatial ability, handedness, and human sexual orientation. *Psychoneuroendocrinology, 20,* 487–497.

Goldfoot, D. A., Wallen, K., Neff, D. A., McBrair, M. C. & Goy, R. W. (1984). Social influence on the display of sexually dimorphic behavior in rhesus monkeys: Isosexual rearing. *Archives of Sexual Behavior, 13,* 395–412.

Goldstein, J. M., Seidman, L. J., Horton, N. J., Makris, N., Kennedy, D. N., Caviness, V. S., Jr., Faraone, S. V. & Tsuang, M. T. (2001). Normal sexual dimorphism of the adult human brain assessed by in vivo magnetic resonance imaging. *Cerebral Cortex, 11,* 490–497.

Gomez-Gil, E., Esteva, I., Carrasco, R., Almaraz, M. C., Pasaro, E., Salamero, M. & Guillamon, A. (2011). Birth order and ratio of brothers to sisters in Spanish transsexuals. *Archives of Sexual Behavior, 40,* 505–510.

Goodenough, E. W. (1957). Interest in persons as an aspect of sex difference in the early years. *Genetic Psychology Monographs, 55,* 287–323.

Gordon, L., Joo, J. E., Powell, J. E., Ollikainen, M., Novakovic, B., Li, X., Andronikos, R., Cruickshank, M. N., Conneely, K. N., Smith, A. K., Alisch, R. S., Morley, R., Visscher, P. M., Craig, J. M. & Saffery, R. (2012). Neonatal DNA methylation profile in human twins is specified by a complex interplay between intrauterine environmental and genetic factors, subject to tissue-specific influence. *Genome Research, 22,* 1395–1406.

Gorski, R. A. (1985). Sexual dimorphisms of the brain. *Journal of Animal Science, 61 Suppl 3,* 38–61.

Gorski, R. A., Gordon, J. H., Shryne, J. E. & Southam, A. M. (1978). Evidence for a morphological sex difference within the medial preoptic area of the rat brain. *Brain Research, 148,* 333–346.

Goto, K., Koizumi, K., Ohta, Y., Hashi, M., Fujii, Y., Ohbo, N., Saika, O., Suzuki, H., Saito, K. & Suzuki, K. (2005). Evaluation of general behavior, memory, learning performance, and brain sexual differentiation in F1 offspring males of rats treated with flutamide during late gestation. *Journal of Toxicological Sciences, 30,* 249–259.

Gouchie, C. & Kimura, D. (1991). The relationship between testosterone levels and cognitive ability patterns. *Psychoneuroendocrinology, 16,* 323–334.

Gower, D. B., Holland, K. T., Mallet, A. I., Rennie, P. J. & Watkins, W. J. (1994). Comparison of 16-androstene steroid concentrations in sterile apocrine sweat and axillary secretions: Interconversions of 16-androstenes by the axillary microflora—a mechanism for axillary odour production in man? *Journal of Steroid Biochemistry and Molecular Biology, 48,* 409–418.

Goy, R. W., Bercovitch, F. B. & McBrair, M. C. (1988). Behavioral masculinization is independent of genital masculinization in prenatally androgenized female rhesus macaques. *Hormones and Behavior, 22,* 552–571.

Green, R. (1987). *The "sissy-boy syndrome" and the development of homosexuality.* Yale University Press.

Green, R. (2000). Birth order and ratio of brothers to sisters in transsexuals. *Psychological Medicine, 30,* 789–795.

Greenfeld, L. A. (1997). *Sex offenses and offenders: An analysis of data on rape and sexual assault.* (http://www.mincava.umn.edu/documents/sexoff/sexoff.pdf)

Grellert, E. A., Newcomb, M. D. & Bentler, P. M. (1982). Childhood play activities of male and female homosexuals and heterosexuals. *Archives of Sexual Behavior, 11,* 451–478.

Grimbos, T., Dawood, K., Burriss, R. P., Zucker, K. J. & Puts, D. A. (2010). Sexual orientation and the second to fourth finger length ratio: A meta-analysis in men and women. *Behavioral Neuroscience, 124,* 278–287.

Grimshaw, G. M., Sitarenios, G. & Finegan, J. A. (1995). Mental rotation at 7 years: Relations with prenatal testosterone levels and spatial play experiences. *Brain and Cognition, 29,* 85–100.

Grosjean, Y., Balakireva, M., Dartevelle, L. & Ferveur, J. F. (2001). PGal4 excision reveals the pleiotropic effects of *Voila,* a *Drosophila* locus that affects development and courtship behaviour. *Genetical Research, 77,* 239–250.

Grosjean, Y., Grillet, M., Augustin, H., Ferveur, J. F. & Featherstone, D. E. (2008). A glial amino-acid transporter controls synapse strength and courtship in *Drosophila*. *Nature Neuroscience, 11*, 54–61.

Grumbach, M. M. & Auchus, R. J. (1999). Estrogen: Consequences and implications of human mutations in synthesis and action. *Journal of Clinical Endocrinology and Metabolism, 84*, 4677–4694.

Habert, R. & Picon, R. (1984). Testosterone, dihydrotestosterone and estradiol-17 beta levels in maternal and fetal plasma and in fetal testes in the rat. *Journal of Steroid Biochemistry, 21*, 193–198.

Haines, M. (2008). Fertility and mortality in the United States. (https://eh.net/encyclopedia/fertility-and-mortality-in-the-united-states/)

Haldeman, D. C. (1994). The practice and ethics of sexual orientation conversion therapy. *Journal of Consulting and Clinical Psychology, 62*, 221–227.

Hall, J. A. Y. & Kimura, D. (1995). Sexual orientation and performance on sexually dimorphic motor tasks. *Archives of Sexual Behavior, 24*, 395–407.

Hall, L. S. (2000). Dermatoglyphic analysis of total finger ridge count of female monozygotic twins discordant for sexual orientation. *Journal of Sex Research, 37*, 315–320.

Hall, L. S. & Love, C. T. (2003). Finger-length ratios in female monozygotic twins discordant for sexual orientation. *Archives of Sexual Behavior, 32*, 23–28.

Hall, P. A. & Schaeff, C. M. (2008). Sexual orientation and fluctuating asymmetry in men and women. *Archives of Sexual Behavior, 37*, 158–165.

Halpern, D. F. (2011). *Sex differences in cognitive abilities (4th ed.).* Psychology Press.

Hamer, D. & Copeland, P. (1994). *The science of desire: The search for the gay gene and the biology of behavior.* Simon and Schuster.

Hamer, D. H., Hu, S., Magnuson, V. L., Hu, N. & Pattatucci, A. M. (1993). A linkage between DNA markers on the X chromosome and male sexual orientation. *Science, 261*, 321–327.

Hampson, E., Ellis, C. L. & Tenk, C. M. (2008). On the relation between 2D:4D and sex-dimorphic personality traits. *Archives of Sexual Behavior, 37*, 133–144.

Hampson, E. & Rovet, J. F. (2015). Spatial function in adolescents and young adults with congenital adrenal hyperplasia: Clinical phenotype and implications for the androgen hypothesis. *Psychoneuroendocrinology, 54*, 60–70.

Harding, R. & Golombok, S. E. (2002). Test–retest reliability of the measurement of penile dimensions in a sample of gay men. *Archives of Sexual Behavior, 31*, 351–357.

Hare, E. H. & Moran, P. A. (1979). Parental age and birth order in homosexual patients: A replication of Slater's study. *British Journal of Psychiatry, 134*, 178–182.

Hare, L., Bernard, P., Sanchez, F. J., Baird, P. N., Vilain, E., Kennedy, T. & Harley, V. R. (2009). Androgen receptor repeat length polymorphism associated with male-to-female transsexualism. *Biological Psychiatry, 65*, 93–96.

Hart, T. A., Wolitski, R. J., Purcell, D. W., Gomez, C. & Halkitis, P. (2003). Sexual behavior among HIV-positive men who have sex with men: What's in a label? *Journal of Sex Research, 40*, 179–188.

Haslam, N. (1997). Evidence that male sexual orientation is a matter of degree. *Journal of Personality and Social Psychology, 73*, 862–870.

Hassan, B. & Rahman, Q. (2007). Selective sexual orientation–related differences in object location memory. *Behavioral Neuroscience, 121*, 625–633.

Hassett, J. M., Siebert, E. R. & Wallen, K. (2008). Sex differences in rhesus monkey toy preferences parallel those of children. *Hormones and Behavior, 54*, 359–364.

Hayes, J., Chakraborty, A. T., McManus, S., Bebbington, P., Brugha, T., Nicholson, S. & King, M. (2012). Prevalence of same-sex behavior and orientation in England: Results from a national survey. *Archives of Sexual Behavior, 41*, 631–639.

Hegarty, P. (2009). Toward an LGBT-informed paradigm for children who break gender norms: Comment on Drummond et al. (2008) and Rieger et al. (2008). *Developmental Psychology, 45*, 895–900.

Henningsson, S., Westberg, L., Nilsson, S., Lundstrom, B., Ekselius, L., Bodlund, O., Lindstrom, E., Hellstrand, M., Rosmond, R., Eriksson, E. & Landen, M. (2005). Sex steroid–related genes and male-to-female transsexualism. *Psychoneuroendocrinology*, *30*, 657–664.

Herdt, G. H. (1981). *Guardians of the flutes: Idioms of masculinity*. McGraw-Hill.

Herlitz, A. & Kabir, Z. N. (2006). Sex differences in cognition among illiterate Bangladeshis: A comparison with literate Bangladeshis and Swedes. *Scandinavian Journal of Psychology*, *47*, 441–447.

Hershberger, S. L. (1997). A twin registry study of male and female sexual orientation. *Journal of Sex Research*, *34*, 212–222.

Hines, M. (2010). Sex-related variation in human behavior and the brain. *Trends in Cognitive Sciences*, *14*, 448–456.

Hines, M., Ahmed, S. F. & Hughes, I. A. (2003a). Psychological outcomes and gender-related development in complete androgen insensitivity syndrome. *Archives of Sexual Behavior*, *32*, 93–101.

Hines, M., Allen, L. S. & Gorski, R. A. (1992). Sex differences in subregions of the medial nucleus of the amygdala and the bed nucleus of the stria terminalis of the rat. *Brain Research*, *579*, 321–326.

Hines, M., Brook, C. & Conway, G. S. (2004). Androgen and psychosexual development: Core gender identity, sexual orientation and recalled childhood gender role behavior in women and men with congenital adrenal hyperplasia (CAH). *Journal of Sex Research*, *41*, 75–81.

Hines, M., Fane, B. A., Pasterski, V. L., Mathews, G. A., Conway, G. S. & Brook, C. (2003b). Spatial abilities following prenatal androgen abnormality: Targeting and mental rotations performance in individuals with congenital adrenal hyperplasia. *Psychoneuroendocrinology*, *28*, 1010–1026.

Hines, M., Golombok, S., Rust, J., Johnston, K. J. & Golding, J. (2002). Testosterone during pregnancy and gender role behavior of preschool children: A longitudinal, population study. *Child Development*, *73*, 1678–1687.

Hiraishi, K., Sasaki, S., Shikishima, C. & Ando, J. (2012). The second to fourth digit ratio (2D:4D) in a Japanese twin sample: Heritability, prenatal hormone transfer, and association with sexual orientation. *Archives of Sexual Behavior*, *41*, 711–724.

Hirschfeld, M. (1914). *Die Homosexualität des Mannes und des Weibes*. Verlag Louis Marcus, Berlin.

Hofman, M. A. & Swaab, D. F. (1989). The sexually dimorphic nucleus of the preoptic area in the human brain: A comparative morphometric study. *Journal of Anatomy*, *164*, 55–72.

Hooker, C. I., Germine, L. T., Knight, R. T. & D'Esposito, M. (2006). Amygdala response to facial expressions reflects emotional learning. *Journal of Neuroscience*, *26*, 8915–8922.

Hu, S., Pattatucci, A. M., Patterson, C., Li, L., Fulker, D. W., Cherny, S. S., Kruglyak, L. & Hamer, D. H. (1995). Linkage between sexual orientation and chromosome Xq28 in males but not in females. *Nature Genetics*, *11*, 248–256.

Hu, S.-H., Wei, N., Wang, Q.-D., Yan, L.-Q., Wei, E.-Q., Zhang, M.-M., Hu, J.-B., Huang, M.-L., Zhou, W.-H. & Xu, Y. (2008). Patterns of brain activation during visually evoked sexual arousal differ between homosexual and heterosexual men. *AJNR American Journal of Neuroradiology*, *29*, 1890–1896.

Huberman, J. & Chivers, M. L. (2016). Gender-specificity of women's genital responses varies with stimulus order. *Archives of Sexual Behavior (in preparation)*.

Hunt, G. L., Jr., Newman, A. L., Warner, M. H., Wingfield, J. C. & Kaiwi, J. (1984). Comparative behavior of male–female and female–female pairs among western gulls prior to egg-laying. *The Condor*, *86*, 157–162.

Hunt, G. L., Jr. & Warner Hunt, M. (1977). Female–female pairing in western gulls (*Larus occidentalis*) in Southern California. *Science*, *196*, 1466–1467.

Hunt, G. L., Jr., Wingfield, J. C., Newman, A. & Farner, D. S. (1980). Sex ratios of gulls on Santa Barbara Island. *The Auk*, *97*, 473–479.

Iemmola, F. & Camperio-Ciani, A. (2009). New evidence of genetic factors influencing sexual orientation in men: Female fecundity increase in the maternal line. *Archives of Sexual Behavior, 38*, 393–399.

Imperato-McGinley, J., Pichardo, M., Gautier, T., Voyer, D. & Bryden, M. P. (1991). Cognitive abilities in androgen-insensitive subjects: Comparison with control males and females from the same kindred. *Clinical Endocrinology, 34*, 341–347.

Ingalhalikar, M., Smith, A., Parker, D., Satterthwaite, T. D., Elliott, M. A., Ruparel, K., Hakonarson, H., Gur, R. E., Gur, R. C. & Verma, R. (2014). Sex differences in the structural connectome of the human brain. *Proceedings of the National Academy of Sciences of the United States of America, 111*, 823–828.

Isay, R. A. (1989). *Being homosexual: Gay men and their development.* Farrar, Straus and Giroux.

Isay, R. A. (1999). Gender development in homosexual boys: Some developmental and clinical considerations. *Psychiatry, 62*, 187–194.

Ito, H., Fujitani, K., Usui, K., Shimizu-Nishikawa, K., Tanaka, S. & Yamamoto, D. (1996). Sexual orientation in *Drosophila* is altered by the satori mutation in the sex-determination gene *fruitless* that encodes a zinc finger protein with a BTB domain. *Proceedings of the National Academy of Sciences of the United States of America, 93*, 9687–9692.

Janssen, E., Carpenter, D. & Graham, C. A. (2003). Selecting films for sex research: Gender differences in erotic film preference. *Archives of Sexual Behavior, 32*, 243–251.

Jansson, J. O., Ekberg, S., Isaksson, O., Mode, A. & Gustafsson, J. A. (1985). Imprinting of growth hormone secretion, body growth, and hepatic steroid metabolism by neonatal testosterone. *Endocrinology, 117*, 1881–1889.

Jeong, J. K., Ryu, B. J., Choi, J., Kim, D. H., Choi, E. J., Park, J. W., Park, J. J. & Lee, B. J. (2008). NELL2 participates in formation of the sexually dimorphic nucleus of the pre-optic area in rats. *Journal of Neurochemistry, 106*, 1604–1613.

Jiang, Y., Costello, P., Fang, F., Huang, M. & He, S. (2006). A gender- and sexual orientation-dependent spatial attentional effect of invisible images. *Proceedings of the National Academy of Sciences of the United States of America, 103*, 17048–17052.

Joel, D., Berman, Z., Tavor, I., Wexler, N., Gaber, O., Stein, Y., Shefi, N., Pool, J., Urchs, S., Margulies, D. S., Liem, F., Hanggi, J., Jancke, L. & Assaf, Y. (2015). Sex beyond the genitalia: The human brain mosaic. *Proceedings of the National Academy of Sciences of the United States of America, 112*(50), 15468–15473.

Johnson, K. L., Gill, S., Reichman, V. & Tassinary, L. G. (2007). Swagger, sway, and sexuality: Judging sexual orientation from body motion and morphology. *Journal of Personality and Social Psychology, 93*, 321–334.

Johnson, K. L. & Tassinary, L. G. (2005). Perceiving sex directly and indirectly: Meaning in motion and morphology. *Psychological Science, 16*, 890–897.

Johnston, V. S., Hagel, R., Franklin, M., Fink, B. & Grammer, K. (2001). Male facial attractiveness: Evidence for hormone mediated adaptive design. *Evolution and Human Behavior, 22*, 251–267.

Jordan-Young, R. M. (2012). Hormones, context, and "brain gender": A review of evidence from congenital adrenal hyperplasia. *Social Science and Medicine, 74*, 1738–1744.

Jozet-Alves, C., Moderan, J. & Dickel, L. (2008). Sex differences in spatial cognition in an invertebrate: The cuttlefish. *Proceedings of the Royal Society of London B: Biological Sciences, 275*, 2049–2054.

Juraska, J. M., Sisk, C. L. & DonCarlos, L. L. (2013). Sexual differentiation of the adolescent rodent brain: Hormonal influences and developmental mechanisms. *Hormones and Behavior, 64*, 203–210.

Juster, R.-P., Hatzenbuehler, M. L., Mendrek, A., Pfaus, J. G., Smith, N. G., Johnson, P. J., Lefebvre-Louis, J.-P., Raymond, C., Marin, M.-F., Sindi, S., Lupien, S. J. & Pruessner, J. C. (2015). Sexual orientation modulates endocrine stress reactivity. *Biological Psychiatry, 77*, 668–676.

Kanazawa, S. (2012). Intelligence and homosexuality. *Journal of Biosocial Science, 44*, 593–623.

Kangassalo, K., Polkki, M. & Rantala, M. J. (2011). Prenatal influences on sexual orientation: Digit ratio (2D:4D) and number of older siblings. *Evolutionary Psychology, 9*, 496–508.

Kargel, C., Massau, C., Weiss, S., Walter, M., Kruger, T. H. & Schiffer, B. (2015). Diminished functional connectivity on the road to child sexual abuse in pedophilia. *Journal of Sexual Medicine, 12,* 783–795.

Kendler, K. S., Thornton, L. M., Gilman, S. E. & Kessler, R. C. (2000). Sexual orientation in a U.S. national sample of twin and nontwin sibling pairs. *American Journal of Psychiatry, 157,* 1843–1846.

Kennedy, E. L. & Davis, M. D. (1983). *Boots of leather, slippers of gold: The history of a lesbian community.* Routledge.

Kerchner, M. & Ward, I. L. (1992). SDN-MPOA volume in male rats is decreased by prenatal stress, but is not related to ejaculatory behavior. *Brain Research, 581,* 244–251.

Kerns, K. A. & Berenbaum, S. A. (1991). Sex differences in spatial ability in children. *Behavior Genetics, 21,* 383–396.

Kimchi, T., Xu, J. & Dulac, C. (2007). A functional circuit underlying male sexual behaviour in the female mouse brain. *Nature, 448,* 1009–1014.

Kimura, D. (1994). Body asymmetry and intellectual pattern. *Personality and Individual Differences, 17,* 53–60.

Kimura, D. (1999). *Sex and cognition.* MIT Press.

Kimura, D. & Carson, M. W. (1995). Dermatoglyphic asymmetry: Relation to sex, handedness and cognitive pattern. *Personality and Individual Differences, 19,* 471–478.

Kimura, K., Hachiya, T., Koganezawa, M., Tazawa, T. & Yamamoto, D. (2008). *Fruitless* and *doublesex* coordinate to generate male-specific neurons that can initiate courtship. *Neuron, 59,* 759–769.

Kindon, H. A., Baum, M. J. & Paredes, R. J. (1996). Medial preoptic/anterior hypothalamic lesions induce a female-typical profile of sexual partner preference in male ferrets. *Hormones and Behavior, 30,* 514–527.

King, M., Green, J., Osborn, D. P., Arkell, J., Hetherton, J. & Pereira, E. (2005). Family size in white gay and heterosexual men. *Archives of Sexual Behavior, 34,* 117–122.

Kinsey, A. C., Pomeroy, W. B. & Martin, C. E. (1948). *Sexual behavior in the human male.* Saunders.

Kirk, K. M., Bailey, J. M., Dunne, M. P. & Martin, N. G. (2000). Measurement models for sexual orientation in a community twin sample. *Behavior Genetics, 30,* 345–356.

Kishida, M. & Rahman, Q. (2015). Fraternal birth order and extreme right-handedness as predictors of sexual orientation and gender nonconformity in men. *Archives of Sexual Behavior, 44,* 1493–1501.

Kite, M. E. & Deaux, K. (1987). Gender belief systems: Homosexuality and the implicit inversion theory. *Psychology of Women Quarterly, 11,* 83–96.

Klar, A. J. S. (2005). Excess of counterclockwise scalp hair-whorl rotation in homosexual men. *Journal of Genetics, 83*(3), 251–255.

Klein, K. O., Baron, J., Colli, M. J., McDonnell, D. P. & Cutler, G. B., Jr. (1994). Estrogen levels in childhood determined by an ultrasensitive recombinant cell bioassay. *Journal of Clinical Investigation, 94,* 2475–2480.

Knecht, M., Lundstrom, J. N., Witt, M., Huttenbrink, K. B., Heilmann, S. & Hummel, T. (2003). Assessment of olfactory function and androstenone odor thresholds in humans with or without functional occlusion of the vomeronasal duct. *Behavioral Neuroscience, 117,* 1135–1141.

Kohl, J. V., Atzmueller, M., Fink, B. & Grammer, K. (2001). Human pheromones: Integrating neuroendocrinology and ethology. *Neuroendocrinology Letters, 22,* 309–321.

Koshibu, K., Levitt, P. & Ahrens, E. T. (2004). Sex specific, postpuberty changes in mouse brain structures revealed by three-dimensional magnetic resonance microscopy. *Neuroimage, 22,* 1636–1645.

Kotrschal, K., Hemetsberger, J. & Weiss, B. M. (2006). Making the best of a bad situation: Homosociality in male greylag geese. In: Sommer, V. & Vasey, P. L. (Eds.), *Homosexual behavior in animals: An evolutionary perspective.* Cambridge University Press, pp. 45–76.

Kouros-Mehr, H., Pintchovski, S., Melnyk, J., Chen, Y. J., Friedman, C., Trask, B. & Shizuya, H. (2001). Identification of non-functional human VNO receptor genes provides evidence for vestigiality of the human VNO. *Chemical Senses, 26,* 1167–1174.

Kraemer, B., Noll, T., Delsignore, A., Milos, G., Schnyder, U. & Hepp, U. (2006). Finger length ratio (2D:4D) and dimensions of sexual orientation. *Neuropsychobiology, 53*, 210–214.

Kraemer, B., Noll, T., Delsignore, A., Milos, G., Schnyder, U. & Hepp, U. (2009). Finger length ratio (2D:4D) in adults with gender identity disorder. *Archives of Sexual Behavior, 38*, 359–363.

Kranz, F. & Ishai, A. (2006). Face perception is modulated by sexual preference. *Current Biology, 16*, 63–68.

Kreukels, B. P. C. & Guillamon, A. (2016). Neuroimaging studies in people with gender incongruence. *International Review of Psychiatry, 28*, 120–128.

Kruijver, F. P., Zhou, J. N., Pool, C. W., Hofman, M. A., Gooren, L. J. & Swaab, D. F. (2000). Male-to-female transsexuals have female neuron numbers in a limbic nucleus. *Journal of Clinical Endocrinology and Metabolism, 85*, 2034–2041.

Kudwa, A. E. & Rissman, E. F. (2003). Double oestrogen receptor alpha and beta knockout mice reveal differences in neural oestrogen-mediated progestin receptor induction and female sexual behaviour. *Journal of Neuroendocrinology, 15*, 978–983.

Kuhle, B. X. & Radtke, S. (2013). Born both ways: The alloparenting hypothesis for sexual fluidity in women. *Evolutionary Psychology, 11*, 304–323.

Lalumière, M. L. (2016). The empirical status of the preparation hypothesis of female genital responses. *Archives of Sexual Behavior (in preparation)*.

Lalumière, M. L., Blanchard, R. & Zucker, K. J. (2000). Sexual orientation and handedness in men and women: A meta-analysis. *Psychological Bulletin, 126*, 575–592.

Lame Deer, J. F. & Erdoes, R. (1972). *Lame Deer: Seeker of visions*. Simon and Schuster.

Lamminmaki, A., Hines, M., Kuiri-Hanninen, T., Kilpelainen, L., Dunkel, L. & Sankilampi, U. (2012). Testosterone measured in infancy predicts subsequent sex-typed behavior in boys and in girls. *Hormones and Behavior, 61*, 611–616.

Långström, N., Rahman, Q., Carlström, E. & Lichtenstein, P. (2010). Genetic and environmental effects on same-sex sexual behavior: A population study of twins in Sweden. *Archives of Sexual Behavior, 39*, 75–80.

Lasco, M. S., Jordan, T. J., Edgar, M. A., Petito, C. K. & Byne, W. (2002). A lack of dimorphism of sex or sexual orientation in the human anterior commissure. *Brain Research, 936*, 95–98.

Laumann, E. O., Gagnon, J. H., Michael, R. T. & Michaels, S. (1994). *The social organization of sexuality: Sexual practices in the United States*. University of Chicago Press.

Lawrence, A. A. (2004). Autogynephilia: A paraphilic model of gender identity disorder. *Journal of Gay and Lesbian Psychotherapy, 8*, 69–87.

Laws, D. R. & O'Donohue, W. T. (2008). *Sexual deviance: Theory, assessment, and treatment (2nd ed.)*. Guilford Press.

Lawson, J. F., James, C., Jannson, A. U.-C., Koyama, N. F. & Hill, R. A. (2014). A comparison of heterosexual and homosexual mating preferences in personal advertisements. *Evolution and Human Behavior, 35*, 408–414.

Leca, J. B., Gunst, N. & Vasey, P. L. (2015). Comparative development of heterosexual and homosexual behaviors in free-ranging female Japanese macaques. *Archives of Sexual Behavior, 44*, 1215–1231.

LeDoux, J. E. (1996). *The emotional brain: The mysterious underpinnings of emotional life*. Simon & Schuster.

Légère, M.-A., Sawatsky, M. & Lalumière, M. L. (2016). Measuring sexual attraction with invisible images. *Archives of Sexual Behavior (in preparation)*.

Lephart, E. D., Call, S. B., Rhees, R. W., Jacobson, N. A., Weber, K. S., Bledsoe, J. & Teuscher, C. (2001). Neuroendocrine regulation of sexually dimorphic brain structure and associated sexual behavior in male rats is genetically controlled. *Biology of Reproduction, 64*, 571–578.

LeVay, S. (1991). A difference in hypothalamic structure between heterosexual and homosexual men. *Science, 253*, 1034–1037.

LeVay, S. (1996). *Queer science: The use and abuse of research into homosexuality*. MIT Press.

Lever, J. (1994). Sexual revelations: The 1994 *Advocate* survey of sexuality and relationships: The men. *The Advocate*, August 23.

Lever, J. (1995). Lesbian sex survey. *The Advocate*, August 22.

Levitt, E. E. & Klassen, A. D. (1974). Public attitudes toward homosexuality: Part of the 1970 national survey by the Institute for Sex Research. *Journal of Homosexuality*, *1*, 29–43.

Lim, A. S., Ellison, B. A., Wang, J. L., Yu, L., Schneider, J. A., Buchman, A. S., Bennett, D. A. & Saper, C. B. (2014). Sleep is related to neuron numbers in the ventrolateral preoptic/ intermediate nucleus in older adults with and without Alzheimer's disease. *Brain*, *137*, 2847–2861.

Linville, S. E. (1998). Acoustic correlates of perceived versus actual sexual orientation in men's speech. *Folia Phoniatrica et Logopedica*, *50*, 35–48.

Lippa, R. A. (2003a). Are 2D:4D finger-length ratios related to sexual orientation? Yes for men, no for women. *Journal of Personality and Social Psychology*, *85*, 179–188.

Lippa, R. A. (2003b). Handedness, sexual orientation, and gender-related personality traits in men and women. *Archives of Sexual Behavior*, *32*, 103–114.

Lippa, R. A. (2005). Sexual orientation and personality. *Annual Review of Sex Research*, *16*, 119–153.

Lippa, R. A. (2006a). Finger lengths, 2D:4D ratios, and their relation to gender-related personality traits and the Big Five. *Biological Psychology*, *71*, 116–121.

Lippa, R. A. (2006b). Is high sex drive associated with increased sexual attraction to both sexes? It depends on whether you are male or female. *Psychological Science*, *17*, 46–52.

Lippa, R. A. (2008a). The relation between childhood gender nonconformity and adult masculinity–femininity and anxiety in heterosexual and homosexual men and women. *Sex Roles*, *59*, 684–693.

Lippa, R. A. (2008b). Sex differences and sexual orientation differences in personality: Findings from the BBC Internet survey. *Archives of Sexual Behavior*, *37*, 173–187.

Lippa, R. A. (2009). Sex differences in sex drive, sociosexuality, and height across 53 nations: Testing evolutionary and social structural theories. *Archives of Sexual Behavior*, *38*, 631–651.

Lippa, R. A. (2013). Men and women with bisexual identities show bisexual patterns of sexual attraction to male and female "swimsuit models." *Archives of Sexual Behavior*, *42*, 187–196.

Lippa, R. (2016). The category specificity of sexual attraction and viewing times in a representative sample of 2825 U.S. adults: Sex, sexual orientation, and demographic effects. *Archives of Sexual Behavior (in preparation)*.

Lippa, R. & Hershberger, S. (1999). Genetic and environmental influences on individual differences in masculinity, femininity, and gender diagnosticity: Analyzing data from a classic twin study. *Journal of Personality*, *67*, 127–155.

Lippa, R., Patterson, T. M. & Marelich, W. D. (2010). Looking at and longing for male and female "swimsuit models": Men are much more category-specific than women. *Social Psychological and Personality Science*, *1*, 238–245.

Liu, T., Dartevelle, L., Yuan, C., Wei, H., Wang, Y., Ferveur, J. F. & Guo, A. (2008). Increased dopamine level enhances male–male courtship in *Drosophila*. *Journal of Neuroscience*, *28*, 5539–5546.

Liu, T., Dartevelle, L., Yuan, C., Wei, H., Wang, Y., Ferveur, J. F. & Guo, A. (2009). Reduction of dopamine level enhances the attractiveness of male *Drosophila* to other males. *PLoS One*, *4*, e4574.

Loehlin, J. C., Jonsson, E. G., Gustavsson, J. P., Stallings, M. C., Gillespie, N. A., Wright, M. J. & Martin, N. G. (2005). Psychological masculinity–femininity via the gender diagnosticity approach: Heritability and consistency across ages and populations. *Journal of Personality*, *73*, 1295–1319.

Loehlin, J. C. & McFadden, D. (2003). Otoacoustic emissions, auditory evoked potentials, and traits related to sex and sexual orientation. *Archives of Sexual Behavior*, *32*, 115–127.

Loehlin, J. C., Medland, S. E. & Martin, N. G. (2009). Relative finger lengths, sex differences, and psychological traits. *Archives of Sexual Behavior*, *38*, 298–305.

Lohman, D. F. & Lakin, J. M. (2009). Consistencies in sex differences on the Cognitive Abilities Test across countries, grades, test forms, and cohorts. *British Journal of Educational Psychology*, *79*, 389–407.

Lombardo, M. V., Ashwin, E., Auyeung, B., Chakrabarti, B., Taylor, K., Hackett, G., Bullmore, E. T. & Baron-Cohen, S. (2012). Fetal testosterone influences sexually dimorphic gray matter in the human brain. *Journal of Neuroscience, 32*, 674–680.

Lovejoy, J. & Wallen, K. (1988). Sexually dimorphic behavior in group-housed rhesus monkeys (*Macaca mulatta*) at 1 year of age. *Psychobiology, 16*, 348–356.

Lübke, K. T., Hoenen, M. & Pause, B. M. (2012). Differential processing of social chemosignals obtained from potential partners in regards to gender and sexual orientation. *Behavioural Brain Research, 228*, 375–387.

Lübke, K. T. & Pause, B. M. (2015). Always follow your nose: The functional significance of social chemosignals in human reproduction and survival. *Hormones and Behavior, 68*, 134–144.

Lübke, K. T., Schablitzky, S. & Pause, B. M. (2009). Male sexual orientation affects sensitivity to androstenone. *Chemosensory Perception, 2*(3), 154–160.

Luders, E., Toga, A. W. & Thompson, P. M. (2014). Why size matters: Differences in brain volume account for apparent sex differences in callosal anatomy: The sexual dimorphism of the corpus callosum. *Neuroimage, 84*, 820–824.

Luine, V. & Dohanich, G. (2007). Sex differences in cognitive function in rodents. In: Becker, J. B. et al. (Eds.), *Sex differences in the brain: From genes to behavior.* Oxford University Press, pp. 217–251.

Lutchmaya, S., Baron-Cohen, S., Raggatt, P., Knickmeyer, R. & Manning, J. T. (2004). 2nd to 4th digit ratios, fetal testosterone and estradiol. *Early Human Development, 77*, 23–28.

Lyons, M., Lynch, A., Brewer, G. & Bruno, D. (2014). Detection of sexual orientation ("gaydar") by homosexual and heterosexual women. *Archives of Sexual Behavior, 43*, 345–352.

Maccoby, E. E. (1998). *The two sexes: Growing up apart, coming together.* Harvard University Press.

Maccoby, E. E., Doering, C. H., Jacklin, C. N. & Kraemer, H. (1979). Concentrations of sex hormones in umbilical-cord blood: Their relation to sex and birth order of infants. *Child Development, 50*, 632–642.

MacCulloch, M. J. & Waddington, J. L. (1981). Neuroendocrine mechanisms and the aetiology of male and female homosexuality. *British Journal of Psychiatry, 139*, 341–345.

Mack, S. & Munson, B. (2012). The influence of /s/ quality on ratings of men's sexual orientation: Explicit and implicit measures of the 'gay lisp' stereotype. *Journal of Phonetics, 40*, 198–212.

Macke, J. P., Hu, N., Hu, S., Bailey, M., King, V. L., Brown, T., Hamer, D. & Nathans, J. (1993). Sequence variation in the androgen receptor gene is not a common determinant of male sexual orientation. *American Journal of Human Genetics, 53*, 844–852.

Madon, S. (1997). What do people believe about gay males? A study of stereotype content and strength. *Sex Roles, 37*, 663–685.

Majdic, G. & Tobet, S. (2011). Cooperation of sex chromosomal genes and endocrine influences for hypothalamic sexual differentiation. *Frontiers in Neuroendocrinology, 32*, 137–145.

Mandiyan, V. S., Coats, J. K. & Shah, N. M. (2005). Deficits in sexual and aggressive behaviors in *Cnga2* mutant mice. *Nature Neuroscience, 8*, 1660–1662.

Manning, J. T., Churchill, A. J. & Peters, M. (2007). The effects of sex, ethnicity, and sexual orientation on self-measured digit ratio (2D:4D). *Archives of Sexual Behavior, 36*, 223–233.

Manning, J. T. & Fink, B. (2008). Digit ratio (2D:4D), dominance, reproductive success, asymmetry, and sociosexuality in the BBC Internet study. *American Journal of Human Biology, 20*, 451–461.

Manning, J. T., Fink, B. & Trivers, R. (2014). Digit ratio (2D:4D) and gender inequalities across nations. *Evolutionary Psychology, 12*, 757–768.

Manning, J. T., Scutt, D., Wilson, J. & Lewis-Jones, D. I. (1998). The ratio of 2nd to 4th digit length: A predictor of sperm numbers and concentrations of testosterone, luteinizing hormone and oestrogen. *Human Reproduction, 13*, 3000–3004.

Mansukhani, V., Adkins-Regan, E. & Yang, S. (1996). Sexual partner preference in female zebra finches: The role of early hormones and social environment. *Hormones and Behavior, 30*, 506–513.

Marcus, E. (1992). *Making history: The struggle for gay and lesbian equal rights.* HarperCollins.

Maresh, M. M. (1955). Linear growth of long bones of extremities from infancy through adolescence; continuing studies. *AMA American Journal of Diseases of Children, 89*, 725–742.

Marmor, J. (1980). The multiple roots of homosexual behavior. In: Marmor, J. (Ed.), *Homosexual behavior: A modern reappraisal*. Basic Books.

Marshall, W. A. & Tanner, J. M. (1974). Puberty. In: Davis, J. A. & Dobbing, J. (Eds.), *Scientific foundations of paediatrics*. William Heinemann Medical Books.

Martin, J. T. & Nguyen, D. H. (2004). Anthropometric analysis of homosexuals and heterosexuals: Implications for early hormone exposure. *Hormones and Behavior, 45*, 31–39.

Martins, Y., Preti, G., Crabtree, C. R., Runyan, T., Vainius, A. A. & Wysocki, C. J. (2005). Preference for human body odors is influenced by gender and sexual orientation. *Psychological Science, 16*, 694–701.

Masek, K. S., Wood, R. I. & Foster, D. L. (1999). Prenatal dihydrotestosterone differentially masculinizes tonic and surge modes of luteinizing hormone secretion in sheep. *Endocrinology, 140*, 3459–3466.

Mast, T. G. & Samuelsen, C. L. (2009). Human pheromone detection by the vomeronasal organ: Unnecessary for mate selection? *Chemical Senses, 34*, 529–531.

McCarthy, M. M. & Konkle, A. T. (2005). When is a sex difference not a sex difference? *Frontiers in Neuroendocrinology, 26*, 85–102.

McCarthy, M. M., Pickett, L. A., VanRyzin, J. W. & Kight, K. E. (2015). Surprising origins of sex differences in the brain. *Hormones and Behavior, 76*, 3–10.

McCormick, C. M. & Witelson, S. F. (1991). A cognitive profile of homosexual men compared to heterosexual men and women. *Psychoneuroendocrinology, 16*, 459–473.

McEwen, B. S. (1998). Multiple ovarian hormone effects on brain structure and function. *Journal of Gender-Specific Medicine, 1*, 33–41.

McFadden, D. (1998). Sex differences in the auditory system. *Developmental Neuropsychology, 14*, 261–298.

McFadden, D. (2000). Masculinizing effects on otoacoustic emissions and auditory evoked potentials in women using oral contraceptives. *Hearing Research, 142*, 23–33.

McFadden, D. & Champlin, C. A. (2000). Comparison of auditory evoked potentials in heterosexual, homosexual, and bisexual males and females. *Journal of the Association for Research in Otolaryngology, 1*, 89–99.

McFadden, D., Loehlin, J. C., Breedlove, S. M., Lippa, R. A., Manning, J. T. & Rahman, Q. (2005). A reanalysis of five studies on sexual orientation and the relative length of the 2nd and 4th fingers (the 2D:4D ratio). *Archives of Sexual Behavior, 34*, 341–356.

McFadden, D., Loehlin, J. C. & Pasanen, E. G. (1996). Additional findings on heritability and prenatal masculinization of cochlear mechanisms: Click-evoked otoacoustic emissions. *Hearing Research, 97*, 102–119.

McFadden, D. & Pasanen, E. G. (1998). Comparison of the auditory systems of heterosexuals and homosexuals: Click-evoked otoacoustic emissions. *Proceedings of the National Academy of Sciences of the United States of America, 95*, 2709–2713.

McFadden, D. & Pasanen, E. G. (1999). Spontaneous otoacoustic emissions in heterosexuals, homosexuals, and bisexuals. *Journal of the Acoustical Society of America, 105*, 2403–2413.

McFadden, D., Pasanen, E. G., Raper, J., Lange, H. S. & Wallen, K. (2006). Sex differences in otoacoustic emissions measured in rhesus monkeys (*Macaca mulatta*). *Hormones and Behavior, 50*, 274–284.

McFadden, D., Pasanen, E. G., Valero, M. D., Roberts, E. K. & Lee, T. M. (2009). Effect of prenatal androgens on click-evoked otoacoustic emissions in male and female sheep (*Ovis aries*). *Hormones and Behavior, 55*, 98–105.

McFadden, D. & Shubel, E. (2002). Relative lengths of fingers and toes in human males and females. *Hormones and Behavior, 42*, 492–500.

McGuire, R. J., Carlisle, J. M. & Young, B. G. (1965). Sexual deviations as conditioned behavior: A hypothesis. *Behavioral Research and Therapy, 2*, 185–190.

McIntyre, M. H. (2003). Digit ratios, childhood gender role behavior, and erotic role preferences of gay men. *Archives of Sexual Behavior, 32*, 495–496.

McIntyre, M. H., Barrett, E. S., McDermott, R., Johnson, D. D. P., Cowden, J. & Rosen, S. P. (2007). Finger length ratio (2D:4D) and sex differences in aggression during a simulated war game. *Personality and Individual Differences, 42*, 755–764.

McKnight, J. & Malcolm, J. (2000). Is male homosexuality maternally linked? *Psychology, Evolution and Gender, 2*, 229–252.

Medland, S. E., Loehlin, J. C., Willemsen, G., Hatemi, P. K., Keller, M. C., Boomsma, D. I., Eaves, L. J. & Martin, N. G. (2008). Males do not reduce the fitness of their female co-twins in contemporary samples. *Twin Research and Human Genetics, 11*, 481–487.

Meek, L. R., Schulz-Wilson, K. M. & Keith, C. A. (2006). Effects of prenatal stress on sexual partner preference in mice. *Physiology and Behavior, 89*, 133–138.

Mehren, E. (2004). Acceptance of gays rises among new generation. *Los Angeles Times*, April 11.

Merker, B. (2007). Consciousness without a cerebral cortex: A challenge for neuroscience and medicine. *Behavioral and Brain Sciences, 30*, 63–81.

Meyer-Bahlburg, H. F. L. (1984). Psychoendocrine research on sexual orientation: Current status and future options. *Progress in Brain Research, 61*, 375–398.

Meyer-Bahlburg, H. F., Dolezal, C., Baker, S. W., Carlson, A. D., Obeid, J. S. & New, M. I. (2004). Prenatal androgenization affects gender-related behavior but not gender identity in 5–12-year-old girls with congenital adrenal hyperplasia. *Archives of Sexual Behavior, 33*, 97–104.

Meyer-Bahlburg, H. F., Dolezal, C., Baker, S. W., Ehrhardt, A. A. & New, M. I. (2006). Gender development in women with congenital adrenal hyperplasia as a function of disorder severity. *Archives of Sexual Behavior, 35*, 667–684.

Meyer-Bahlburg, H. F., Dolezal, C., Baker, S. W. & New, M. I. (2008). Sexual orientation in women with classical or non-classical congenital adrenal hyperplasia as a function of degree of prenatal androgen excess. *Archives of Sexual Behavior, 37*, 85–99.

Miller, E. M. (2000). Homosexuality, birth order, and evolution: Toward an equilibrium reproductive economics of homosexuality. *Archives of Sexual Behavior, 29*, 1–34.

Mock, S. E. & Eibach, R. P. (2012). Stability and change in sexual orientation identity over a 10-year period in adulthood. *Archives of Sexual Behavior, 41*, 641–648.

Mohr, M. A. & Sisk, C. L. (2013). Pubertally born neurons and glia are functionally integrated into limbic and hypothalamic circuits of the male Syrian hamster. *Proceedings of the National Academy of Sciences of the United States of America, 110*, 4792–4797.

Money, J. & Ehrhardt, A. E. (1971). *Man and woman, boy and girl: The differentiation and dimorphism of gender identity from conception to maturity.* Johns Hopkins University Press.

Money, J., Hampson, J. G. & Hampson, J. L. (1957). Imprinting and the establishment of gender role. *Archives of Neurology and Psychiatry, 77*, 333–336.

Money, J. & Russo, A. J. (1979). Homosexual outcome of discordant gender identity/role: Longitudinal follow-up. *Journal of Pediatric Psychology, 4*, 29–41.

Moore, D. S. & Johnson, S. P. (2008). Mental rotation in human infants: A sex difference. *Psychological Science, 19*, 1063–1066.

Morgan, C. P. & Bale, T. L. (2011). Early prenatal stress epigenetically programs dysmasculinization in second-generation offspring via the paternal lineage. *Journal of Neuroscience, 31*, 11748–11755.

Mori, H., Matsuda, K., Pfaff, D. W. & Kawata, M. (2008). A recently identified hypothalamic nucleus expressing estrogen receptor alpha. *Proceedings of the National Academy of Sciences of the United States of America, 105*, 13632–13637.

Morris, J. A., Jordan, C. L. & Breedlove, S. M. (2008a). Sexual dimorphism in neuronal number of the posterodorsal medial amygdala is independent of circulating androgens and regional volume in adult rats. *Journal of Comparative Neurology, 506*, 851–859.

Morris, J. A., Jordan, C. L., King, Z. A., Northcutt, K. V. & Breedlove, S. M. (2008b). Sexual dimorphism and steroid responsiveness of the posterodorsal medial amygdala in adult mice. *Brain Research, 1190*, 115–121.

Moskowitz, D. A. (2015). From top to bottom: Assessing the debut, construction, and mutability of anal penetrative orientation of gay and bisexual men. *Archives of Sexual Behavior (in preparation).*

Moskowitz, D. A. & Hart, T. A. (2011). The influence of physical body traits and masculinity on anal sex roles in gay and bisexual men. *Archives of Sexual Behavior, 40*, 835–841.

Moskowitz, D. A., Rieger, G. & Roloff, M. E. (2008). Tops, bottoms and versatiles. *Sexual and Relationship Therapy, 23*, 191–202.

Munson, B. (2007). The acoustic correlates of perceived masculinity, perceived femininity, and perceived sexual orientation. *Language and Speech, 50*, 125–142.

Munson, B., McDonald, E. C., DeBoe, N. L. & White, A. R. (2006). The acoustic and perceptual bases of judgments of women and men's sexual orientation from read speech. *Journal of Phonetics, 34*, 202–240.

Murnen, S. K. & Stockton, M. (1997). Gender and self-reported sexual arousal in response to sexual stimuli: A meta-analytic review. *Sex Roles, 37*, 135–153.

Murray, S. O. (2000). *Homosexualities*. University of Chicago Press.

Mustanski, B. S., Bailey, J. M. & Kaspar, S. (2002). Dermatoglyphics, handedness, sex, and sexual orientation. *Archives of Sexual Behavior, 31*, 113–132.

Mustanski, B. S., Dupree, M. G., Nievergelt, C. M., Bocklandt, S., Schork, N. J. & Hamer, D. H. (2005). A genomewide scan of male sexual orientation. *Human Genetics, 116*, 272–278.

Nanda, S. (1998). *Neither man nor woman: The hijras of India (2nd ed.)*. Cengage Learning.

Copen, C. E., Chandra, A., & Febo-Vazquez, I. (2016). *Sexual behavior, sexual attraction, and sexual orientation among adults aged 18–44 in the United States: Data from the 2011–2013 National Survey of Family Growth*. National Health Statistics Reports no. 8. (http://www.cdc.gov/nchs/data/nhsr/nhsr088.pdf)

National Library of Medicine (2008). *Androgen insensitivity syndrome*. (http://ghr.nlm.nih.gov/condition=androgeninsensitivitysyndrome)

Neave, N., Menaged, M. & Weightman, D. R. (1999). Sex differences in cognition: The role of testosterone and sexual orientation. *Brain and Cognition, 41*, 245–262.

Neglia, A. (2009). Comedian Carol Leifer on her mid-life change. (http://documents.mx/documents/comedian-carol-leifer-on-her-mid-life-change.html)

Nettle, D. (2007). Empathizing and systemizing: What are they, and what do they contribute to our understanding of psychological sex differences? *British Journal of Psychology, 98*, 237–255.

Nicolosi, J. & Nicolosi, L. A. (2002). *A parent's guide to preventing homosexuality*. InterVarsity Press.

Nielsen, H. S., Mortensen, L., Nygaard, U., Schnor, O., Christiansen, O. B. & Andersen, A. M. (2008). Brothers and reduction of the birth weight of later-born siblings. *American Journal of Epidemiology, 167*, 480–484.

Norris, A. L., Marcus, D. K. & Green, B. A. (2015). Homosexuality as a discrete class. *Psychological Science, 26(12)*, 1843–1853.

Norton, R. (1999). *Mother Clap's molly house: The gay subculture in England, 1700–1830*. Heretic Books.

Novakova, L., Varella Valentova, J. & Havlicek, J. (2013). Olfactory performance is predicted by individual sex-atypicality, but not sexual orientation. *PLoS One, 8*, e80234.

Nugent, B. M., Wright, C. L., Shetty, A. C., Hodes, G. E., Lenz, K. M., Mahurkar, A., Russo, S. J., Devine, S. E. & McCarthy, M. M. (2015). Brain feminization requires active repression of masculinization via DNA methylation. *Nature Neuroscience, 18*, 690–697.

Ökten, A., Kalyoncu, M. & Yaris, N. (2002). The ratio of second- and fourth-digit lengths and congenital adrenal hyperplasia due to 21-hydroxylase deficiency. *Early Human Development, 70*, 47–54.

Olvera-Hernandez, S., Chavira, R. & Fernandez-Guasti, A. (2015). Prenatal letrozole produces a subpopulation of male rats with same-sex preference and arousal as well as female sexual behavior. *Physiology and Behavior, 139*, 403–411.

Oosterhuis, H. & Kennedy, H. (1991). *Homosexuality and male bonding in pre-Nazi Germany*. Harrington Park Press.

Organisation Internationale des Intersexués (2009). *Androgen insensitivity syndrome*. (http://www.intersexualite.org/AIS.html)

Pallone, D. & Steinberg, A. (1990). *Behind the mask: My double life in baseball*. Viking.

Papadatou-Pastou, M., Martin, M., Munafo, M. R. & Jones, G. V. (2008). Sex differences in left-handedness: A meta-analysis of 144 studies. *Psychological Bulletin, 134*, 677–699.

Paredes, R. G. & Baum, M. J. (1995). Altered sexual partner preference in male ferrets given excitotoxic lesions of the preoptic area/anterior hypothalamus. *Journal of Neuroscience, 15*, 6619–6630.

Paredes, R. G., Tzschentke, T. & Nakach, N. (1998). Lesions of the medial preoptic area/anterior hypothalamus (MPOA/AH) modify partner preference in male rats. *Brain Research, 813*, 1–8.

Pasterski, V., Acerini, C. L., Dunger, D. B., Ong, K. K., Hughes, I. A., Thankamony, A. & Hines, M. (2015a). Postnatal penile growth concurrent with mini-puberty predicts later sex-typed play behavior: Evidence for neurobehavioral effects of the postnatal androgen surge in typically developing boys. *Hormones and Behavior, 69*, 98–105.

Pasterski, V., Geffner, M. E., Brain, C., Hindmarsh, P., Brook, C. & Hines, M. (2011). Prenatal hormones and childhood sex segregation: Playmate and play style preferences in girls with congenital adrenal hyperplasia. *Hormones and Behavior, 59*, 549–555.

Pasterski, V., Hindmarsh, P., Geffner, M., Brook, C., Brain, C. & Hines, M. (2007). Increased aggression and activity level in 3- to 11-year-old girls with congenital adrenal hyperplasia (CAH). *Hormones and Behavior, 52*, 368–374.

Pasterski, V., Zucker, K. J., Hindmarsh, P. C., Hughes, I. A., Acerini, C., Spencer, D., Neufeld, S. & Hines, M. (2015b). Increased cross-gender identification independent of gender role behavior in girls with congenital adrenal hyperplasia: Results from a standardized assessment of 4- to 11-year-old children. *Archives of Sexual Behavior, 44*, 1365–1375.

Pattatucci, A. M. & Hamer, D. H. (1995). Development and familiality of sexual orientation in females. *Behavior Genetics, 25*, 407–420.

Paulhus, D. L., Trapnell, P. D. & Chen, D. (1999). Birth order effects on personality and achievement within families. *Psychological Science, 10*, 482–488.

Pearcey, S. M., Docherty, K. J. & Dabbs, J. M., Jr. (1996). Testosterone and sex role identification in lesbian couples. *Physiology and Behavior, 60*, 1033–1035.

Pei, M., Matsuda, K., Sakamoto, H. & Kawata, M. (2006). Intrauterine proximity to male fetuses affects the morphology of the sexually dimorphic nucleus of the preoptic area in the adult rat brain. *European Journal of Neuroscience, 23*, 1234–1240.

Penton-Voak, I. S. & Perrett, D. I. (2000). Female preference for male faces changes cyclically: Further evidence. *Evolution and Human Behavior, 21*, 39–48.

Perkins, A., Fitzgerald, J. A. & Moss, G. E. (1995). A comparison of LH secretion and brain estradiol receptors in heterosexual and homosexual rams and female sheep. *Hormones and Behavior, 29*, 31–41.

Perry, D., Walder, K., Hendler, T. & Shamay-Tsoory, S. G. (2013). The gender you are and the gender you like: Sexual preference and empathic neural responses. *Brain Research, 1534*, 66–75.

Peters, M., Manning, J. T. & Reimers, S. (2007). The effects of sex, sexual orientation, and digit ratio (2D:4D) on mental rotation performance. *Archives of Sexual Behavior, 36*, 251–260.

Petrulis, A. (2013). Chemosignals, hormones and mammalian reproduction. *Hormones and Behavior, 63*, 723–741.

Petterson, L. J., Dixson, B. J., Little, A. C. & Vasey, P. L. (2015). Viewing time measures of sexual orientation in Samoan cisgender men who engage in sexual interactions with fa'afafine. *PLoS One, 10*, e0116529.

Phoenix, C. H., Goy, R. W., Gerall, A. A. & Young, W. C. (1959). Organizing action of prenatally administered testosterone propionate on the tissues mediating mating behavior in the female guinea pig. *Endocrinology, 65*, 369–382.

Pierrehumbert, J. B., Bent, T., Munson, B., Bradlow, A. R. & Bailey, J. M. (2004). The influence of sexual orientation on vowel production. *Journal of the Acoustical Society of America, 116*, 1905–1908.

Pillard, R. C. (1990). The Kinsey scale: Is it familial? In: McWhirter, D. P. et al. (Eds.), *Homosexuality/heterosexuality: Concepts of sexual orientation*. Oxford University Press.

Pillard, R. C., Poumadere, J. & Carretta, R. A. (1981). Is homosexuality familial? A review, some data, and a suggestion. *Archives of Sexual Behavior, 10*, 465–475.

Pillard, R. C., Poumadere, J. & Carretta, R. A. (1982). A family study of sexual orientation. *Archives of Sexual Behavior, 11*, 511–520.

Pillard, R. C. & Weinrich, J. D. (1986). Evidence of familial nature of male homosexuality. *Archives of General Psychiatry, 43*, 808–812.

Plöderl, M. (2014). Bayesian advice for gaydar-based picking up: Commentary on Lyons, Lynch, Brewer, and Bruno (2013). *Archives of Sexual Behavior, 43*, 7–9.

Plöderl, M. & Fartacek, R. (2008). Childhood gender nonconformity and harassment as predictors of suicidality among gay, lesbian, bisexual, and heterosexual Austrians. *Archives of Sexual Behavior, 38*, 400–410.

Ponseti, J., Bosinski, H. A., Wolff, S., Peller, M., Jansen, O., Mehdorn, H. M., Buchel, C. & Siebner, H. R. (2006). A functional endophenotype for sexual orientation in humans. *Neuroimage, 33*, 825–833.

Ponseti, J., Granert, O., Jansen, O., Wolff, S., Mehdorn, H., Bosinski, H. & Siebner, H. (2009). Assessment of sexual orientation using the hemodynamic brain response to visual sexual stimuli. *Journal of Sexual Medicine, 6*, 1628–1634.

Ponseti, J., Siebner, H. R., Kloppel, S., Wolff, S., Granert, O., Jansen, O., Mehdorn, H. M. & Bosinski, H. A. (2007). Homosexual women have less grey matter in perirhinal cortex than heterosexual women. *PLoS One, 2*, e762.

Poston, D. L. & Baumle, A. K. (2010). Patterns of asexuality in the United States. *Demographic Research, 36*, 509–530.

Prause, N. & Graham, C. A. (2007). Asexuality: Classification and characterization. *Archives of Sexual Behavior, 36*, 341–356.

Preti, G., Wysocki, C. J., Barnhart, K. T., Sondheimer, S. J. & Leyden, J. J. (2003). Male axillary extracts contain pheromones that affect pulsatile secretion of luteinizing hormone and mood in women recipients. *Biology of Reproduction, 68*, 2107–2113.

Purcell, D. W., Blanchard, R. & Zucker, K. J. (2000). Birth order in a contemporary sample of gay men. *Archives of Sexual Behavior, 29*, 349–356.

Puts, D. A., Gaulin, S. J. C., Sporter, R. J. & McBurney, D. H. (2004). Sex hormones and finger length: What does 2D:4D indicate? *Evolution and Human Behavior, 25*, 182–199.

Quigley, C. A. (2002). The postnatal gonadotropin and sex steroid surge: Insights from the androgen insensitivity syndrome. *Journal of Clinical Endocrinology and Metabolism, 87*, 24–28.

Quinn, P. C. & Liben, L. S. (2008). A sex difference in mental rotation in young infants. *Psychological Science, 19*, 1067–1070.

Rahman, Q. (2005). Fluctuating asymmetry, second to fourth finger length ratios and human sexual orientation. *Psychoneuroendocrinology, 30*, 382–391.

Rahman, Q., Abrahams, S. & Wilson, G. D. (2003a). Sexual-orientation-related differences in verbal fluency. *Neuropsychology, 17*, 240–246.

Rahman, Q., Andersson, D. & Govier, E. (2005). A specific sexual orientation–related difference in navigation strategy. *Behavioral Neuroscience, 119*, 311–316.

Rahman, Q., Bhanot, S., Emrith-Small, H., Ghafoor, S. & Roberts, S. (2012). Gender nonconformity, intelligence, and sexual orientation. *Archives of Sexual Behavior, 41*, 623–630.

Rahman, Q., Clarke, K. & Morera, T. (2009). Hair whorl direction and sexual orientation in human males. *Behavioral Neuroscience, 123*, 252–256.

Rahman, Q., Collins, A., Morrison, M., Orrells, J. C., Cadinouche, K., Greenfield, S. & Begum, S. (2008). Maternal inheritance and familial fecundity factors in male homosexuality. *Archives of Sexual Behavior, 37*, 962–969.

Rahman, Q. & Hull, M. S. (2005). An empirical test of the kin selection hypothesis for male homosexuality. *Archives of Sexual Behavior, 34*, 461–467.

Rahman, Q., Kumari, V. & Wilson, G. D. (2003b). Sexual orientation–related differences in prepulse inhibition of the human startle response. *Behavioral Neuroscience, 117*, 1096–1102.

Rahman, Q. & Wilson, G. D. (2003a). Large sexual-orientation-related differences in performance on mental rotation and judgment of line orientation tasks. *Neuropsychology, 17*, 25–31.

Rahman, Q. & Wilson, G. D. (2003b). Sexual orientation and the 2nd to 4th finger length ratio: Evidence for organising effects of sex hormones or developmental instability? *Psychoneuroendocrinology, 28,* 288–303.

Rahman, Q., Wilson, G. D. & Abrahams, S. (2003c). Sexual orientation related differences in spatial memory. *Journal of the International Neuropsychological Society, 9,* 376–383.

Rahman, Q. & Yusuf, S. (2015). Lateralization for processing facial emotions in gay men, heterosexual men, and heterosexual women. *Archives of Sexual Behavior, 44,* 1405–1413.

Ramagopalan, S. V., Dyment, D. A., Handunnetthi, L., Rice, G. P. & Ebers, G. C. (2010). A genome-wide scan of male sexual orientation. *Journal of Human Genetics, 55,* 131–132.

Rametti, G., Carrillo, B., Gomez-Gil, E., Junque, C., Segovia, S., Gomez, A. & Guillamon, A. (2011a). White matter microstructure in female to male transsexuals before cross-sex hormonal treatment. A diffusion tensor imaging study. *Journal of Psychiatric Research, 45,* 199–204.

Rametti, G., Carrillo, B., Gomez-Gil, E., Junque, C., Zubiarre-Elorza, L., Segovia, S., Gomez, A. & Guillamon, A. (2011b). The microstructure of white matter in male to female transsexuals before cross-sex hormonal treatment. A DTI study. *Journal of Psychiatric Research, 45,* 949–954.

Raznahan, A., Shaw, P. W., Lerch, J. P., Clasen, L. S., Greenstein, D., Berman, R., Pipitone, J., Chakravarty, M. M. & Giedd, J. N. (2014). Longitudinal four-dimensional mapping of subcortical anatomy in human development. *Proceedings of the National Academy of Sciences of the United States of America, 111,* 1592–1597.

Reddy, R. C., Amodei, R., Estill, C. T., Stormshak, F., Meaker, M. & Roselli, C. E. (2015). Effect of testosterone on neuronal morphology and neuritic growth of fetal lamb hypothalamus-preoptic area and cerebral cortex in primary culture. *PLoS One, 10,* e0129521.

Reiner, W. G. & Gearhart, J. P. (2004). Discordant sexual identity in some genetic males with cloacal exstrophy assigned to female sex at birth. *New England Journal of Medicine, 350,* 333–341.

Rendall, D., Vasey, P. L. & McKenzie, J. (2008). The Queen's English: An alternative, biosocial hypothesis for the distinctive features of "gay speech." *Archives of Sexual Behavior, 37,* 188–204.

Reynolds, M. (2002). Kandahar's lightly veiled homosexual habits. *Los Angeles Times,* April 3.

Rhees, R. W., Shryne, J. E. & Gorski, R. A. (1990a). Onset of the hormone-sensitive perinatal period for sexual differentiation of the sexually dimorphic nucleus of the preoptic area in female rats. *Journal of Neurobiology, 21,* 781–786.

Rhees, R. W., Shryne, J. E. & Gorski, R. A. (1990b). Termination of the hormone-sensitive period for differentiation of the sexually dimorphic nucleus of the preoptic area in male and female rats. *Brain Research Developmental Brain Research, 52,* 17–23.

Rice, G., Anderson, C., Risch, N. & Ebers, G. (1999). Male homosexuality: Absence of linkage to microsatellite markers at Xq28. *Science, 284,* 665–667.

Rieger, G., Cash, B. M., Merrill, S. M., Jones-Rounds, J., Dharmavaram, S. M. & Savin-Williams, R. C. (2015a). Sexual arousal: The correspondence of eyes and genitals. *Biological Psychology, 104,* 56–64.

Rieger, G., Chivers, M. L. & Bailey, J. M. (2005). Sexual arousal patterns of bisexual men. *Psychological Science, 16,* 579–584.

Rieger, G., Gygax, L., Linsenmeier, J. A., Siler-Knogl, A., Moskowitz, D. A. & Bailey, J. M. (2011). Sex typicality and attractiveness in childhood and adulthood: Assessing their relationships from videos. *Archives of Sexual Behavior, 40,* 143–154.

Rieger, G., Linsenmeier, J. A., Gygax, L. & Bailey, J. M. (2008). Sexual orientation and childhood gender nonconformity: Evidence from home videos. *Developmental Psychology, 44,* 46–58.

Rieger, G., Linsenmeier, J. A., Gygax, L., Garcia, S. & Bailey, J. M. (2010). Dissecting "gaydar": Accuracy and the role of masculinity–femininity. *Archives of Sexual Behavior, 39,* 124–140.

Rieger, G., Rosenthal, A. M., Cash, B. M., Linsenmeier, J. A., Bailey, J. M. & Savin-Williams, R. C. (2013). Male bisexual arousal: A matter of curiosity? *Biological Psychology, 94,* 479–489.

Rieger, G. & Savin-Williams, R. C. (2012). The eyes have it: Sex and sexual orientation differences in pupil dilation patterns. *PLoS One*, 7, e40256.

Rieger, G., Savin-Williams, R. C., Chivers, M. L. & Bailey, J. M. (2015b). Sexual arousal and masculinity–femininity of women. *Journal of Personality and Social Psychology, Online before print, October 26.*

Rind, B. (2013). Homosexual orientation—from nature, not abuse: A critique of Roberts, Glymour, and Koenen (2013). *Archives of Sexual Behavior*, 42, 1653–1664.

Ristori, J. & Steensma, T. D. (2016). Gender dysphoria in childhood. *International Review of Psychiatry*, 28, 13–20.

Rivas, M. P., Moreira, L. M., Santo, L. D., Marques, A. C., El-Hani, C. N. & Toralles, M. B. (2014). New studies of second and fourth digit ratio as a morphogenetic trait in subjects with congenital adrenal hyperplasia. *American Journal of Human Biology*, 26, 559–561.

Roberts, A. L., Austin, S. B., Corliss, H. L., Vandermorris, A. K. & Koenen, K. C. (2010). Pervasive trauma exposure among US sexual orientation minority adults and risk of posttraumatic stress disorder. *American Journal of Public Health*, 100, 2433–2441.

Roberts, A. L., Glymour, M. M. & Koenen, K. C. (2013). Does maltreatment in childhood affect sexual orientation in adulthood? *Archives of Sexual Behavior*, 42, 161–171.

Roberts, A. L., Glymour, M. M. & Koenen, K. C. (2014). Considering alternative explanations for the associations among childhood adversity, childhood abuse, and adult sexual orientation: Reply to Bailey and Bailey (2013) and Rind (2013). *Archives of Sexual Behavior*, 43, 191–196.

Roberts, A. L., Rosario, M., Corliss, H. L., Koenen, K. C. & Austin, S. B. (2012). Elevated risk of posttraumatic stress in sexual minority youths: Mediation by childhood abuse and gender nonconformity. *American Journal of Public Health*, 102, 1587–1593.

Roberts, E. K., Flak, J. N., Ye, W., Padmanabhan, V. & Lee, T. M. (2009). Juvenile rank can predict male-typical adult mating behavior in female sheep treated prenatally with testosterone. *Biology of Reproduction*, 80, 737–742.

Roberts, S. (2014). Tom Daley: I'm definitely gay not bisexual. (http://www.pinknews.co.uk/2014/04/03/tom-daley-im-definitely-gay-not-bisexual/)

Robinson, S. J. & Manning, J. T. (2000). The ratio of 2nd to 4th digit length and male homosexuality. *Evolution and Human Behavior*, 21, 333–345.

Rodeck, C. H., Gill, D., Rosenberg, D. A. & Collins, W. P. (1985). Testosterone levels in midtrimester maternal and fetal plasma and amniotic fluid. *Prenatal Diagnosis*, 5, 175–181.

Romeo, R. D. (2003). Puberty: A period of both organizational and activational effects of steroid hormones on neurobehavioural development. *Journal of Neuroendocrinology*, 15, 1185–1192.

Roselli, C. E., Larkin, K., Resko, J. A., Stellflug, J. N. & Stormshak, F. (2004a). The volume of a sexually dimorphic nucleus in the ovine medial preoptic area/anterior hypothalamus varies with sexual partner preference. *Endocrinology*, 145, 478–483.

Roselli, C. E., Larkin, K., Schrunk, J. M. & Stormshak, F. (2004b). Sexual partner preference, hypothalamic morphology and aromatase in rams. *Physiology and Behavior*, 83, 233–245.

Roselli, C. E., Reddy, R. C. & Kaufman, K. R. (2011). The development of male-oriented behavior in rams. *Frontiers in Neuroendocrinology*, 32, 164–169.

Roselli, C. E., Schrunk, J. M., Stadelman, H. L., Resko, J. A. & Stormshak, F. (2006). The effect of aromatase inhibition on the sexual differentiation of the sheep brain. *Endocrine*, 29, 501–511.

Roselli, C. E., Stadelman, H., Reeve, R., Bishop, C. V. & Stormshak, F. (2007). The ovine sexually dimorphic nucleus of the medial preoptic area is organized prenatally by testosterone. *Endocrinology*, 148, 4450–4457.

Roselli, C. E. & Stormshak, F. (2010). The ovine sexually dimorphic nucleus, aromatase, and sexual partner preferences in sheep. *Journal of Steroid Biochemistry and Molecular Biology*, 118, 252–256.

Rosenthal, A. M., Sylva, D., Safron, A. & Bailey, J. M. (2011). Sexual arousal patterns of bisexual men revisited. *Biological Psychology*, 88, 112–115.

Rostker, B. D., Hosek, S. D. & Vaina, M. E. (2011). Gays in the military: Eventually, new facts conquer old taboos. (http://www.rand.org/pubs/periodicals/rand-review/issues/2011/spring/gays.html)

Rudder, C. (2010). The big lies people tell in online dating. (http://blog.okcupid.com/index.php/the-biggest-lies-in-online-dating/)

Rudder, C. (2014). *Dataclysm: Who we are when we think no one's looking.* Crown.

Ruigrok, A. N., Salimi-Khorshidi, G., Lai, M. C., Baron-Cohen, S., Lombardo, M. V., Tait, R. J. & Suckling, J. (2014). A meta-analysis of sex differences in human brain structure. *Neuroscience and Biobehavioral Reviews 39,* 34–50.

Rule, N. O. (2016). Perceiving sexual orientation from minimal cues. *Archives of Sexual Behavior (in preparation).*

Rullo, J. E., Strassberg, D. S. & Israel, E. (2010). Category-specificity in sexual interest in gay men and lesbians. *Archives of Sexual Behavior, 39,* 874–879.

Rullo, J. E., Strassberg, D. S. & Miner, M. H. (2014). Gender-specificity in sexual interest in bisexual men and women. *Archives of Sexual Behavior, Online ahead of print, October 17.*

Rust, J., Golombok, S., Hines, M., Johnston, K. & Golding, J. (2000). The role of brothers and sisters in the gender development of preschool children. *Journal of Experimental Child Psychology, 77,* 292–303.

Ryner, L. C., Goodwin, S. F., Castrillon, D. H., Anand, A., Villella, A., Baker, B. S., Hall, J. C., Taylor, B. J. & Wasserman, S. A. (1996). Control of male sexual behavior and sexual orientation in *Drosophila* by the *fruitless* gene. *Cell, 87,* 1079–1089.

Sachs, J., Lieberman, P. & Erickson, D. (1973). Anatomical and cultural determinants of male and female speech. In: Shuy, W. & Fasold, R. W. (Eds.), *Language attitudes: Current trends and prospects.* Georgetown University Press.

Safron, A., Barch, B., Bailey, J. M., Gitelman, D. R., Parrish, T. B. & Reber, P. J. (2007). Neural correlates of sexual arousal in homosexual and heterosexual men. *Behavioral Neuroscience, 121,* 237–248.

Sagarin, B. J., Martin, A. L., Coutinho, S. A., Edlund, J. E., Patel, L., Skowronski, J. J. & Zengel, B. (2012). Sex differences in jealousy: A meta-analytic examination. *Evolution and Human Behavior, 33,* 595–614.

Sakuma, Y. (2009). Gonadal steroid action and brain sex differentiation in the rat. *Journal of Neuroendocrinology, 21,* 410–414.

Salais, D. & Fischer, R. B. (1995). Sexual preference and altruism. *Journal of Homosexuality, 28,* 185–196.

Sanders, A. R., Martin, E. R., Beecham, G. W., Guo, S., Dawood, K., Rieger, G., Badner, J. A., Gershon, E. S., Krishnappa, R. S., Kolundzija, A. B., Duan, J., Gejman, P. V. & Bailey, J. M. (2015). Genome-wide scan demonstrates significant linkage for male sexual orientation. *Psychological Medicine, 45,* 1379–1388.

Sanders, G. & Wright, M. (1997). Sexual orientation differences in cerebral asymmetry and in the performance of sexually dimorphic cognitive and motor tasks. *Archives of Sexual Behavior, 26,* 463–480.

Saper, C. B. & Lowell, B. B. (2014). The hypothalamus. *Current Biology, 24,* R1111–R1116.

Sato, K. & Yamamoto, D. (2014). An epigenetic switch of the brain sex as a basis of gendered behavior in *Drosophila.* In: Yamamoto, D. (Ed.), *Epigenetic shaping of sociosexual interactions: From plants to humans.* Academic Press.

Savic, I., Berglund, H., Gulyas, B. & Roland, P. (2001). Smelling of odorous sex hormone-like compounds causes sex-differentiated hypothalamic activations in humans. *Neuron, 31,* 661–668.

Savic, I., Berglund, H. & Lindström, P. (2005). Brain response to putative pheromones in homosexual men. *Proceedings of the National Academy of Sciences of the United States of America, 102,* 7356–7361.

Savic, I., Heden-Blomqvist, E. & Berglund, H. (2009). Pheromone signal transduction in humans: What can be learned from olfactory loss. *Human Brain Mapping, 30,* 3057–3065.

Savic, I. & Lindström, P. (2008). PET and MRI show differences in cerebral asymmetry and functional connectivity between homo- and heterosexual subjects. *Proceedings of the National Academy of Sciences of the United States of America, 105,* 9403–9408.

Savin-Williams, R. C. & Vrangalova, Z. (2013). Mostly heterosexual as a distinct sexual orientation group: A systematic review of the empirical evidence. *Developmental Review, 33,* 58–88.

Sawatsky, M. L., Dawson, S. J. & Lalumière, M. L. (2016). Vaginal lubrication: A cue-specific sexual response in women? *Archives of Sexual Behavior (in preparation).*

Saxton, T. K., Lyndon, A., Little, A. C. & Roberts, S. C. (2008). Evidence that androstadienone, a putative human chemosignal, modulates women's attributions of men's attractiveness. *Hormones and Behavior, 54,* 597–601.

Schiffer, B., Peschel, T., Paul, T., Gizewski, E., Forsting, M., Leygraf, N., Schedlowski, M. & Krueger, T. H. (2007). Structural brain abnormalities in the frontostriatal system and cerebellum in pedophilia. *Journal of Psychiatric Research, 41,* 753–762.

Schiller, G. & Rosenberg, R. (1986). *Before Stonewall: The making of a gay and lesbian community* (documentary film).

Schiltz, K., Witzel, J., Northoff, G., Zierhut, K., Gubka, U., Fellmann, H., Kaufmann, J., Tempelmann, C., Wiebking, C. & Bogerts, B. (2007). Brain pathology in pedophilic offenders: Evidence of volume reduction in the right amygdala and related diencephalic structures. *Archives of General Psychiatry, 64,* 737–746.

Schmidt, G. & Clement, U. (1990). Does peace prevent homosexuality? *Archives of Sexual Behavior, 19,* 183–187.

Schmitt, D. P. (2003). Universal sex differences in the desire for sexual variety: Tests from 52 nations, 6 continents, and 13 islands. *Journal of Personality and Social Psychology, 85,* 85–104.

Schmitt, D. P., Jonason, P. K., Byerley, G. J., Flores, S. D., Illbeck, B. E., O'Leary, K. N. O. & Qudrat, A. (2012). A reexamination of sex differences in sexuality: New studies reveal old truths. *Current Directions in Psychological Science, 21,* 135–139.

Schmitt, D. P., Realo, A., Voracek, M. & Allik, J. (2008). Why can't a man be more like a woman? Sex differences in Big Five personality traits across 55 cultures. *Journal of Personality and Social Psychology, 94,* 168–182.

Schneider, S., Peters, J., Bromberg, U., Brassen, S., Menz, M. M., Miedl, S. F., Loth, E., Banaschewski, T., Barbot, A., Barker, G., Conrod, P. J., Dalley, J. W., Flor, H., Gallinat, J., Garavan, H., Heinz, A., Itterman, B., Mallik, C., Mann, K., Artiges, E., Paus, T., Poline, J. B., Rietschel, M., Reed, L., Smolka, M. N., Spanagel, R., Speiser, C., Strohle, A., Struve, M., Schumann, G. & Buchel, C. (2011). Boys do it the right way: Sex-dependent amygdala lateralization during face processing in adolescents. *Neuroimage, 56,* 1847–1853.

Schwartz, G., Kim, R. M., Kolundzija, A. B., Rieger, G. & Sanders, A. R. (2010). Biodemographic and physical correlates of sexual orientation in men. *Archives of Sexual Behavior, 39,* 83–109.

Scott, N., Prigge, M., Yizhar, O. & Kimchi, T. (2015). A sexually dimorphic hypothalamic circuit controls maternal care and oxytocin secretion. *Nature, 525,* 519–522.

Searles, R. V., Yoo, M. J., He, J. R., Shen, W. B. & Selmanoff, M. (2000). Sex differences in GABA turnover and glutamic acid decarboxylase (GAD(65) and GAD(67)) mRNA in the rat hypothalamus. *Brain Research, 878,* 11–19.

Segal, N. (2000). *Entwined lives: Twins and what they tell us about human behavior.* Plume.

Segal, N. L. & Diamond, M. (2014). Identical reared apart twins concordant for transsexuality. *Journal of Experimental and Clinical Medicine, 6,* 74.

Semon, T., Smith, M. & Bailey, M. (2016). Dimensions of male asexuality: Sexual interests, behaviors, and arousal patterns. *Archives of Sexual Behavior (in preparation).*

Serbin, L. A., Poulin-Dubois, D., Colburne, K. A., Sen, M. G. & Eichstedt, J. A. (2001). Gender stereotyping in infancy: Visual preferences for and knowledge of gender-stereotyped toys in the second year. *International Journal of Behavioral Development, 25,* 7–15.

Sergeant, M. J. T., Dickins, T. E., Davies, M. N. O. & Griffiths, M. D. (2006). Aggression, empathy and sexual orientation in males. *Personality and Individual Differences, 40,* 475–486.

Seto, M. C. (2012). Is pedophilia a sexual orientation? *Archives of Sexual Behavior, 41*, 231–236.

Shah, N. M., Pisapia, D. J., Maniatis, S., Mendelsohn, M. M., Nemes, A. & Axel, R. (2004). Visualizing sexual dimorphism in the brain. *Neuron, 43*, 313–319.

Shelp, S. G. (2002). Gaydar: Visual detection of sexual orientation among gay and straight men. *Journal of Homosexuality, 44*, 1–14.

Shidlo, A. & Schroeder, M. (2002). Changing sexual orientation: A consumers' report. *Professional Psychology: Research and Practice, 33*, 249–259.

Shirangi, T. R., Taylor, B. J. & McKeown, M. (2006). A double-switch system regulates male courtship behavior in male and female *Drosophila melanogaster. Nature Genetics, 38*, 1435–1439.

Signoret, J. P. (1970). Reproductive behaviour of pigs. *Journal of Reproduction and Fertility, Suppl 11*, 105–117.

Simerly, R. B. (2002). Wired for reproduction: Organization and development of sexually dimorphic circuits in the mammalian forebrain. *Annual Review of Neuroscience, 25*, 507–536.

Simmons, J. L. (1965). Public stereotypes of deviants. *Social Problems, 13*, 223–232.

Simpson, E. A., Nicolini, Y., Shetler, M., Suomi, S. J., Ferrari, P. F. & Paukner, A. (2016). Experience-independent sex differences in newborn macaques: Females are more social than males. *Scientific Reports, 6*, 19669.

Singh, D., Vidaurri, M., Zambarano, R. J. & Dabbs, J. M., Jr. (1999). Lesbian erotic role identification: Behavioral, morphological, and hormonal correlates. *Journal of Personality and Social Psychology, 76*, 1035–1049.

Sisk, C. L. & Berenbaum, S. A. (2013). Editorial for the special issue of *Hormones and Behavior* on puberty and adolescence. *Hormones and Behavior, 64*, 173–174.

Skidmore, W. C., Linsenmeier, J. A. & Bailey, J. M. (2006). Gender nonconformity and psychological distress in lesbians and gay men. *Archives of Sexual Behavior, 35*, 685–697.

Skorska, M. N., Geniole, S. N., Vrysen, B. M., McCormick, C. M. & Bogaert, A. F. (2015). Facial structure predicts sexual orientation in both men and women. *Archives of Sexual Behavior, 44*, 1377–1394.

Slater, E. (1962). Birth order and maternal age of homosexuals. *Lancet, 1*, 69–71.

Smith, A. M., Rissel, C. E., Richters, J., Grulich, A. E. & de Visser, R. O. (2003). Sex in Australia: Sexual identity, sexual attraction and sexual experience among a representative sample of adults. *Australian and New Zealand Journal of Public Health, 27*, 138–145.

Smyth, R., Jacobs, G. & Rogers, H. (2003). Male voices and perceived sexual orientation: An experimental and theoretical approach. *Language in Society, 32*, 329–350.

Smyth, R. & Rogers, H. (2008). Do gay-sounding men speak like women? *Toronto Working Papers in Linguistics, 27*, 129–144.

Snihur, A. W. & Hampson, E. (2011). Sex and ear differences in spontaneous and click-evoked otoacoustic emissions in young adults. *Brain and Cognition, 77*, 40–47.

Snihur, A. W. & Hampson, E. (2012a). Click-evoked otoacoustic emissions: Response amplitude is associated with circulating testosterone levels in men. *Behavioral Neuroscience, 126*, 325–331.

Snihur, A. W. & Hampson, E. (2012b). Oral contraceptive use in women is associated with defeminization of otoacoustic emission patterns. *Neuroscience, 210*, 258–265.

Socarides, C. W. (1978). *Homosexuality.* J. Aronson.

Sommer, I. E., Aleman, A., Somers, M., Boks, M. P. & Kahn, R. S. (2008). Sex differences in handedness, asymmetry of the planum temporale and functional language lateralization. *Brain Research, 1206*, 76–88.

Sommer, V. & Vasey, P. L. (Eds.) (2006). *Homosexual behaviour in animals: An evolutionary perspective.* Cambridge University Press.

Spape, J., Timmers, A. D., Yoon, S., Ponseti, J. & Chivers, M. L. (2014). Gender-specific genital and subjective sexual arousal to prepotent sexual features in heterosexual women and men. *Biological Psychology, 102*, 1–9.

Spelke, E. S. (2005). Sex differences in intrinsic aptitude for mathematics and science? A critical review. *American Psychologist, 60*, 950–958.

Spengler, A. (1977). Manifest sadomasochism of males: Results of an empirical study. *Archives of Sexual Behavior, 6*, 441–456.

Sperling, M. A. (2008). *Pediatric endocrinology (3rd ed.).* Saunders.

Spitzer, R. L. (2012). Spitzer reassesses his 2003 study of reparative therapy of homosexuality. *Archives of Sexual Behavior, 41*, 757.

Statistics Canada (2004). *Canadian Community Health Survey 2003.* (http://www.statcan.gc.ca/daily-quotidien/040615/dq040615b-eng.htm)

Steensma, T. D., van der Ende, J., Verhulst, F. C. & Cohen-Kettenis, P. T. (2013). Gender variance in childhood and sexual orientation in adulthood: A prospective study. *Journal of Sexual Medicine, 10*, 2723–2733.

Stellflug, J. N. & Berardinelli, J. G. (2002). Ram mating behavior after long-term selection for reproductive rate in Rambouillet ewes. *Journal of Animal Science, 80*, 2588–2593.

Stenstrom, E., Saad, G., Nepomuceno, M. V. & Mendenhall, Z. (2011). Testosterone and domain-specific risk: Digit ratios (2D:4D and *rel2*) as predictors of recreational, financial, and social risk-taking behaviors. *Personality and Individual Differences, 51*, 412–416.

Stephens-Davidowitz, S. (2013). How many American men are gay? *New York Times*, December 7.

Stief, M. C., Rieger, G. & Savin-Williams, R. C. (2014). Bisexuality is associated with elevated sexual sensation seeking, sexual curiosity, and sexual excitability. *Personality and Individual Differences, 66*, 193–198.

Stoleru, S., Fonteille, V., Cornelis, C., Joyal, C. & Moulier, V. (2012). Functional neuroimaging studies of sexual arousal and orgasm in healthy men and women: A review and meta-analysis. *Neuroscience and Biobehavioral Reviews, 36*, 1481–1509.

Stowers, L., Holy, T. E., Meister, M., Dulac, C. & Koentges, G. (2002). Loss of sex discrimination and male–male aggression in mice deficient for TRP2. *Science, 295*, 1493–1500.

Sulloway, F. J. (1996). *Born to rebel: Birth order, family dynamics, and creative lives.* Pantheon Books.

Sulpizio, S., Fasoli, F., Maass, A., Paladino, M. P., Vespignani, F., Eyssel, F. & Bentler, D. (2015). The sound of voice: Voice-based categorization of speakers' sexual orientation within and across languages. *PLoS One, 10*, e0128882.

Suschinsky, K. D., Lalumière, M. L. & Chivers, M. L. (2009). Sex differences in patterns of genital sexual arousal: Measurement artifacts or true phenomena? *Archives of Sexual Behavior, 38*, 559–573.

Svetec, N., Houot, B. & Ferveur, J. F. (2005). Effect of genes, social experience, and their interaction on the courtship behaviour of transgenic *Drosophila* males. *Genetical Research, 85*, 183–193.

Swaab, D. F. (1995). Development of the human hypothalamus. *Neurochemical Research, 20*, 509–519.

Swaab, D. F. & Fliers, E. (1985). A sexually dimorphic nucleus in the human brain. *Science, 228*, 1112–1115.

Swaab, D. F., Gooren, L. J. & Hofman, M. A. (1992). Gender and sexual orientation in relation to hypothalamic structures. *Hormone Research, 38 Suppl 2*, 51–61.

Swaab, D. F. & Hofman, M. A. (1988). Sexual differentiation of the human hypothalamus: Ontogeny of the sexually dimorphic nucleus of the preoptic area. *Brain Research Developmental Brain Research, 44*, 314–318.

Swaab, D. F. & Hofman, M. A. (1990). An enlarged suprachiasmatic nucleus in homosexual men. *Brain Research, 537*, 141–148.

Swanson, L. W. (2003). The amygdala and its place in the cerebral hemisphere. *Annals of the New York Academy of Sciences, 985*, 174–184.

Swerdlow, N. R., Auerbach, P., Monroe, S. M., Hartston, H., Geyer, M. A. & Braff, D. L. (1993). Men are more inhibited than women by weak prepulses. *Biological Psychiatry, 34*, 253–260.

Sylva, D., Safron, A., Rosenthal, A. M., Reber, P. J., Parrish, T. B. & Bailey, J. M. (2013). Neural correlates of sexual arousal in heterosexual and homosexual women and men. *Hormones and Behavior, 64*, 673–684.

Talarovicova, A., Krskova, L. & Blazekova, J. (2009). Testosterone enhancement during pregnancy influences the 2D:4D ratio and open field motor activity of rat siblings in adulthood. *Hormones and Behavior, 55*, 235–239.

Taylor, A. (1983). Conceptions of masculinity and femininity as a basis for stereotypes of male and female homosexuals. *Journal of Homosexuality, 9*, 37–53.

Taylor, J. (1992). *Born that way?* (documentary film). Windfall Films, London.

Tobet, S. A., Zahniser, D. J. & Baum, M. J. (1986). Differentiation in male ferrets of a sexually dimorphic nucleus of the preoptic/anterior hypothalamic area requires prenatal estrogen. *Neuroendocrinology, 44*, 299–308.

Tollison, C. D., Adams, H. E. & Tollison, J. W. (1979). Cognitive and physiological indices of sexual arousal in homosexual, bisexual, and heterosexual males. *Journal of Behavioral Assessment, 1*, 305–314.

Tomassilli, J. C., Golub, S. A., Bimbi, D. S. & Parsons, J. T. (2009). Behind closed doors: An exploration of kinky sexual behaviors in urban lesbian and bisexual women. *Journal of Sex Research, 46*, 438–445.

Tomeo, M. E., Templer, D. I., Anderson, S. & Kotler, D. (2001). Comparative data of childhood and adolescence molestation in heterosexual and homosexual persons. *Archives of Sexual Behavior, 30*, 535–541.

Tooby, J. & Cosmides, L. (1992). The psychological foundations of culture. In: Barkow, J. H. et al. (Eds.), *The adapted mind.* Oxford University Press, pp. 19–136.

Toro-Morn, M. & Sprecher, S. (2003). A cross-cultural comparison of mate preferences among university students: The United States vs. the People's Republic of China (PRC). *Journal of Comparative Family Studies, 34*, 151–174.

Tortorice, J. (2001). Gender identity, sexual orientation, and second-to-fourth digit ratio in females. *Human Behavior and Evolution Society Abstracts, 13*, 35.

Tracy, E. C., Bainter, S. A. & Satariano, N. P. (2015). Judgments of self-identified gay and heterosexual male speakers: Which phonemes are most salient in determining sexual orientation? *Journal of Phonetics, 52*, 13–25.

Trimble, M. R., Mendez, M. F. & Cummings, J. L. (1997). Neuropsychiatric symptoms from the temporolimbic lobes. In: Salloway, S. et al. (Eds.), *The neuropsychiatry of limbic and subcortical disorders.* American Psychiatric Publishing.

Trivers, R. L. (1974). Parent–offspring conflict. *American Zoologist, 14*, 249–264.

Trotier, D., Eloit, C., Wassef, M., Talmain, G., Bensimon, J. L., Doving, K. B. & Ferrand, J. (2000). The vomeronasal cavity in adult humans. *Chemical Senses, 25*, 369–380.

Valentova, J. V. & Havlicek, J. (2013). Perceived sexual orientation based on vocal and facial stimuli is linked to self-rated sexual orientation in Czech men. *PLoS One, 8*, e82417.

Valentova, J. V., Kleisner, K., Havlicek, J. & Neustupa, J. (2014). Shape differences between the faces of homosexual and heterosexual men. *Archives of Sexual Behavior, 43*, 353–361.

van Anders, S. M. (2015). Beyond sexual orientation: Integrating gender/sex and diverse sexualities via sexual configurations theory. *Archives of Sexual Behavior, 44*, 1177–1213.

van Anders, S. M., Hamilton, L. D., Schmidt, N. & Watson, N. V. (2007). Associations between testosterone secretion and sexual activity in women. *Hormones and Behavior, 51*, 477–482.

van Anders, S. M. & Hampson, E. (2005). Testing the prenatal androgen hypothesis: Measuring digit ratios, sexual orientation, and spatial abilities in adults. *Hormones and Behavior, 47*, 92–98.

van Anders, S. M., Vernon, P. A. & Wilbur, C. J. (2006). Finger-length ratios show evidence of prenatal hormone-transfer between opposite-sex twins. *Hormones and Behavior, 49*, 315–319.

van Anders, S. M. & Watson, N. V. (2006). Relationship status and testosterone in North American heterosexual and non-heterosexual men and women: Cross-sectional and longitudinal data. *Psychoneuroendocrinology, 31*, 715–723.

van Anders, S. M. & Watson, N. V. (2007). Testosterone levels in women and men who are single, in long-distance relationships, or same-city relationships. *Hormones and Behavior, 51*, 286–291.

van Beijsterveldt, C. E., Hudziak, J. J. & Boomsma, D. I. (2006). Genetic and environmental influences on cross-gender behavior and relation to behavior problems: A study of Dutch twins at ages 7 and 10 years. *Archives of Sexual Behavior, 35*, 647–658.

VanderLaan, D. P., Garfield, Z. H., Garfield, M. J., Leca, J.-B., Vasey, P. L. & Hames, R. B. (2014). The "female fertility–social stratification–hypergyny" hypothesis of male homosexuality: Factual, conceptual and methodological errors in Barthes et al. *Evolution and Human Behavior, 35*, 445–447.

VanderLaan, D. P. & Vasey, P. L. (2009). Patterns of sexual coercion in heterosexual and non-heterosexual men and women. *Archives of Sexual Behavior, 38*, 987–999.

VanderLaan, D. P. & Vasey, P. L. (2012). Relationship status and elevated avuncularity in Samoan *fa'afafine. Personal Relationships, 19*, 326–339.

VanderLaan, D. P. & Vasey, P. L. (2013). Birth order and avuncular tendencies in Samoan men and *fa'afafine. Archives of Sexual Behavior, 42*, 371–379.

Vasey, P. L. (2006). The pursuit of pleasure: An evolutionary history of female homosexual behavior in Japanese macaques. In: Sommer, V. & Vasey, P. L. (Eds.), *Homosexual behavior in animals: An evolutionary perspective.* Cambridge University Press, pp. 191–219.

Vasey, P. L. & Bartlett, N. H. (2007). What can the Samoan *"fa'afafine"* teach us about the Western concept of gender identity disorder in childhood? *Perspectives in Biology and Medicine, 50*, 481–490.

Vasey, P. L., Parker, J. L. & VanderLaan, D. P. (2014). Comparative reproductive output of androphilic and gynephilic males in Samoa. *Archives of Sexual Behavior, 43*, 363–367.

Vasey, P. L. & Pfaus, J. G. (2005). A sexually dimorphic hypothalamic nucleus in a macaque species with frequent female–female mounting and same-sex sexual partner preference. *Behavioural Brain Research, 157*, 265–272.

Vasey, P. L., Pocock, D. S. & Vanderlaan, D. P. (2007). Kin selection and male androphilia in Samoan *fa'afafine. Evolution and Human Behavior, 28*, 159–167.

Vasey, P. L. & VanderLaan, D. P. (2007). Birth order and male androphilia in Samoan *fa'afafine. Proceedings of the Royal Society of London B: Biological Sciences, 274*, 1437–1442.

Vasey, P. L. & Vanderlaan, D. P. (2008). Avuncular tendencies and the evolution of male androphilia in Samoan *fa'afafine. Archives of Sexual Behavior, 39*, 821–830.

Vasey, P. L. & VanderLaan, D. P. (2010a). An adaptive cognitive dissociation between willingness to help kin and nonkin in Samoan *fa'afafine. Psychological Science, 21*, 292–297.

Vasey, P. L. & VanderLaan, D. P. (2010b). Monetary exchanges with nieces and nephews: A comparison of Samoan men, women, and *fa'afafine. Evolution and Human Behavior, 31*, 373–380.

Veale, D., Miles, S., Bramley, S., Muir, G. & Hodsoll, J. (2015). Am I normal? A systematic review and construction of nomograms for flaccid and erect penis length and circumference in up to 15 521 men. *BJU International, 115*, 978–986.

Veale, J. F., Clarke, D. E. & Lomax, T. C. (2010). Biological and psychosocial correlates of adult gender-variant identities: A review. *Personality and Individual Differences, 48*, 357–366.

Vega Matuszczyk, J., Fernandez-Guasti, A. & Larsson, K. (1988). Sexual orientation, proceptivity, and receptivity in the male rat as a function of neonatal hormonal manipulation. *Hormones and Behavior, 22*, 362–378.

Vingerhoets, G., Acke, F., Alderweireldt, A. S., Nys, J., Vandemaele, P. & Achten, E. (2012). Cerebral lateralization of praxis in right- and left-handedness: Same pattern, different strength. *Human Brain Mapping, 33*, 763–777.

vom Saal, F. S. & Bronson, F. H. (1980). Sexual characteristics of adult female mice are correlated with their blood testosterone levels during prenatal development. *Science, 208*, 597–599.

Voracek, M. & Dressler, S. G. (2007). Digit ratio (2D:4D) in twins: Heritability estimates and evidence for a masculinized trait expression in women from opposite-sex pairs. *Psychological Reports, 100*, 115–126.

Voracek, M., Manning, J. T. & Ponocny, I. (2005). Digit ratio (2D:4D) in homosexual and heterosexual men from Austria. *Archives of Sexual Behavior, 34*, 335–340.

Vrangalova, Z. & Savin-Williams, R. C. (2012). Mostly heterosexual and mostly gay/lesbian: Evidence for new sexual orientation identities. *Archives of Sexual Behavior, 41*, 85–101.

Wallen, K. (1996). Nature needs nurture: The interaction of hormonal and social influences on the development of behavioral sex differences in rhesus monkeys. *Hormones and Behavior, 30*, 364–378.

Wallien, M. S., Zucker, K. J., Steensma, T. D. & Cohen-Kettenis, P. T. (2008). 2D:4D finger-length ratios in children and adults with gender identity disorder. *Hormones and Behavior*, *54*, 450–454.

Wang, B., Zhou, S., Hong, F., Wang, J., Liu, X., Cai, Y., Wang, F., Feng, T. & Ma, X. (2012). Association analysis between the tag SNP for *sonic hedgehog* rs9333613 polymorphism and male sexual orientation. *Journal of Andrology*, *33*, 951–954.

Wang, P. Y., Protheroe, A., Clarkson, A. N., Imhoff, F., Koishi, K. & McLennan, I. S. (2009). Mullerian inhibiting substance contributes to sex-linked biases in the brain and behavior. *Proceedings of the National Academy of Sciences of the United States of America*, *106*, 7203–7208.

Ward, I. L. (1972). Prenatal stress feminizes and demasculinizes the behavior of males. *Science*, *175*, 82–84.

Ward, I. L. & Stehm, K. E. (1991). Prenatal stress feminizes juvenile play patterns in male rats. *Physiology and Behavior*, *50*, 601–605.

Ward, I. L. & Weisz, J. (1984). Differential effects of maternal stress on circulating levels of corticosterone, progesterone, and testosterone in male and female rat fetuses and their mothers. *Endocrinology*, *114*, 1635–1644.

Wassersug, R., Walker, L. & Robinson, J. (2014). *Androgen deprivation therapy: An essential guide for prostate cancer patients and their loved ones*. Demos Health.

Wegesin, D. J. (1998a). A neuropsychologic profile of homosexual and heterosexual men and women. *Archives of Sexual Behavior*, *27*, 91–108.

Wegesin, D. J. (1998b). Relation between language lateralisation and spatial ability in gay and straight women and men. *Laterality*, *3*, 227–239.

Wegesin, D. & Meyer-Bahlburg, H. F. L. (2000). Top/bottom self-label, anal sex practices, HIV risk and gender role identity in gay men in New York City. *Journal of Psychology and Human Sexuality*, *12*, 43–62.

Weinrich, J. D. (1978). Nonreproduction, homosexuality, transsexualism, and intelligence: I. A systematic literature search. *Journal of Homosexuality*, *3*, 275–289.

Weinrich, J. D. (1987a). A new sociobiological theory of homosexuality applicable to societies with universal marriage. *Behavioral Ecology and Sociobiology*, *8*, 37–47.

Weinrich, J. D. (1987b). *Sexual landscapes: Why we are what we are, why we love whom we love*. Scribner's.

Weinrich, J. D., Grant, I., Jacobson, D. L., Robinson, S. R. & McCutchan, J. A. (1992). Effects of recalled childhood gender nonconformity on adult genitoerotic role and AIDS exposure. HNRC Group. *Archives of Sexual Behavior*, *21*, 559–585.

Wellings, K., Field, J., Johnson, A. M. & Wadsworth, J. (1994). *Sexual behavior in Britain: The National Survey of Sexual Attitudes and Lifestyles*. Penguin.

Wheelwright Schmitt, S. & Baron-Cohen, S. (2011). Systemizing and empathizing. In: Fein, D. A. (Ed.), *The neuropsychology of autism*. Oxford University Press.

Whishaw, I. Q. & Kolb, B. (1985). The mating movements of male decorticate rats: Evidence for subcortically generated movements by the male but regulation of approaches by the female. *Behavioural Brain Research*, *17*, 171–191.

Whitam, F. L. (1983). Culturally invariant properties of male homosexuality: Tentative conclusions from cross-cultural research. *Archives of Sexual Behavior*, *12*, 207–226.

Whitam, F. L., Diamond, M. & Martin, J. (1993). Homosexual orientation in twins: A report on 61 pairs and three triplet sets. *Archives of Sexual Behavior*, *22*, 187–206.

White, M. (1994). *Stranger at the gate: To be gay and Christian in America*. Simon and Schuster.

Whitelaw, N. C., Chong, S. & Whitelaw, E. (2010). Tuning in to noise: Epigenetics and intangible variation. *Developmental Cell*, *19*, 649–650.

Wilhelm, D., Palmer, S. & Koopman, P. (2007). Sex determination and gonadal development in mammals. *Physiological Reviews*, *87*, 1–28.

Williams, C. L. & Meck, W. H. (1991). The organizational effects of gonadal steroids on sexually dimorphic spatial ability. *Psychoneuroendocrinology*, *16*, 155–176.

Williams, M. A., Morris, A. P., McGlone, F., Abbott, D. F. & Mattingley, J. B. (2004). Amygdala responses to fearful and happy facial expressions under conditions of binocular suppression. *Journal of Neuroscience, 24*, 2898–2904.

Williams, T. J., Pepitone, M. E., Christensen, S. E., Cooke, B. M., Huberman, A. D., Breedlove, N. J., Breedlove, T. J., Jordan, C. L. & Breedlove, S. M. (2000). Finger-length ratios and sexual orientation. *Nature, 404*, 455–456.

Williams, W. L. (1986). *The spirit and the flesh: Sexual diversity in American Indian culture.* Beacon Press.

Wilson, E. O. (1975). *Sociobiology: The new synthesis.* Harvard University Press.

Wisniewski, A. B. (2015). Cognitive and behavioral impact of androgen disorders in females: Learning from complete androgen insensitivity syndrome and congenital adrenal hyperplasia. In: Plouffe, L. & Rizk, B. R. M. B. (Eds.), *Androgens in gynecological practice.* Cambridge University Press.

Wisniewski, A. B., Espinoza-Varas, B., Aston, C. E., Edmundson, S., Champlin, C. A., Pasanen, E. G. & McFadden, D. (2014). Otoacoustic emissions, auditory evoked potentials and self-reported gender in people affected by disorders of sex development (DSD). *Hormones and Behavior, 66*, 467–474.

Wisniewski, A. B., Migeon, C. J., Malouf, M. A. & Gearhart, J. P. (2004). Psychosexual outcome in women affected by congenital adrenal hyperplasia due to 21-hydroxylase deficiency. *Journal of Urology, 171*, 2497–2501.

Witelson, S. F., Kigar, D. L., Scamvougeras, A., Kideckel, D. M., Buck, B., Stanchev, P. L., Bronskill, M. & Black, S. (2008). Corpus callosum anatomy in right-handed homosexual and heterosexual men. *Archives of Sexual Behavior, 37*, 857–863.

Wittmann, W. & McLennan, I. S. (2013). Anti-mullerian hormone may regulate the number of calbindin-positive neurons in the sexually dimorphic nucleus of the preoptic area of male mice. *Biology of Sex Differences, 4*, 18.

Wong, W. I., Pasterski, V., Hindmarsh, P. C., Geffner, M. E. & Hines, M. (2013). Are there parental socialization effects on the sex-typed behavior of individuals with congenital adrenal hyperplasia? *Archives of Sexual Behavior, 42*, 381–391.

Woolery, L. M. (2007). Gaydar: A social-cognitive analysis. *Journal of Homosexuality, 53*, 9–17.

Wright, C. L., Burks, S. R. & McCarthy, M. M. (2008). Identification of prostaglandin E2 receptors mediating perinatal masculinization of adult sex behavior and neuroanatomical correlates. *Developmental Neurobiology, 68*, 1406–1419.

Xu, Y. & Zheng, Y. (2015a). Does sexual orientation precede childhood sexual abuse? Childhood gender nonconformity as a risk factor and instrumental variable. *Sexual Abuse, Online ahead of print, November 29.*

Xu, Y. & Zheng, Y. (2015b). The relationship between digit ratio (2D:4D) and sexual orientation in men from China. *Archives of Sexual Behavior, Online ahead of print, May 10.*

Yamamoto, D. (2007). The neural and genetic substrates of sexual behavior in *Drosophila. Advances in Genetics, 59*, 39–66.

Yang, S. L., Chen, Y. Y., Hsieh, Y. L., Jin, S. H., Hsu, H. K. & Hsu, C. (2004). Perinatal androgenization prevents age-related neuron loss in the sexually dimorphic nucleus of the preoptic area in female rats. *Developmental Neuroscience, 26*, 54–60.

Yankelovich Partners (1994). *A Yankelovich MONITOR perspective on gays/lesbians.* Yankelovich Partners.

Yonker, J. E., Eriksson, E., Nilsson, L. G. & Herlitz, A. (2006). Negative association of testosterone on spatial visualization in 35 to 80 year old men. *Cortex, 42*, 376–386.

YouGov (2015). A third of young Americans say they aren't 100% heterosexual. (https://today.yougov.com/news/2015/08/20/third-young-americans-exclusively-heterosexual/)

YouGov UK (2015). 1 in 2 young people say they are not 100% heterosexual. (https://yougov.co.uk/news/2015/08/16/half-young-not-heterosexual/)

Yule, M. A., Brotto, L. A. & Gorzalka, B. B. (2014). Biological markers of asexuality: Handedness, birth order, and finger length ratios in self-identified asexual men and women. *Archives of Sexual Behavior, 43*, 299–310.

Yule, M. A., Brotto, L. A. & Gorzalka, B. B. (2016). Sexual fantasy and masturbation among asexual individuals. *Archives of Sexual Behavior (in preparation)*.

Zietsch, B. P., Morley, K. I., Shekar, S. N., Verweij, K. H., Keller, M. C., Macgregor, S., Wright, M. J., Bailey, J. M. & Martin, N. G. (2008). Genetic factors predisposing to homosexuality may increase mating success in heterosexuals. *Evolution and Human Behavior, 29*, 424–433.

Zucker, K. J. & Blanchard, R. (1994). Reanalysis of Bieber et al.'s 1962 data on sibling sex ratio and birth order in male homosexuals. *Journal of Nervous and Mental Disease, 182*, 528–530.

Zucker, K. J., Bradley, S. J., Oliver, G., Blake, J., Fleming, S. & Hood, J. (1996). Psychosexual development of women with congenital adrenal hyperplasia. *Hormones and Behavior, 30*, 300–318.

Zuger, B. (1984). Early effeminate behavior in boys: Outcome and significance for homosexuality. *Journal of Nervous and Mental Disease, 172*, 90–97.

Zuloaga, D. G., Puts, D. A., Jordan, C. L. & Breedlove, S. M. (2008). The role of androgen receptors in the masculinization of brain and behavior: What we've learned from the testicular feminization mutation. *Hormones and Behavior, 53*, 613–626.

AUTHOR INDEX

SUBJECT INDEX

References to figures and footnotes are denoted by an italicized *f* and *n*